THE SCIENCE OF TRANSITIONING

THE SCIENCE OF TRANSITIONING

A Complete Guide to Hair Care for Transitioners and New Naturals

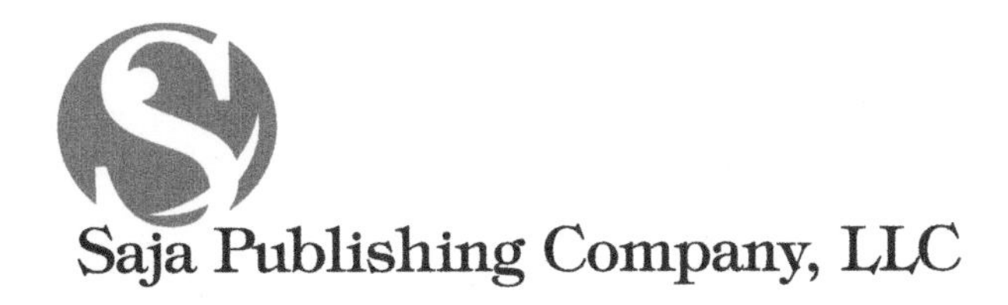

AUDREY DAVIS-SIVASOTHY

www.blackhairscience.com

Published in 2014 by
SAJA Publishing Company
P. O. Box 2383
Stafford, Texas 77497
www.sajapublishing.com

Printed in the United States of America.
Page and book design by Velin Saramov
Cover design by Rachel Lindley

Cover Images courtesy of ©iStockphoto.com/m-imagephotography, Ondine32, and Studio-ThreeDots.

Illustrations provided by Marah Piña and Ana-Gabriela Stroe

Ordering Information: Special discounts are available on quantity purchases by salons, book clubs, bookstores, wholesalers, corporations, associations, and others. For details, contact the publisher at info@sajapublishing.com.

Publisher's Cataloging-in-Publication Data

Davis-Sivasothy, Audrey, 1984—
The science of transitioning: a complete guide to hair care for transitioners and new naturals/
Audrey Sivasothy.
p. cm.

Includes bibliographical references and index.

ISBN-978-1-938266-07-2 (paperback)
ISBN-978-1-938266-08-9 (ebook)

1. Hair—Care and hygiene. 2. African-American women—Health and hygiene. 3. Hairdressing of Blacks. I. Title.

2014919482

First Edition

"I will praise thee; for I am fearfully and wonderfully made: marvelous are thy works . . ."

— Psalm 139:14 (KJV)

Dedication

To all of us—who dare look into the mirror and find absolute beauty in the person staring back at us. And for Pepper, whom I will always love.

Contents

nat•u•ral

naCHərəl/

adjective

1. existing in or caused by nature; not made or caused by humankind.
2. of or in agreement with the character or makeup of, or circumstances surrounding, someone or something.

Our hair's default state is *natural.*
And do to it what you may,
It's *always striving* to get back there.

- The Science of Black Hair

@blackhair101

Introduction

What is the one thing that all of us—no matter our age, nationality, skin color, ethnicity, hair texture or financial status—have in common? *We all come into this world with our hair in its natural state.* But for a majority of women with naturally kinky, coily and curly hair, things changed somewhere along the line. We lost touch with our natural texture. We found new and creative ways to fight against those spirals, coils and waves. And when those resilient strands faithfully returned just weeks after having been straightened, what did we do? We quickly sent them back on their way. That's relaxer psychology for you: a lifetime spent going from two weeks of freshly done to several more weeks of working diligently to cover up the roots. In all of our zeal to fix our roots, we didn't realize that we were missing out on an entire world of amazing hair.

Today, things are slowly changing—and your reading this book is a sign of that change. Many of us are finally starting to see our beauty in a new light, and with new eyes. We are finding that we no longer have to go into harm's way every few weeks to permanently change something about ourselves that is simply beautiful as is. We are learning that our hair is good enough on its own. We are transitioning our minds and our hair!

So, how did simply wearing our hair the way it naturally grows from the scalp become an issue worthy of books, blogs, video tutorials and even lawsuits? Why do we have to *learn* how to work with something we came into this world with?

The Natural Minority

We have to learn because so many of us simply do not know what to do with our own natural hair! Some of us have had relaxed hair for so

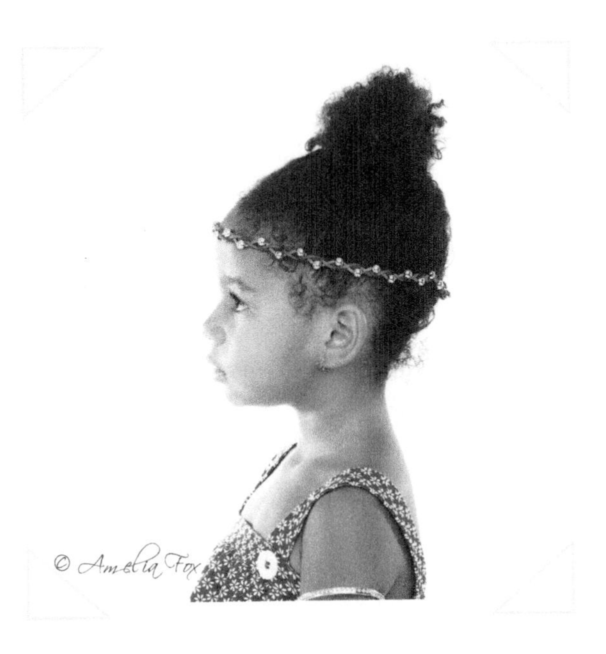

long that our relaxed hair is what *feels natural* to us. Relaxed hair, in many ways, is pretty much our default texture! It's how our hair has *always* been. Relaxed hair, for many of us, is natural. In fact, most of us are trained from almost an elementary age in the art of caring for straight hair.

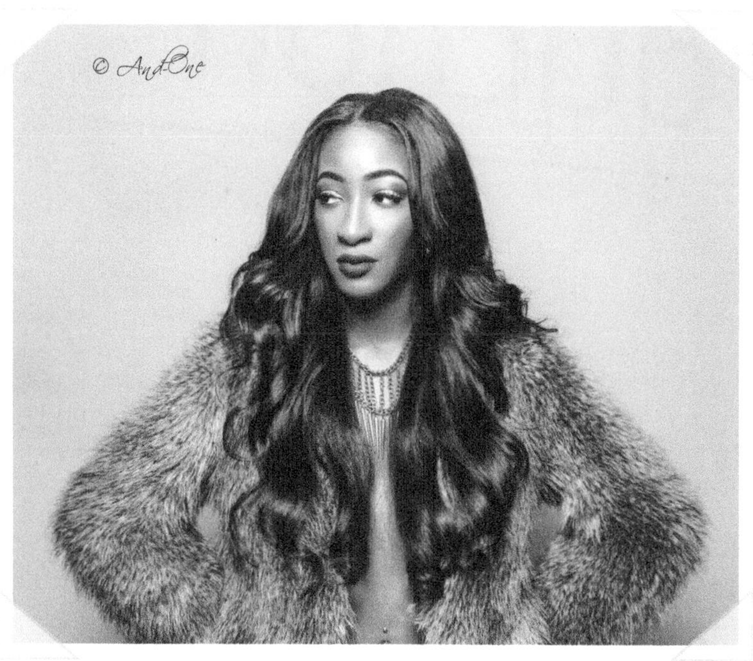

Seeing ourselves with straight hair is a training that starts so early and is reinforced so deeply that we almost have trouble seeing it. It just feels normal. When something feels normal, everything else becomes abnormal.

We normalize this picture—*brown face, straight hair*—until we can't see any other possibilities. That picture is even reinforced with the toys and dolls we play with until, eventually, it is us. We become so used to seeing various shades of beautiful black and brown faces—with straight hair—that the natural combination of those faces with their natural hair looks wrong.

Children in our community are not always aware that relaxers are an *optional* category of hair product. As a child, you may have heard comments from people about how so-and-so "needs a touch up" or simply taken note of the fact that relaxers are sold side-by-side with shampoos, conditioners, lotions, deodorants and other basic grooming must-haves. How much more normal could relaxers get? In fact, relaxers are so normal in our community that many of us truly believe that the natural state of our hair is a peculiar mix of stick-straightness with a constant pillow-puffiness at the roots.

We have been taught early on, through all types of messages, that our hair is not ideal. Many of us were taught that relaxers are also a "rite of passage"—a mature choice. For our young girls who are growing up today, trading in their ponytails, braids and barrettes for the long, straight, flowing hair that they see glorified in magazines and on television almost seems like a no-brainer. Our mothers' and grandmothers' tug-of-war with our hair on wash days also let many of us know early on that our hair must be "problematic." In the absence of positive messages, many of us have learned contempt and even shame about our hair in the place of pride.

So, what we have today is a real natural-hair minority. Yes, despite the rosy picture painted in the blogosphere, the growing number of YouTube channels, the overflowing natural-hair-product shelves and the hundreds of thousands of women who turn out for natural-hair meet-ups and shows each year, only about three of every ten American women of African descent wears her hair in its natural state. Wearing hairstyles that celebrate and display highly textured hair in its natural state is uncommon. When not even half of us wear our hair in its natural state, it's definitely a big deal to one day end your long-term relationship with your relaxer!

Even in places where natural hair is more common, we still suffer from a lack of knowledge

©Moneca

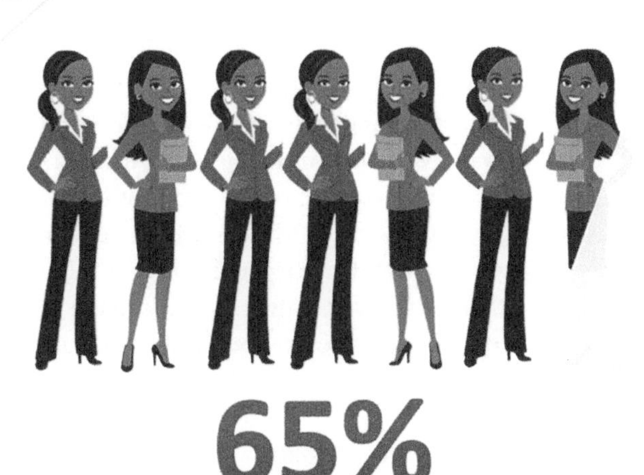

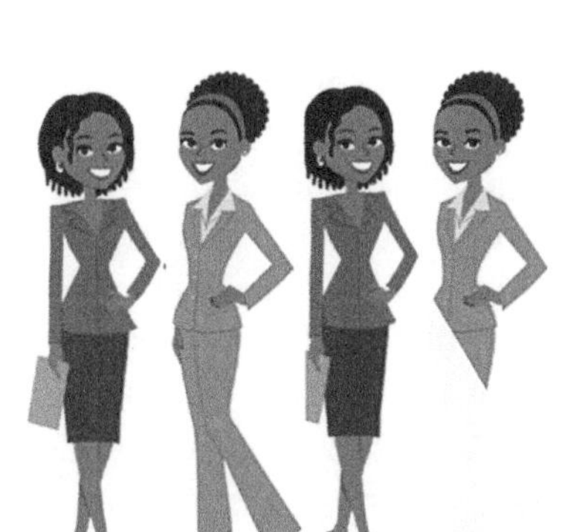

Almost 7 out of every 10 US women chemically relax their hair.

surrounding our hair. Our own hair has become a lost art, just like the native languages, customs and knowledge of home and self that our ancestors possessed. We are so conditioned to understand the challenges and needs of straight hair that anything else is difficult. We simply haven't been taught how to work with, or what to expect from, our natural hair. In fact, we usually don't have much exposure to it beyond a few incredibly dry centimeters of length. For many of us, relaxers have become our standard and the basis by which we judge everything. Even our stylists are trained almost exclusively to care for relaxed hair or natural hair that is worn straight.

If you think about us, we're like songbirds that have never learned to sing. Although we were born to sing, when we try to carry a tune—we just can't. This book is going to teach you how to sing again!

In this book we'll discuss the two basic ways by which you can return to your natural hair:

1. the *Big Chop* (cutting off your relaxed hair and then growing in your natural hair)

   or by

2. *slowly transitioning your hair* (growing in your natural hair while your relaxed hair remains, and then cutting off your relaxed ends slowly over time).

We will spend the most time on the process of transitioning, since it is by far the most popular (and the most time-intensive!) way to "go natural."

Getting Your Hair Done

Think about your earliest experiences at the salon. If you are like most people, you were conditioned from very early on to associate your hair's "doneness" with straightness. Our minds are conditioned to see kinky-curly hair going into the salon and silky, flat, straight hair coming out. How different would our outlook be if we regularly saw kinky-curly hair going into the salon and saw the same kinky-curly hair—styled in a way that celebrates its texture and nature—coming out?

Defining Natural

As you make steps along your natural journey, you'll quickly find that there are lots of definitions of *natural*. In the truest sense, natural hair is hair that has never been chemically processed—ever. Chemical processing includes both permanent color treatments and straightening treatments.

In this book, we use a very texture-focused definition of the word *natural*. We define natural very simply as hair that is free from any *deliberate* means of chemical straightening without regard for whether or not the hair is color treated.

What To Expect When You Are Expecting (Natural Hair)

If you're a mom, no doubt you've heard of the wildly popular book series *What To Expect When You're Expecting*. In a way, you could say that going natural is like expecting a baby! The transitioning process is like the pregnancy that eventually brings you face to face with your new bundle of joy.

The nine months of pregnancy are an important time. This time gives the mother-to-be a chance to get comfortable with the idea of becoming a mother. It's a preparatory period that gives her time to choose a name for the little one, decide how she'll raise the child and figure out how she'll share her worldview with this new little person. The mother learns how to sacrifice some of her own comforts and some of her old ways of doing things for the benefit of another person. Some days are better for her than others; she might even have to field the occasional well-intentioned but awkward comment. But pregnancy is a time that builds the mother-in-waiting's confidence and teaches her about herself, her body and her limits. Just imagine if pregnancy were an overnight process and mothers magically woke up one day with a baby in their arms! Some mothers would take right off and be just fine, while others would certainly struggle with the new challenge. And, the rest of the family would need time to adjust to the changes, too!

Transitioning to natural hair is very similar to a pregnancy. For many women who do need a bit more time and encouragement to get going, taking on the Big Chop right away is like waking up with the baby in your arms on day one! Some women could wake up fully natural and be able to take right off on their natural journeys, while others would need a bit more motivation, support and time to get to that point. Transitioning can level the playing field between the two groups so that just about everyone does well.

Transitioning not only allows time for the hair to grow, but for the transitioning woman to grow as well. The weeks, months or years of transitioning give the natural-to-be a chance to get comfortable with the idea of returning to her natural hair. Like a mother-to-be, the natural-to-be learns how to sacrifice her own comforts and old ways of doing things for the benefit of her hair and herself. And just like the mom-to-be, some moments are better for her than others. The natural-in-waiting too will very likely have to deal with occasional well-intentioned but unhelpful comments—and her family also may have to adjust.

No Time Like the Present

The good thing for you is that you are in the right place at the right time! Transitioning your relaxed hair back to its natural, unprocessed state is just as much a liberating experience as it is a terrifying one—but there is no time like today

The Science of Black Hair Super Survey

Throughout this book, you will see references to some of the results we collected from our informal opinion poll on hair attitudes, trends and practices. More than five hundred respondents who were at various points in their hair journeys completed the poll. We are pretty sure that you'll find the survey info very interesting!

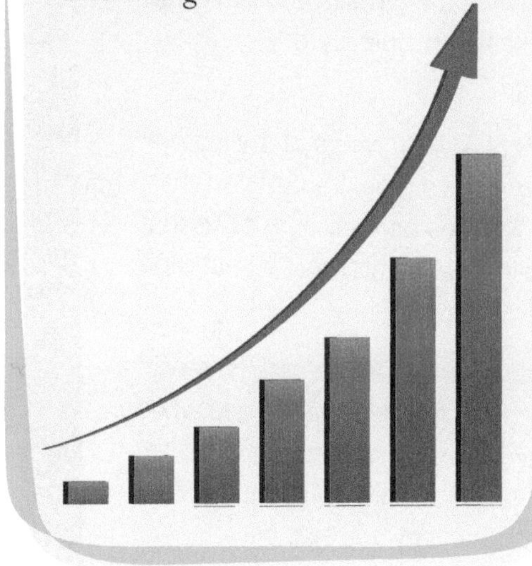

to try your natural hair again. The Internet has all but pushed the revolution into overdrive and made it that much easier to get on board! Inspirational photos, tips and techniques for caring for our hair make it from one side of the world to the other in seconds, and products for moisturizing, defining and bringing kinks and curls to life continue to spring up every single day. When you embark on this journey, you help normalize natural hair for others who are watching you find your way back to natural. And that's amazing! Everywhere you turn, there is new inspiration and love—so much so that you will likely feel overwhelmed by all of the resources and information. This guide is here simply to help you sort through the excitement and fall in love with your hair again.

How This Book Will Help You

You may be considering transitioning to your natural hair because you want to try something new, because you like natural hairstyles and their versatility or because you've simply been forced to make a change due to damage from chemical relaxers. No matter what brings you to this journey, let me tell you one thing: You are certainly in for an amazing, even a life-changing experience!

But change is not always easy. When you decide one day to just abruptly back away from relaxers and allow the hair that you've laid down on schedule every six to eight weeks to just . . . *be*—friends, coworkers and even family members may not understand what you are doing and why. And, of course, it is not always easy to charge forward when the ones you care about most seem to care very little for what they are hoping is just your new hair phase. This book will help you reason through those moments. You will learn that, in many ways, transitioning is not a solo event; it's a very public one. Those around you will also be transitioning in their own way, and you'll need to allow them the space and opportunity for that.

The path to natural hair is also just as much a journey back as it is a journey forward. You'll have to challenge some old thinking along the way. You'll have to unlearn some things and relearn others. This path is a process, that's for sure, and the journey is different for everyone. Are you ready?

How do you make the transition from relaxed to natural hair? What's involved in the process, and what should you consider? This book is designed to answer these questions for you and expand upon the original transitioning discussion provided in my first book, *The Science of Black Hair: A Comprehensive Guide to Textured Hair Care.*

Top Reasons Why You Should Definitely Go Au Naturel

Here's why you are making a great hair care choice:

1. **It's healthy.** Wearing your hair in its natural state is best for your hair's long-term health and maintenance. Hair simply thrives better when we get out of its way and let it grow the way it was originally designed to!
2. **No chemical risk.** Going natural means no more chemical exposure for your scalp and hair. The alkalinity and aggressiveness of both lye and no-lye relaxers can leave the scalp chronically dry and your hair vulnerable to breakage and splitting.
3. **Styling versatility.** Natural hair offers a wide range of styling options: Hair can be worn straight one day, curly the next and, if your hair type allows, in super-textured kinky hairstyles as well. Any style that you can create with relaxed hair can be replicated on natural hair—and often with a much fuller, lusher result!
4. **Improved strength.** If you constantly battle breakage problems with your relaxed hair, you'll find much of this random breakage alleviated when you experience your natural hair—provided you follow a proactive, healthy hair-care regimen. When we wear our textured hair in its natural state, these fragile fibers are truly the strongest that they will ever be.
5. **A real shot at reaching terminal length.** Over time, improved strength translates to longer hair and increases the chances that your hair will reach its terminal length—that is, the longest length your hair can potentially grow given your genetic makeup. Reaching terminal length takes anywhere from four to ten years, and if your hair-care practices have created a favorable environment for growth during this time, you'll see the healthiest, longest (and biggest, since most natural hair grows up and out) hair of your life!
6. **You are beautiful as you are.** And that's final. You are wonderfully and perfectly made. Every single wave, kink and coil upon your head.

Your Journey, Your Way

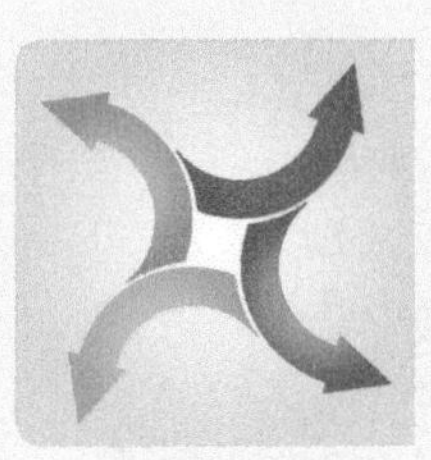

If you've already done your Big Chop or are newly natural, you may skip ahead to page 115, "Living the Natural Life," for more hands-on information that is relevant to your stage of this process. If at any time you feel like you need some work and extra encouragement to get yourself emotionally prepared to enjoy the natural life, feel free to refer to Chapter 7 (page 100), "Your Mind in Transition," for some great tips!

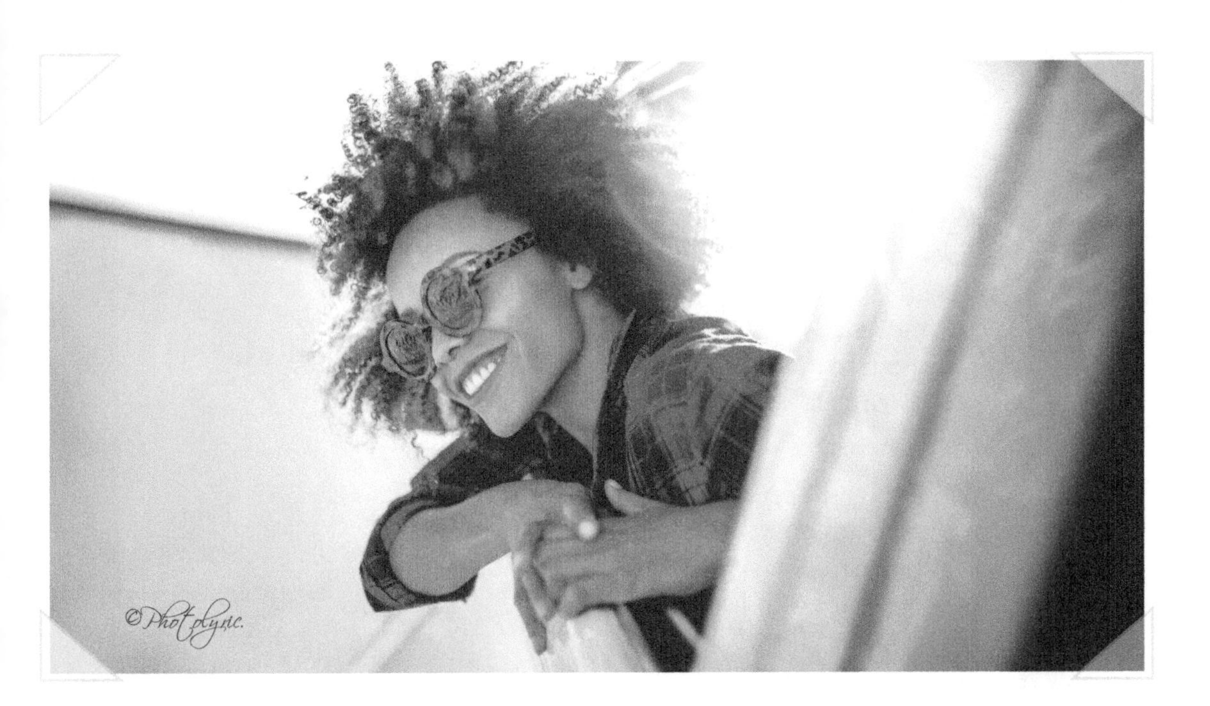

Déjà vu?

Now, some of you may be thinking, We've done this all before. And we have. We only need to look back to the 1960s and '70s to see moments when big, full manes of healthy natural hair reigned supreme. Like today, those were times when sales of relaxer products and services were down, and natural hair was very much in! But that first movement did not stay with us. Relaxers came back into vogue during the '80s, and once again, straight soon became the default style for kinky-curly girls. Fortunately, there are some pretty significant things that we have going in our favor these days that will probably give this new renaissance more staying power! Here's where we are strong:

Education is King!

Today's movement is rooted in education. In fact, what we suffer from these days is information overload and having to sift through a huge store of experiences and opinions. There are more workshops, meet-ups, books and websites dedicated to expanding natural-hair education today than ever before. Our sisters who traveled this path before us did not have the luxury of information overload, education and a "virtual family" to support their journeys—although the movement certainly blossomed and moved right along just fine without these things!

We're Wired

Natural hair journeys these days are taking place amidst a whirlwind of technological activity. Where would many of us be if we could not scroll through [insert your favorite social media network] feeds for styling inspiration or visit blogs and hair-care forums for tips? If I had to make a guess, I'd say: Lost!

Videos, blogs, websites and books have helped us to reimagine our hair and have created a community with new language around it. Who'd have thought that you could take a photo of your hair or jot down a paragraph on your blog and have women the world over like it, share it and feel inspired enough by it to march into their bathrooms and cut off their own hair? That's the movement today! Sisters before us did not have the luxury of logging on to chat and sharing ideas with their extended international family, but they pressed on anyway (no pun intended!). They had to rely on what was immediately around them: their families, their friends and the sometimes narrow images of black beauty that television and magazines provided.

Increased Product Offerings and Innovation

There is no shortage of hair-care products for naturalistas these days. Our hair salons and cosmetology schools are working overtime to adapt to the needs of a changing clientele, while product manufacturers scramble to reengineer, repackage and create hair products to support the natural-hair renaissance. Sisters in earlier decades couldn't stroll down the aisles of their local grocery stores and find an overwhelming selection of products formulated with them in mind, or watch step-by-step product videos from women around the world on how to build a good hair-care regimen with those products. Sure, products were available—but not with anything near the accessibility and variety of today.

Explosion in Entrepreneurship

Finally, we can't forget about the entrepreneurship and economic opportunities this movement has made available to just about any woman with a computer or a camera who is willing to share her thoughts. Bloggers, vloggers, event planners, marketing divas, inspirational speakers, artists, nutrition gurus, clothing and apparel makers have all found a place where their creativity can be tapped and used for the better. And what about books like this one and the others my fellow hair mavens have written? Or the "kitchenticians" and former-kitchenticians-turned-commercial-product-makers who have provided us with amazing hair-care products designed especially for our hair? Or the stylists who've added natural styling and care to their lists of skills and services? Our work is economically viable because this movement is amazingly ALIVE!

Things are looking up, but we do have to be careful. Although the movement is maturing and seems to have firmly put down its roots, believing that the current renaissance will be immune to the fate of the previous one makes it even more vulnerable to the same demise. There are others outside of our community who see the economic power of this movement, and they are ready and willing to capitalize on our efforts if we do not fiercely protect what we have.

unit 1

The Risks of Chemical Dependency

Why Is This Section Important?

It may seem odd to start off a book for transitioners and new naturals with a primer on relaxers, but this discussion is necessary for a few reasons. Many of you have already made the decision to return to your natural hair, but for those of you who are still relaxed and are on the fence about making a move away from relaxers, you may not be fully aware of how relaxing affects the hair. It's so important for you to have some background about what relaxers are, how they work and what they do. Arming yourself with this knowledge will ensure that you are walking into your relaxer/no-relaxer hair care decision with open eyes.

For those of you who are already well into your transition to natural hair or are newly natural, this section is also important for you. Should you ever start feeling doubtful about your decision to make the transition or simply to maintain your natural hair, this section will serve as a reminder of the very many good reasons to continue avoiding these products in your hair-care journey.

Teaching in Love

Remember, it's difficult to present the negatives of any choice in a balanced way. While it is healthy to challenge one another, we should always strive to encourage and teach one another in love. Our goal in this book is not to bash chemical relaxers or those who use them. However, we will certainly explore the very many reasons why we should think twice about including them in our healthy hair-care journeys. Making informed choices about your hair care is always the goal—no matter what you ultimately decide to do with your hair.

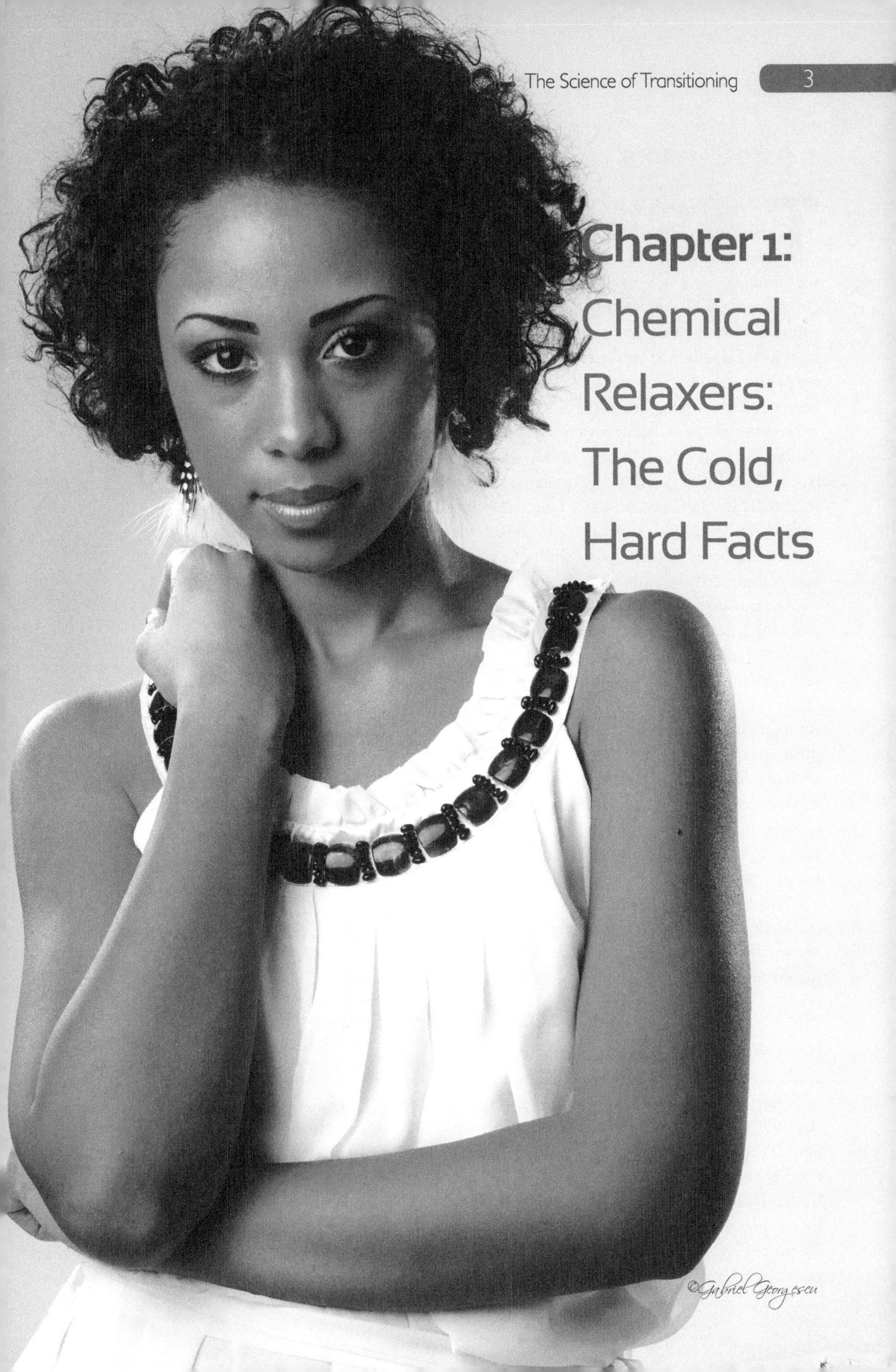

Chapter 1: Chemical Relaxers: The Cold, Hard Facts

1. A Brief History

The very first chemical relaxer was discovered by accident. Garrett Morgan, an African-American sewing machine mechanic, was looking for a way to polish his sewing machine needles and had already developed a liquid solution that showed some promise. One day, he wiped his solution onto a wool cloth and was surprised the next day to find that the woolly fibers had been straightened. He experimented with the solution on his neighbor's dog (an Airedale terrier) and then, finally, on his own curly hair. After a bit of tweaking, Morgan soon began to market the new product as a hair straightening gel. In 1913, G. A. Morgan Hair Refining Cream was born. Because of its ability to quickly and permanently straighten the hair, the relaxer easily surpassed the popular "hot plate" and "hot combing" methods of the early 1900s to become the preferred choice for straightening highly textured hair.

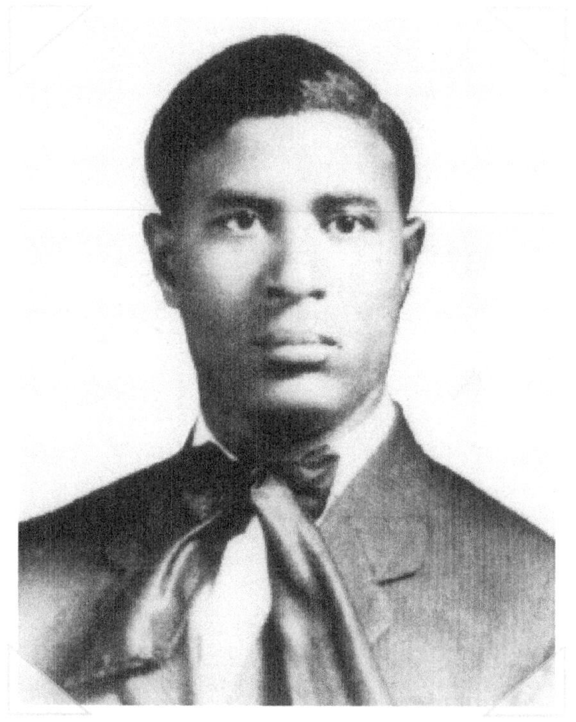

Fig. 1.0: Garrett A. Morgan. In addition to developing the earliest chemical relaxer formula, Garrett Morgan also gave us inventions such as the three-way traffic signal and gas mask.

Relaxers have evolved quite a bit since the beginning of the twentieth century and the days of Morgan's first crude relaxer cream. The first modern hair relaxer was released onto the commercial market in the 1950's but, like the formulas in Morgan's day, these formulas were still very harsh. Consumer demand pushed product manufacturers to explore safer ways to remove the kinks and curls from textured tresses, and eventually newer chemical compounds that produced similar straightening results with less irritation were introduced.

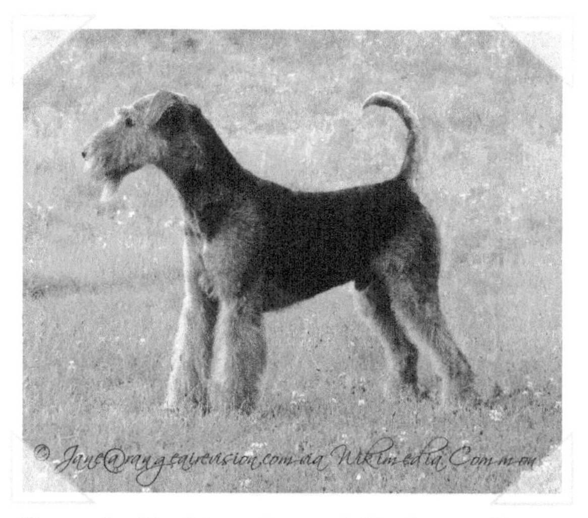

Fig. 1.1: An Airedale terrier much like the one Garrett Morgan used for his hair-straightening experiments.

However, despite improvements in formulation, application and safety, reports of hair breakage, hair loss and thinning continued to mount. In the 1970s, the U.S. Federal Trade Commission (FTC) required that warning labels be added to relaxer products. Ayana Byrd and Lori Tharpe's book, Hair Story, provides interesting background into the FTC warning label story. At first, the FTC required only the makers of Ultra Sheen relaxer (a black-owned company) to add a warning label to its product, while its major competitor, Revlon, was allowed to market its relaxers—which contained the same ingredients—warning free. During this time, Revlon was able to gain a greater market share because

> **Did You Know?**
>
> Contrary to popular belief, women of African descent are not the only users of chemical relaxers—but they are the most prevalent.

they were able to market their relaxers as safer products. Nearly two years passed before other companies were required to add a warning label.

These warnings are important because chemical relaxing is by far the harshest basic styling process that a hair strand will encounter in its lifetime. Relaxers alter the hair's texture through a process of "controlled damage" to the hair's inner protein structure. During the relaxer process, the hair's outer protective layer is attacked, and the bonds that hold the strand together are seized, broken apart and physically rearranged. Multiply this process many times over a lifetime, and you can imagine the stress and trauma our hair and scalp must regularly endure for curly-kinky tresses to be kept straight.

1.1 Modern Relaxer Chemistry

Despite the advancements in relaxer formulas over the years, today's chemical relaxers are still hard on the hair. Relaxers remain extremely alkaline hair-care products that penetrate our hair and skin tissues quickly and immediately begin the work of breaking down the hair fiber.

What really makes relaxers problematic is the pH level to which they must be formulated in order to work on the hair. We can't discuss the real impact of chemical relaxing without knowing something about pH. A substance's pH is measured on a scale that runs from 0 to 14. Substances that measure higher than 7 on the pH scale are considered alkaline (basic), while substances that measure lower than 7 on the scale are considered acidic. Our hair and skin both carry a slightly acidic pH of 4.5 to 5.5, which is near the lower end of the pH scale. Most hair products are also formulated to have a low pH to help keep our hair within the healthy range.

We run into problems when we use products like relaxers and permanent hair colors that take us far out of our pH safety zone and into the alkaline range. Chemical relaxers are formulated

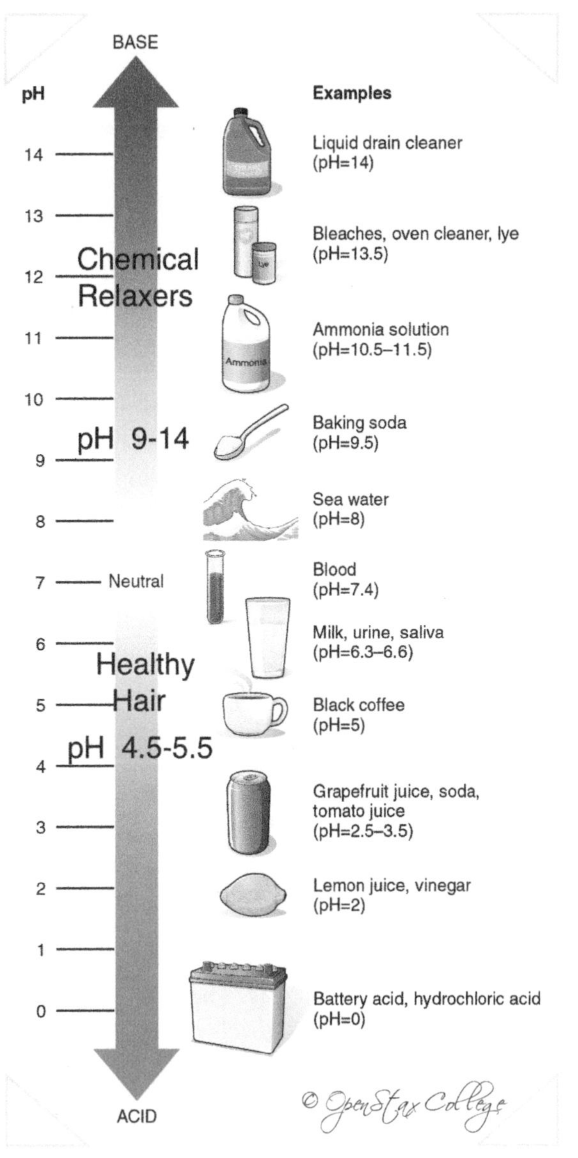

Fig. 1.2: The pH Scale.

at pH ranges that are often one million times more alkaline than hair at its resting pH. How is this so? The pH scale is *logarithmic*. Each step on the pH scale represents a **ten-fold** increase in strength. This means that a product formulated at a pH of 5 is ten times more alkaline than a product formulated at pH 4, and one hundred times more alkaline than a product formulated at pH 3. Relaxers' high pH range puts them in the company of other caustic products such as ammonia, bleach and drain cleaners. We will talk more about the importance of pH in our hair care when we discuss our other hair products in Chapter 4 (pages 47-51).

Breaking Down Your Basic Relaxer

Most people are surprised to learn that only a very small percentage of the relaxer cream is active. Relaxer creams are mostly oil, water, thickeners and emulsifiers (ingredients that keep oil and water from separating) by concentration. The active ingredient is usually some form of hydroxide. In both lye and no-lye relaxers, the hydroxide active ingredients are so potent that very little is required in formulation to achieve straightening results. Relaxers are mostly made up of heavy oils for two reasons: 1) to buffer and protect the hair from the harsh active ingredient, while still allowing it to be in close contact with the hair and 2) to help hold the hair in a straightened position to achieve a straighter end result.

Lye vs. No-Lye Relaxers

Lye relaxers are *sodium hydroxide*-based systems. These types of relaxers process the hair very quickly and are the preferred type of relaxer for professional cosmetologists. These relaxers usually have the highest pH levels (between pH 12 and 14) and tend to be the most aggressive. In general, the concentration of sodium hydroxide in a relaxer rarely exceeds 2.5 percent, even in the strongest formulas. Lye relaxers are said to be "easy on the hair and hard on the scalp" because unlike "no-lye" relaxers, they do not leave mineral buildup behind on the hair. However, they can be extremely aggressive on the scalp if contact occurs inadvertently.

No-lye relaxer systems are the variety you'll find on shelves for DIY consumers. These include *potassium hydroxide-, lithium hydroxide-* and *guanidine hydroxide*-based relaxer products. These no-lye relaxers are formulated at a slightly lower pH than lye relaxers, usually between pH 9 and 11. Although the concentration of active ingredient in no-lye relaxers is somewhat higher than in lye relaxers (5 to 9 percent), their lower pH means that they still tend to be less aggressive and don't pack as hard a punch. No-lye relaxers are said to be "easy on the scalp and hard on the hair" because while they do not aggravate the scalp as quickly as lye relaxers, they can leave calcium mineral deposits behind on the hair shaft. These mineral deposits can make the hair feel extremely dry and brittle.

1.2 How Relaxers Affect Your Scalp

The chemical relaxing process takes its toll on our skin, and exposing the scalp to these products can lead to temporary—and sometimes permanent—adverse health effects. When relaxers come in contact with our delicate skin, they "defat" and dehydrate the scalp. Defatting occurs when chemicals dissolve the skin's natural fatty acids and sebum (the oil our scalp naturally produces). Proteins in the skin are also denatured, or broken down, by the relaxing process. Without these much-needed layers of protection, the scalp is more likely to lose its natural moisture and feel chronically dry. Common adverse effects include scalp tightness, redness, dryness, itchiness, weeping, scabbing, and discomfort. Unfortunately, we can experience these side effects of relaxer use even when these products are applied correctly.

Greenwashing

In 2011, a California environmental group sued 26 natural product companies and forced them to re-label their products. The reason for the lawsuit? The companies had "greenwashed" their products. Greenwashing occurs when a company claims that their product is natural, organic or environmentally-friendly, but the company's practices or ingredients just don't measure up to their claims. In the case of the popular natural companies, many of them had included the word "organic" in their product names. Unfortunately, their products and ingredients simply did not meet the criteria for organic products.

Because chemical relaxers are not products that actually benefit the hair, relaxer companies often rely on greenwashing to help market them. They may use greenwashed terms in the product's name, labels or other marketing. Have you seen any of these words used on your relaxer boxes? If so, they've been greenwashed!

- Botanical
- Fresh
- Inspired by Nature
- Organic
- Pure
- Conditioning
- Green
- Natural
- Sustainable
- Wholesome
- Exotic
- Innovative
- Nourishes
- Vegan

Companies also greenwash by:

- Emphasizing natural oils (coconut oil, olive oil, argan oil, etc) or ingredients that barely figure into the formula. (Ex: calling a product mango butter relaxer when mango butter is 13th on the ingredients list and less than one percent of the product.)

- Using earthy colors on packaging and ads, and putting natural things like leaves and berries on the box.

- Using their own natural/organic ingredient logo certifications or quality logos rather than established 3rd party certifications.

Now, doing these kinds of things is not greenwashing IF the product is legitimate and actually lives up to the claims. It's only greenwashing when these types of things are done just to make a product look greener, safer or more natural than it really is. In the case of chemical relaxers, green terms are almost always an attempt to play down the negatives of an inherently damaging product.

Fortunately, for many users the effects of chemical relaxing are mild and heal quickly after the relaxer service. Many of these negative effects can be treated with time and regular conditioning. Unfortunately, this ability to easily patch up the damage from relaxers also creates a certain tolerance or acceptance for these negative effects. Since many of us are introduced to chemical relaxers at an early age, the negatives have been pretty much normalized as "just the cost of doing business."

For many users who have only experienced the temporary side effects of chemical relaxing, the perceived benefits of relaxing still outweigh the risks. However, prolonged chemical relaxing may also lead to more permanent problems. These effects include scarring of the scalp skin, hair breakage or loss, and increased sensitivity for our delicate scalp skin. Prolonged contact with relaxers can result in dermatitis and permanent damage to the scalp and hair follicles. In fact, chemically relaxing the hair increases the risk of developing traction alopecia—a condition in which repetitive tension on the hair follicle results in irreversible hair loss.

Transitional Hair (a.k.a. "Scab Hair")

Yet another way that relaxers may have an effect on the scalp can be heard in the natural hair community's debates about the myth or reality of "scab hair." If you are a frequent visitor of hair-care websites, you've no doubt heard of *scab hair*. (NOTE: Because scab hair is a misnomer—there are no scabs, skin or crusts involved whatsoever—we will refer to this hair from here on out as *transitional hair*.) Transitional hair is a phenomenon that many new naturals experience at their Big Chop, and it is defined as a combination of wiry, dry and semi-straight natural hair that does not have a defined curl or coil pattern. This transitional hair is usually isolated to the first few inches of new growth that emerge after chemical relaxing has been stopped. No one knows what causes these hair changes—but there are some really good theories, one of which we'll discuss here.

Follicle Shape Change Theory

According to "Follicle Shape-Change Theory," extra-dry, unpredictable transitional hair is caused by changes to the hair follicles' structure as a result of the long-term use of chemical relaxers. Transitional hair is a temporary hair situation that is usually resolved as the follicle recovers and the hair grows and settles into its permanent natural arrangement. Some naturals are convinced that it is a hair-care myth cooked up by transitioners and new naturals to explain away hair textures they don't like. But for those who feel they have experienced transitional hair firsthand, it is definitely as real as real gets. Since there is no scientific research to prove or disprove the existence of transitional hair, theories are all we have to work with.

Hair Follicles are Living Structures

In order to understand where transitional hair might come from, we need to understand how hair grows and how its shape is ultimately determined. Our hair follicles are self-renewing and are the only live parts of the hair shaft. Since the hair follicle is constantly generating new hair cells, changes in the follicle's size and shape can affect the way hair is presented or grown out. When the follicle changes shape and size, the hair that pushes through it will also change shape and texture. Although the original shape and position of our hair follicles is predetermined by hormones and genetics, damage from day-to-day environmental stressors such as heat, tension and chemical relaxers can also affect our hair follicles.

Waxing is a prime example of an external stressor that can lead to follicle shape change. Waxing and tweezing thin out hair over time because these practices stress the hair follicle and cause it to miniaturize, or shrink. This change in follicle size causes thinner, finer hair to grow up from the follicle.

Traction alopecia is another great example of follicle shape change. Tension placed on delicate follicles leads to inflammation under the skin and, eventually, to follicle miniaturization. Hair follicles produce thinner and thinner hair shafts until eventually no new hairs are produced. Follicle miniaturization is largely irreversible. Once a follicle shrinks, it is usually out for the count! But there is a grace period. If caught in its earliest stages, before the scalp is permanently damaged, this form of hair loss is temporary and reversible. Removing the stressor (tight hair styles) allows the hair follicle to recover so that it can produce hairs once again as intended.

In the case of chemical relaxing, changes to the follicle shape are also temporary and reversible—if the stressor (relaxing) is discontinued before any permanent damage to the scalp occurs. When relaxers do permanently damage the scalp and hair follicles, we experience complete hair loss. As the follicle begins to recover in the weeks following the last relaxer, the immediate new growth we produce is pushed out as transitional hair. Once the follicle is fully reestablished, we lose the hybrid texture and see our true natural texture.

To date there is no literature or scientific evidence available either proving or disproving this hair texture-change phenomenon. This should not be surprising, given that the science of textured hair in general, whether relaxed or natural, is light-years behind the science of European and Asian hair. I like Follicle Change Theory as a potential explanation for transitional hair because it accepts the amazing permeability of skin layers as fact but avoids the pitfalls of "Relaxed Scalp Theory," which suggests that relaxer chemicals seep into the scalp and continue to actively process hair, even before the hair actually emerges from the scalp. Follicle Change Theory also underscores the ability of environmental stressors to influence our biology and affect our health. When we consider the fact that many women have chemical relaxers in contact (or near contact) with their scalps every eight to ten weeks for five or more decades, it is very possible that this regular contact could sensitize and affect the structures of the scalp skin.

Without scientific data to prove or disprove that Follicle Change Theory is the cause of transitional hair textures, we are all still left guessing. Certainly, more research is needed in this area.

1.3 How Relaxers Affect Your Hair

Our hair is made up mostly of very strong proteins, but even the most robust proteins don't fare well in alkaline pH environments. When alkaline relaxers and other chemicals are used on the hair, they must destroy the hair's protein in order to make the cosmetic changes we desire. Although many of us work diligently to protect the scalp with petroleum bases and other oil-based products, we can't protect and account for every inch of skin. Relaxers still make regular contact with our scalps, especially during the "smoothing" stage of the relaxing process, when the stylist physically straightens the relaxer-coated fibers. Chemical relaxers are able to work because their alkalinity gives them the power to break down and dissolve our hair's proteins. If the hair's protein structure is under attack for long enough, the strand will weaken, swell and eventually disintegrate.

This tendency for hair proteins to break down in alkaline environments is the same one that allows liquid drain cleaning products, which are like super-concentrated relaxers without the extra conditioning oil bases, to unclog and remove hair from drains. These products simply break down the proteins they find—much more aggressively than a relaxer, of course—and turn them into mush. Once the proteins are broken down into mush, the force of water easily tears through the compromised protein structure and pushes the hair down the drain.

If we look at the steps in the chemical relaxing process and how chemical relaxers actually straighten our hair, we see that the potential for damage is great and—if the relaxer is going to really straighten as we want it to—unavoidable. Let's go through the steps to see what happens when we relax our hair:

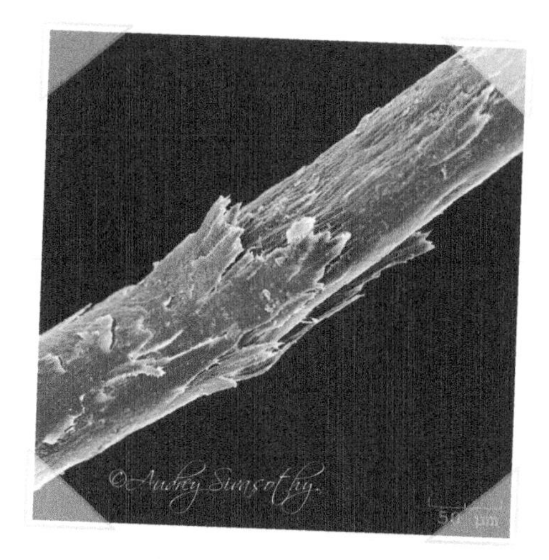

Step 1: The relaxer must penetrate the hair fiber.

When relaxers come in contact with the hair, the first thing they must do is raise its pH environment. The hair's pH rises from a comfortable pH of 4 or 5 to a much higher pH of 10 or more. This causes the hair fiber to swell and allows the relaxer's active ingredient to gain entry into the hair's inner cortex. Research has shown that hair fibers can swell as much as 60 to 80 percent of their normal diameter during the chemical-relaxing process. Because the cuticle layer is less flexible and isn't able to expand at the same rate as the inner layers, it simply cracks and fractures along the length of the hair strand in much the same way that a tight sausage skin splits and peels when the sausage is cooked. Lye relaxers are formulated near the pinnacle of the pH scale and therefore swell the hair shaft quickly and more significantly than other relaxer types.

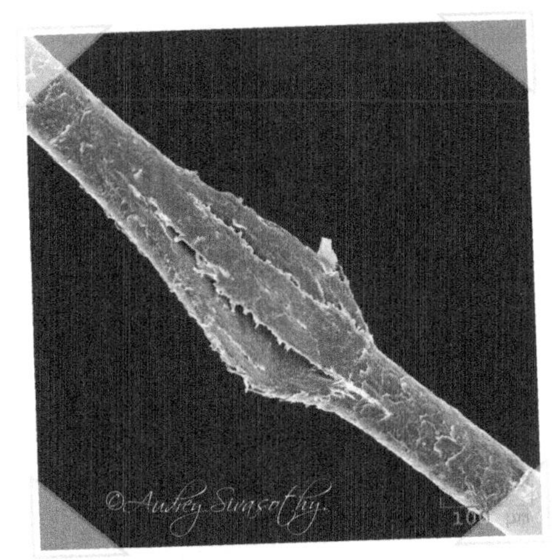

Step 2: The relaxer must start breaking bonds.

Most of the damage we encounter with chemical relaxing comes from this step in the relaxing process. Our hair is held together by a network of bonds called disulfide bonds. These bonds are what reinforce our hair's curly shape, and give it its strength and texture. These bonds are so strong that they cannot be broken by water or heat. Chemicals are the only substances powerful enough to break down and disrupt disulfide bonds.

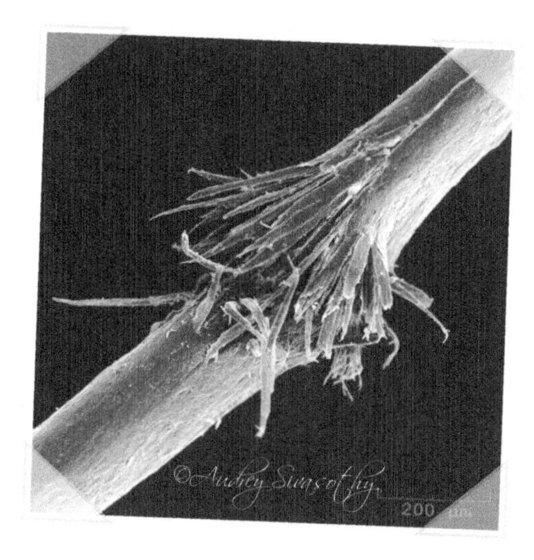

Fig. 1.3: Microscopic images of my own chemically relaxed hair strands. This hair survived ten months of transitioning and was harvested from the hair I cut during my Big Chop. Note the severe cracking and erosion of my hair's outer protective layer.

Each disulfide bond in our hair contains two sulfur atoms. During the relaxing process, millions of cross-linked disulfide bonds are dismantled. New bonds that contain just one sulfur atom are created in their place. These new, weaker bonds are called *lanthionine bonds*, and they are what hold the hair fiber in its new, straight configuration. The chemical relaxing process also affects the hair's protein linkages and hydrogen bonds. These bonds contribute strength to the hair and help it maintain optimal levels of moisturization.

With each new relaxer, the potential for overlapping relaxer chemicals onto previously relaxed cuticle layers (and the scalp) is high because most new growth is still quite short and compact. This is especially true at six to eight weeks after a relaxer, when most people schedule their touchups. Unfortunately, the points where the relaxer has overlapped onto previously relaxed hair become weak points along the hair strand that are extremely prone to breakage.

Overlapping leads to unintentional damage from overprocessing. Hair that has been overprocessed by chemical relaxers has a difficult time holding onto its moisture, is extremely porous and lacks elasticity. (See, Chapter 4, pages 47-51 for more on hair porosity and elasticity.) If the hair is not addressed and treated quickly, chronic breakage will occur. Those with finer hair strands and color-treated hair tend to have the most immediate negative impact from chemical relaxing. This is why processing times for fine and colored hair types tend to be much shorter than for other types of hair. Since the hairline and edges tend to have finer overall strands, processing times there tend to be shorter as well.

Step 3: The hair's bonds must be rearranged.

Did you know that the active ingredient in chemical relaxers is not responsible for the physical straightening of our hair? A relaxer's job is to hold the hair still while it raises the pH environment around the hair so that the fiber swells and the hair's disulfide bonds break. But breaking bonds isn't the end of the story. Once these bonds are broken, the hair still isn't straight. The hair has to be arranged into its new, desired shape. This is where the smoothing process comes in.

Relaxer Trauma: A Matter of Degrees

When chemical relaxers come in contact with the hair, they swell the hair shaft and strip away its outermost protective layer (the cuticle). Hair that is relaxed to near complete straightness (pin-straight), or that is overlapped on a regular basis, receives more cuticle trauma than hair that has been relaxed to a lesser degree or has not been relaxed at all.

Relaxer products are formulated to be thick, heavy creams, so that they can hold the hair in place. These paste-like products keep the hair immobile while kinks, coils and curls are extended for straightening. This process is highly damaging to textured hair fibers and great care must be taken during the smoothing stage to ensure that manipulation is kept to a minimum and that the relaxer cream isn't overlapped. Aggressive smoothing or combing the hair during the relaxing process can damage and thin out a hair strand by stretching it beyond what it can tolerate. In some cases, the strand simply breaks immediately under the pressure. But even when the strand remains intact, it's often an overextended, much weaker strand that will eventually break later on with normal day-to-day styling.

Step 4: The hair's pH must be neutralized.

In the final step, neutralization, the pH of the hair is ushered back down with the help of water and a low pH shampoo, lotion or conditioner.

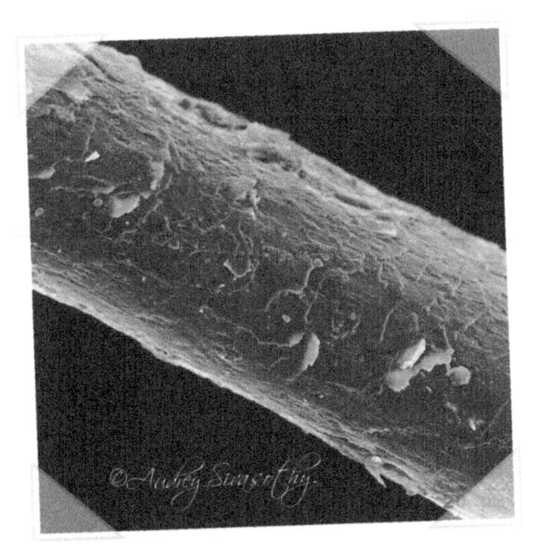

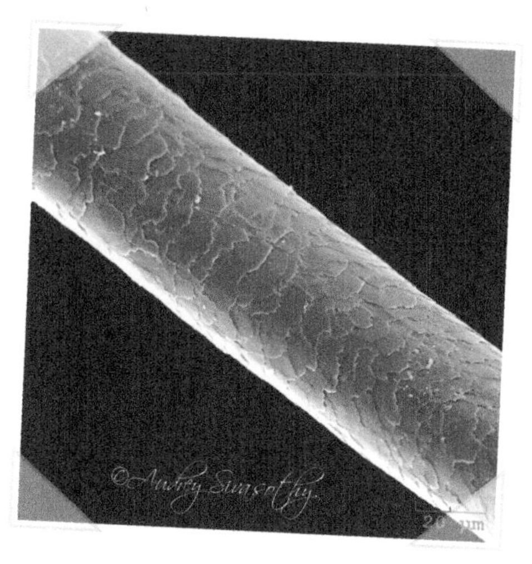

Fig 1.4: Top photo shows hair that has been chemically relaxed. Bottom photo shows a strand of untreated, natural hair. Notice how the cuticle scales are all still present and intact on the natural strand. On the relaxed strand, cuticles show extreme lift, pitting and damage—especially along the top portion of the strand.

Decreasing the pH in this manner permanently "freezes" the hair's bonds into the new, straight shape. Once the pH of the hair is brought back down to the normal range, disulfide bond breakage slows, and the relaxing process ends. Damage can occur during the neutralizing stage if the hair is not neutralized in a timely fashion. This stage also should be one of the longest steps in the process. Bond breakage occurs at the very heart of the hair strand, and if the hair is not properly neutralized at its very core, additional bond breakage can continue long after you've moved on from the process. The more bond breakage that occurs, the weaker the strand will be.

Relaxers: Not Quite Kid Stuff?

When we asked our relaxed, transitioning and natural-haired survey respondents about what they considered to be an "appropriate" age for relaxing a child's hair, most of the responses followed the same line of thinking. Across all groups in the survey, there seemed to be some agreement that if hair relaxing were to be done, it should take place only in the latest years of childhood (after 13 years old). No one in our poll selected "under 5 years old" as an answer choice for the first chemical relaxer. Here's a sampling of some of the anonymous comments we received for this question:

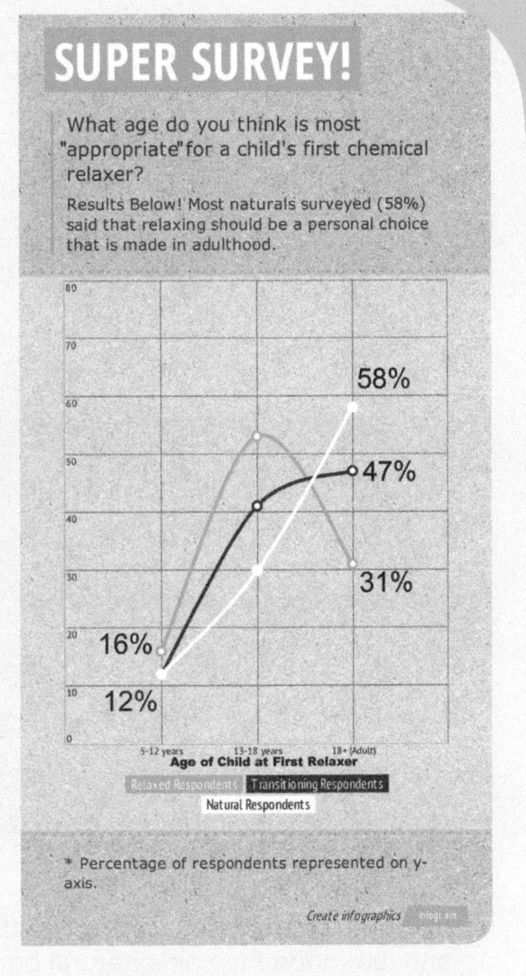

"After what I have gone through: Don't do it at all."

"It's never 'appropriate' to apply damaging chemicals to the hair just to alter its texture. Never 'appropriate' to compromise hair health. Never 'appropriate' for Blacks to change their features to conform to Eurocentric ideals of beauty!"

"Depends upon the manageability of the hair and the effort required to make it presentable."

I don't think little girls should have relaxers at all. Would we allow them to color their hair as well? It reinforces the idea that relaxers are "for big girls" and a "sign of growing up"—which most little girls are itching to do!

What we learned: Among the women we polled, we found that the farther removed a respondent was from relaxing her own hair, the less likely she was to agree to relaxing a child's hair at any age. Our relaxed group of respondents overwhelmingly selected 13 to 18 years old as their top choice for first-time relaxing. Transitioners—and naturals, to an even greater extent—were more likely to agree that chemical relaxing should be a choice made in adulthood—by the individual herself, not a parent. We also allowed written comments for this question, and it was not surprising that naturals and transitioners also tended to favor "Never" as a response to this question.

Your Chapter 1 Take-Aways

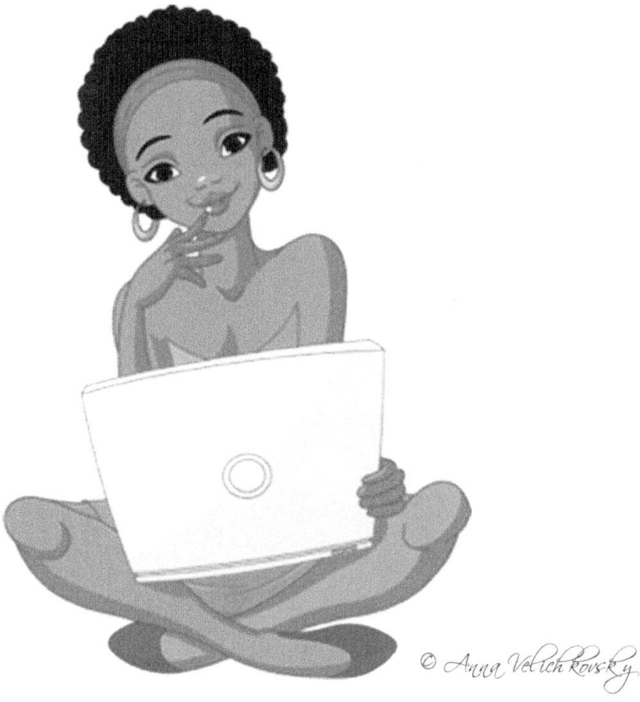

- ✓ Natural hair is hair that has never been processed by chemical straightening treatments.
- ✓ Relaxers are alkaline hair products that permanently break down and rearrange the hair's natural bonds to straighten the hair.
- ✓ Most of the damage from relaxers comes from their aggressively high pH levels.
- ✓ Chemical relaxers straighten the hair in four basic steps: penetration, bond breakage, bond rearrangement and neutralization.
- ✓ Increased thinning, breakage, hair damage, burning, irritation, scabbing and hair loss are all very real problems that can be attributed to long-term use of relaxers, even when applied professionally.

In the next chapter, we will discuss the various stages of the "back to natural" process. How do we get from not ever really thinking about being natural to one day cutting off our hair? Find out in Chapter 2!

unit 2

The Journey Back

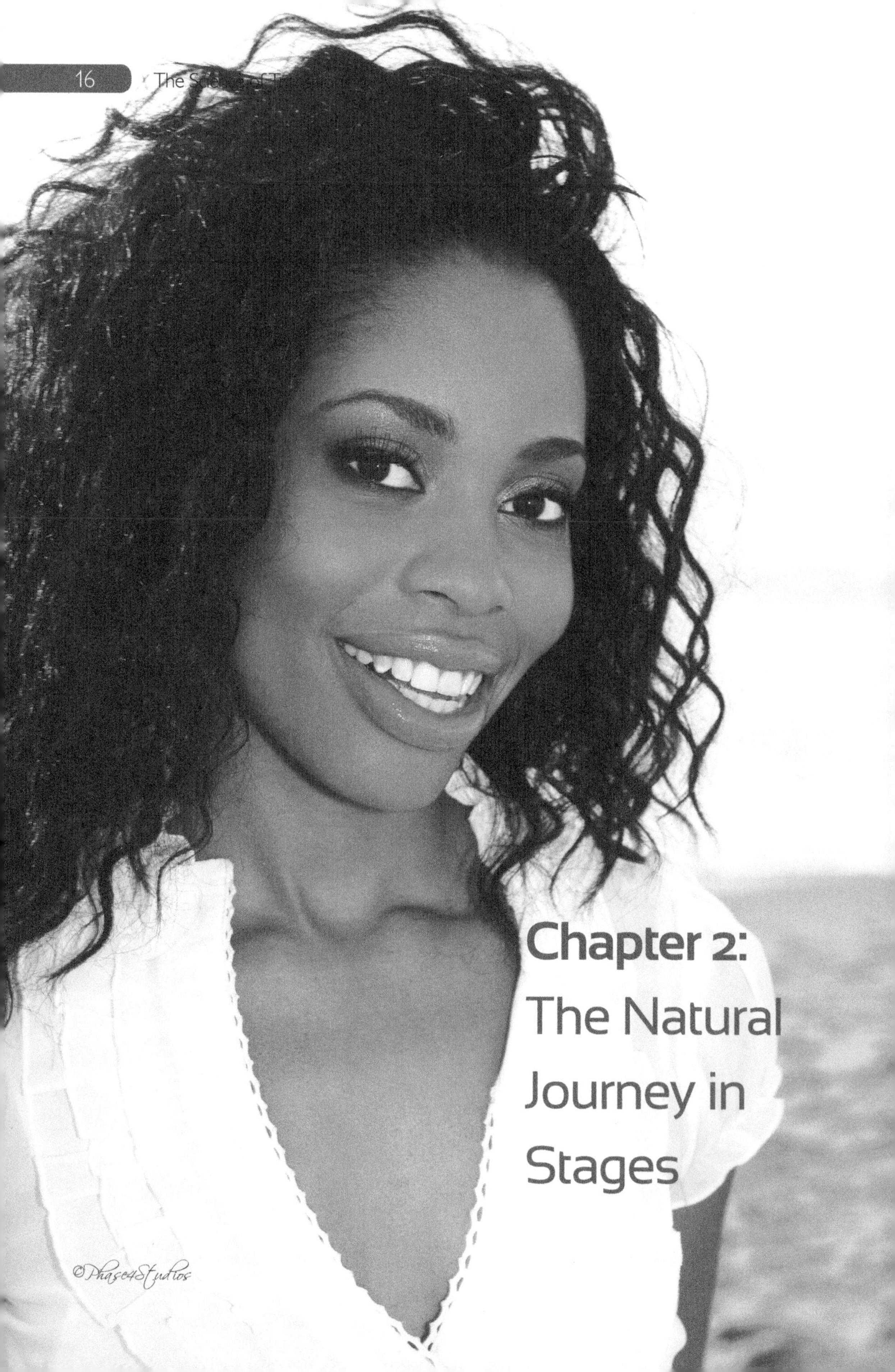

Chapter 2: The Natural Journey in Stages

2. The Stages of Change

When we first really start thinking about returning to our natural textures, or "going natural," things can seem pretty overwhelming. That's because when you decide to embark on this journey, you are essentially leaving behind a dedicated, long-term relationship—the relationship between you and your relaxer. When you leave any long-term relationship, there will be some issues that come up. We can break the entire transitioning process down into five stages:

1. **Pre-transitioning** is a phase in which we are dismissive or show very little interest in natural hair, and may be unaware of the consequences of continuing to relax the hair.

2. **Early transitioning** is the phase in which we are aware of the consequences of continuing to relax our hair, but we are not quite ready to give up relaxers.

3. **Preparation** is the stage in which thoughts about being natural meet action! This is the stage in which we either decide to transition or cut straight to the chase and do our Big Chop. Transitioners have an extended preparation phase, while Big Choppers quickly bypass preparation and head straight into the Action phase.

4. **Action** is the stage during which we perform the Big Chop and have crossed the threshold from relaxed to natural.

5. **Maintenance** is the stage in which we maintain our change to natural hair.

We can break the stages down into "thinking" stages and "action" stages. The first two stages are all about thinking, worrying and wondering about the "hows, whys and whats" of being natural. The final three stages are where we start to act and make decisions. The time you'll spend in each stage will vary, and you may or may not experience them all. We'll cover these five stages in the next few chapters.

Your Journey, Your Way

If you've already done your Big Chop or are newly natural, you may skip ahead to page 115, "Living the Natural Life," for more hands-on information that is relevant to your stage of this process. If at any time you feel like you need some work and extra encouragement to get yourself emotionally prepared to enjoy the natural life, feel free to refer to Chapter 7 (page 100),, "Your Mind in Transition," for some great tips!

Stage 1: The Pre-Transitioning Stage

Going natural? Who me? With this hair? Um, not in this lifetime.

As you may have guessed, this stage is one that comes before the actual decision to transition to natural hair. We're discussing it here because it's a very real first step in the journey to natural hair for many people. Many of us start off our journey to natural hair in a phase where we are dismissive or show very little interest in natural hair. In this stage, our thinking is

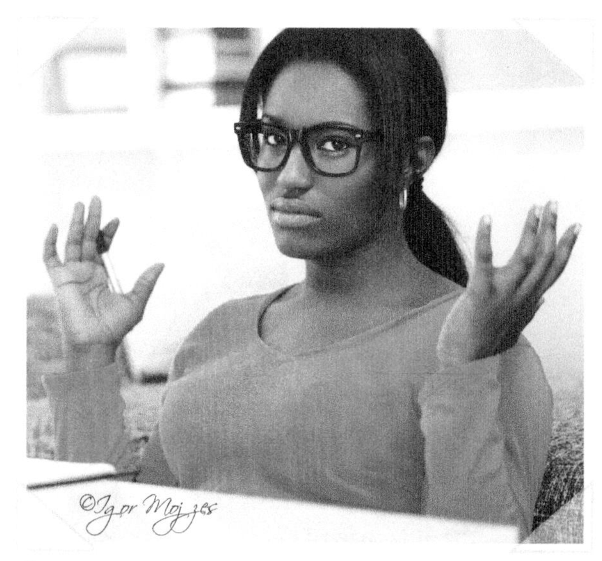

Fig 2.0: Pre-transitioners show very little interest in natural hair.

something like this: *We've had this relationship with our relaxed hair, and we are okay with it. It's working for us. We've heard about the "going natural" thing, and it seems to have some benefits, but it also seems to be a lot more trouble than it's worth.* When you're in this stage, you don't give going natural much more than casual thought. Natural hair is just not for you, for a million and one reasons. We all know someone who is firmly in Stage 1—in fact, some of us live our entire lifetimes in this stage.

Stage 1 pre-transitioners (PTs) tend not to know much about the consequences of relaxing or about trying natural hair as an alternative. When they do find out, they are indifferent or still do not give the consequences much thought. They are often happy with the status quo and aren't thinking about making a change any time soon. They routinely avoid reading or listening to anything that challenges their current comfort level with relaxing. It's just not that big a deal to them. They are happy. Their hair is fine as is, and they just don't want to hear it!

> The **pre-transitioning stage** is marked by dismissiveness or lack of interest in transitioning to natural hair.

Pre-transitioners do not see chemical relaxing as a real problem or concern that they need to address in any way. This is especially true if the PT has never personally experienced any of the negative consequences of chemical straightening. For many PTs, transitioning and letting go of relaxers would simply be answers to a problem that they just don't have yet. Even when PTs have had major issues with chemical relaxing (burns, hair loss, thinning), they still believe the risks to be mostly worth it.

Many of the detractors we encounter during natural hair journeys are Stage 1 pre-transitioners who are simply acting their stage. Given the education, exposure and desire, they too may eventually find themselves in the stage we'll talk about next.

Stage 2: The Early Transitioning Stage

Going natural? If I knew what to do with this hair, I might consider it.

Now, as time passes by, we may decide it's time for a style change . . . or we may have had a negative experience with relaxing that brings natural hair to the table again. We continue to see and hear more and more about natural hair, and our curiosity grows. At this point, we've entered the second phase of the journey, the one in which we attempt to imagine ourselves fully natural for the first time. In this stage, your mind tries to make sense of natural hair and what a natural journey would mean for you. You fly through the possibilities:

Is it worth it to give up what I have now?
Can this work?
What's my backup plan if this doesn't work?

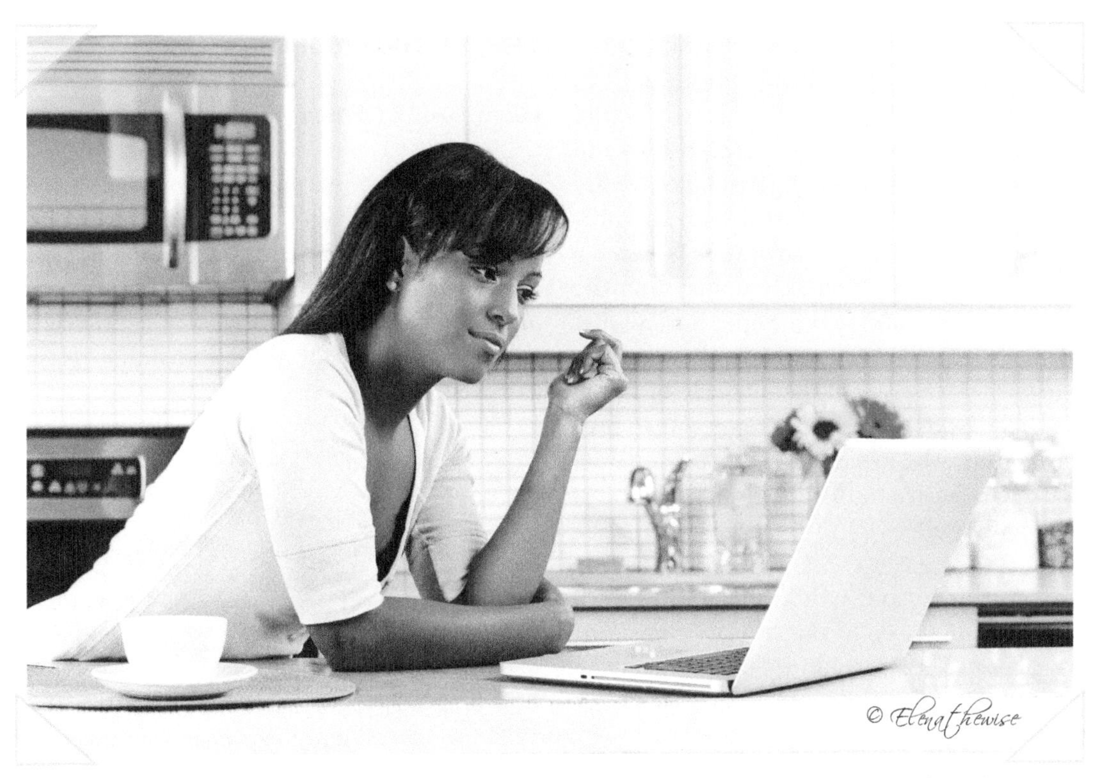

Fig 2.1: Early transitioners are aware of possible dangers but aren't quite ready to commit to change.

Who will this decision affect?

In the early transitioning stage, you are aware that continuing to relax is harmful to your hair. You are thinking about kicking the chemicals to the curb, but you're not quite ready yet. Early transitioners (ETs) straddle the fence for a variety of reasons. It may be because they don't think that they would look good with natural hair, they don't think they can handle natural hair or they don't believe the dangers of continuing to relax their hair are significant enough for them to stop. Women in this stage will often look for ways to minimize the risks of chemical relaxing as much as possible while continuing the behavior. They may opt to reduce or cut back their exposure to relaxers by using gentler formulas or stretching out the time between applications, but transitioning is often still not on the radar.

Early transitioners are especially concerned about how transitioning will affect their family and work lives, too. Husbands, mothers, children, coworkers and others' beliefs and ideas about their choice weigh heavily on their decision to start or continue with the back-to-natural process.

Can my stylist do my hair when I'm natural?
Will my boyfriend like my natural hair?
How will my coworkers react?
Will I even like it myself?
Can I do this?

It is not uncommon for people to linger in the early transitioning phase for years.

The good thing about ETs is that they are much more open to feedback and informa-

The **early transitioning stage** is marked by some interest in transitioning to natural hair, but the commitment isn't total.

tion about transitioning from friends, family, stylists and others than those who are still in the pre-transitioning stage. In fact, you'll find major attitude differences between PTs and ETs. Just try convincing a girlfriend or family member who is still comfortably in the pre-transitioning stage to go natural or "stretch a relaxer," and you will quickly understand the difference! We found in our Super Survey that early transitioners were more likely to report having other naturals in their "circle of influence" (family, friends and coworkers) than pre-transitioners. The more naturals you know, the more open you are to the possibility of natural hair for yourself.

Pre-transitioning and early transitioning mark the beginning stages of the transitioning process. These are the "thinking" stages you hang out in before you ever decide to take the physical plunge!

Stage 3: The Preparation Stage

Okay, I think I'm ready to do this natural thing.

After some time, we eventually make a decision about whether we will continue to relax or not. If we decide to move forward in our natural journey, we go through a third stage in which we begin to prepare for the change and get ourselves ready to cut away all of the remaining relaxed hair we still have.

> The **preparation stage** is marked by small steps that lead to big actions!

This prep stage is where thoughts meet actions. When you move into the preparation stage, you have to decide how you are going to go from a full head of relaxed hair to a full head of natural

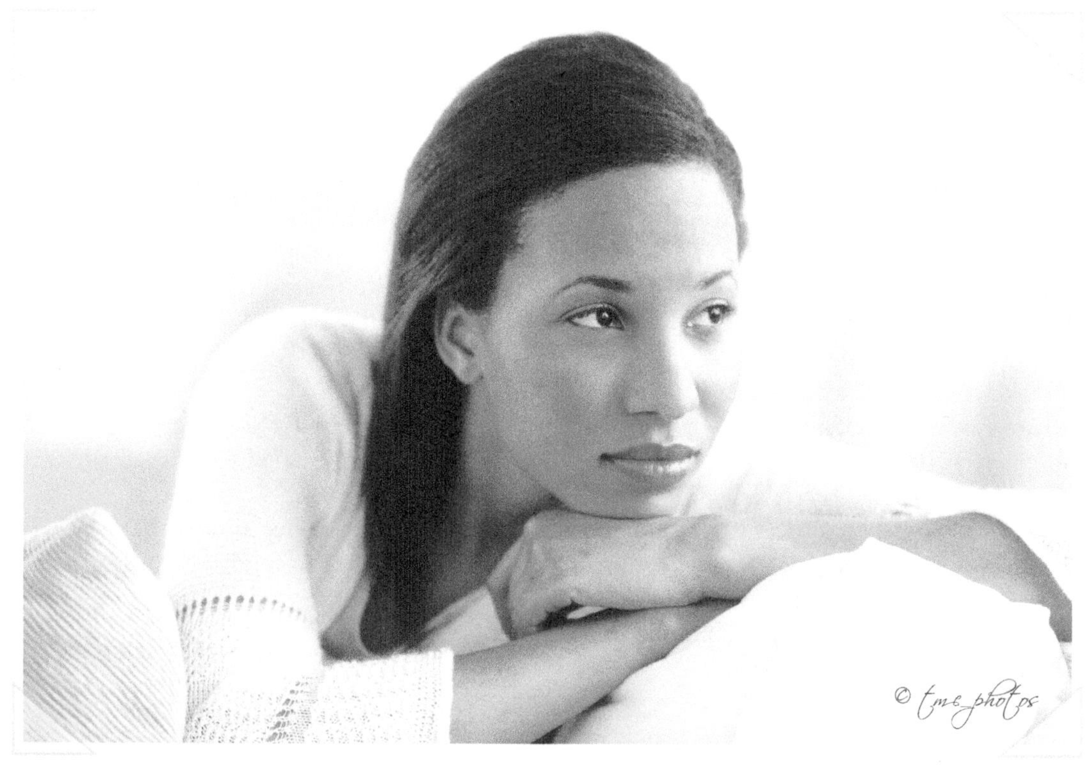

Fig 2.2: "Preparers" have made a decision to return back to their natural hair.

hair. This book is especially for those of you who are in this preparation stage!

Where Do I Start?

Up until now, the road to natural hair has been mostly lots of thinking, wondering and worrying, but now you're ready to take action. During the preparation stage, you take the first really public steps toward being natural. But where do you start?

Since relaxers permanently straighten the hair, they cannot be "stripped out," reversed or undone with hair products, natural remedies or by any other means (you'd be surprised what's floating around out there!). To "go natural," relaxed hair must be cut off or grown out and replaced by new, unprocessed hair. The good news about this is that your hair begins its transition back to its natural state almost immediately after you apply your relaxer. Our hair's default state is natural, and it's always striving to get back there!

The length of time spent in this stage depends entirely on you. Your preparation period can be as long as a few years—or as short as a few minutes. Ultimately, *how you decide to go natural* is what determines how long your preparation period lasts.

The fastest, most no-nonsense way to go natural is by simply cutting off all the relaxed hair right away with what many naturals refer to as a "Big Chop," "Big Cut or, simply, a "BC." When you do a Big Chop, you drastically shorten the preparation stage and launch right into the action phase! Contrast this with slowly *transitioning* into your hair—following the process of allowing your chemically relaxed hair to gradually grow out until it is completely replaced by your incoming, unprocessed hair. If you decide to continue your journey to natural hair with a transition rather than with an immediate Big Chop, your preparation period will last much longer.

Path A: The Big Chop

The Big Chop method involves cutting all of your relaxed hair from the head in one session. It's fast, and it's bold! Depending on how long the new growth is, a Big Chop or BC can result in hair as short as a low fade or longer. Big Chopping is best for those who want to be completely natural right away and do not want to bother with handling relaxed and natural textures together. Nearly 36 percent of the naturals in our hair survey reported that they did a Big Chop right away with no transitioning time whatsoever.

Big Chops are major cuts that occur very soon (usually less than three months) after a relaxer application and completely remove all relaxed hair. These cuts usually result in natural hair that is less than two to three inches long when stretched.

Why Should You Big Chop?

1. You are natural right away! You get a jump start on learning the ins and outs of your new hair.

2. You avoid the infamous "battle of the textures."

3. You see your face in a new way. There's nowhere to hide!

4. You save lots of time because of the carefree styling Big Chopping often gives. There's less combing, less styling and less hassle on wash day.

5. It's a fresh, new start. Any hair damage or problems you may have had previously will all soon be cut away.

Big Chop Benefits

Many women find that their eyes, lips and cheekbones come to life after a Big Chop. Big Chops often reveal and bring out the beauty in our facial features that our longer hair can hide. Many new choppers also find that earrings and other accessories become indispensable at this time.

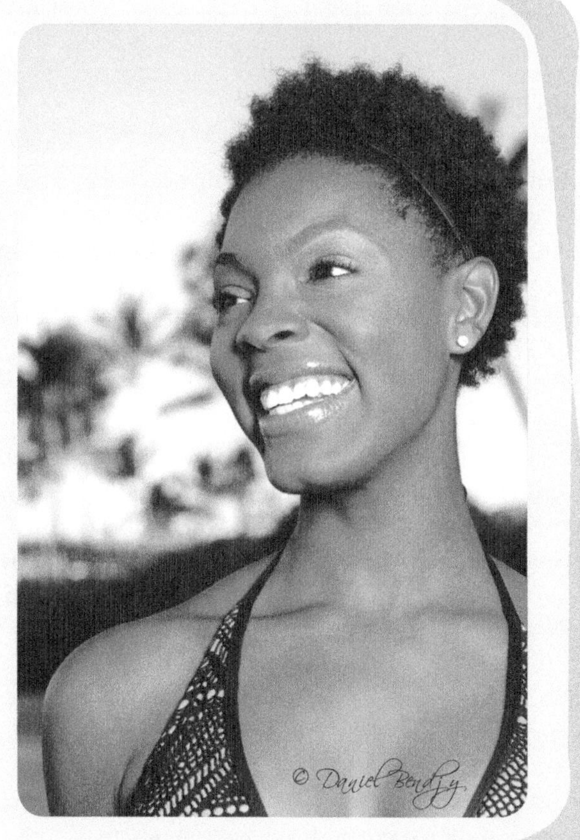

The Big Chop is often a liberating experience!

Big Chopping: Five Things To Think About

Most of the challenges new naturals face with Big Chopping arise from simply having shorter hair.

1. **You may miss your old hair.** Some Big Choppers may find that they miss having lots of hair. If your relaxed hair was long, going natural via a Big Chop can feel like a drastic change. Even if your relaxed hair wasn't very long, a Big Chop can still feel like a complete overhaul.

> **The Science of Black Hair Super Survey**
>
> **Survey Says!** Of the natural women polled in our super survey, nearly **36%** said they did a Big Chop with no transition at all.

2. **There may be some texture shock.** It is also normal to feel some "texture shock" after chopping and seeing your new hair for the first time. Natural hair that grows under relaxed hair looks and behaves much differently than natural hair on its own. What you long believed were waves may very well be tight ringlets, corkscrews or lots of beautiful, freeform compacted frizz!

3. **Big Chopping often means shorter hair with restrictions.** Your styling options may be somewhat limited with shorter hair, especially if you Big Chop very soon after your last relaxer. While short hairstyles

can be accessorized, some styles may still be outside of your reach for a while until you can grow your hair and add length. Depending on how soon after your relaxer you chop, you may have to give it several months before you can try braids, twists, puffs and other styles that require length. Fortunately, this is just a temporary situation that can be solved by simply allowing your hair to grow out for a few months before your Big Chop.

4. **You'll have to deal with immediate shrinkage!** When your hair is natural, you'll have to learn a certain appreciation for shorter-looking hair. If you are looking for cascading locks with natural hair, you may be in for a long wait—especially if your hair has a tighter texture. Shrinkage is an everyday part of the natural life. Even with shoulder-length or waist-length natural hair, your long hair may be your own little secret! For those with the tightest textures and greatest shrinkage, it's not uncommon to have near waist-length natural hair that only falls to shoulder length. You'll need to stretch or blow out your hair to see its true length.

5. **It's you—but it's a new you.** Big Chopping will thrust you right into a new you—or, more correctly, the original version of you! But, while being natural is all about embracing and learning to love what you have, that doesn't mean that you'll love it immediately. Your hair may have to grow on you (literally!) before you fully take to it. Keep in mind that it'll also be a very new look for the people around you as well, so you may have to field some interesting feedback and comments.

If you think you are ready to Big Chop, just skip right on ahead to Chapter 8, page 116, for tips on doing the perfect Big Chop!

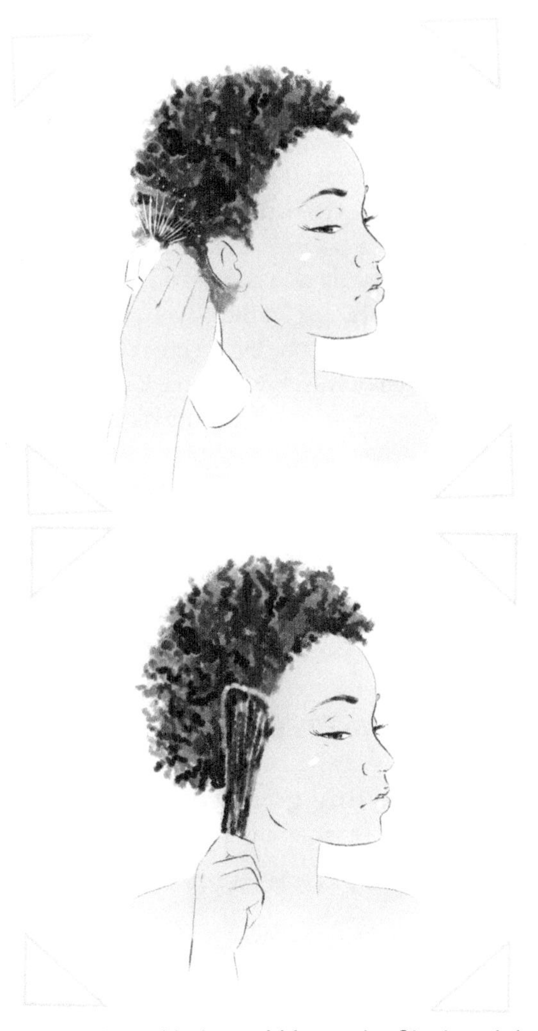

Fig 2.3: Natural hair can hide much of its length in its shrinkage.

When the Big Chop Is Too Big a Change

Now, it almost goes without saying that cutting off a lot of hair at once can require a confidence and strength that not everyone is equipped with at the outset of a hair-care journey. For others, short hair just isn't a plausible option. When this is the case, deliberate transitioning (complete with Mini Chops) may be a necessary part of the back-to-natural process. In this book, we will focus on this "transitioning-followed-by-a-chop" method.

Path B: Transitioning

When early transitioners make the decision to continue on their natural journey without a Big Chop, they enter into an extended preparatory stage. They are now bona fide transitioners! This path to natural hair is best for those who are still on the fence about going natural and for those who prefer not to part with their hair in one big event. While transitioning also typically ends with some kind of major chop at the end to get rid of any final relaxed pieces, for most people, a chop after transitioning is not as dramatic as an immediate Big Chop with little to no transitioning beforehand. In some hair-care circles, chops that occur at the end of a transitioning period are called "transitioning chops" rather than Big Chops.

Why Should You Transition?

1. **Transitioning gives you the benefit of time.** Transitioning to natural gives you time to really think about going natural. *Is this something you can do?* (Yes!) Transitioning gives you time to bring your heart and mind into alignment and allows you to get somewhat accustomed to your natural texture. We used the word *somewhat* here because, again, you won't really know your hair's true texture or behavior until the relaxed ends are completely gone.

2. **Transitioning buys you a bit more privacy in your journey.** Big Chopping is often a very public process and event, but transitioning allows you to go natural in a discreet way. You can embark on your natural hair journey without added pressure or prying questions from friends, family and coworkers, at least in the very beginning.

3. **Your hair is healthier after a transition, even if you don't stick it out to the end.** Now, in a book about transitioning to natural hair it may seem odd to talk about what happens when you feel

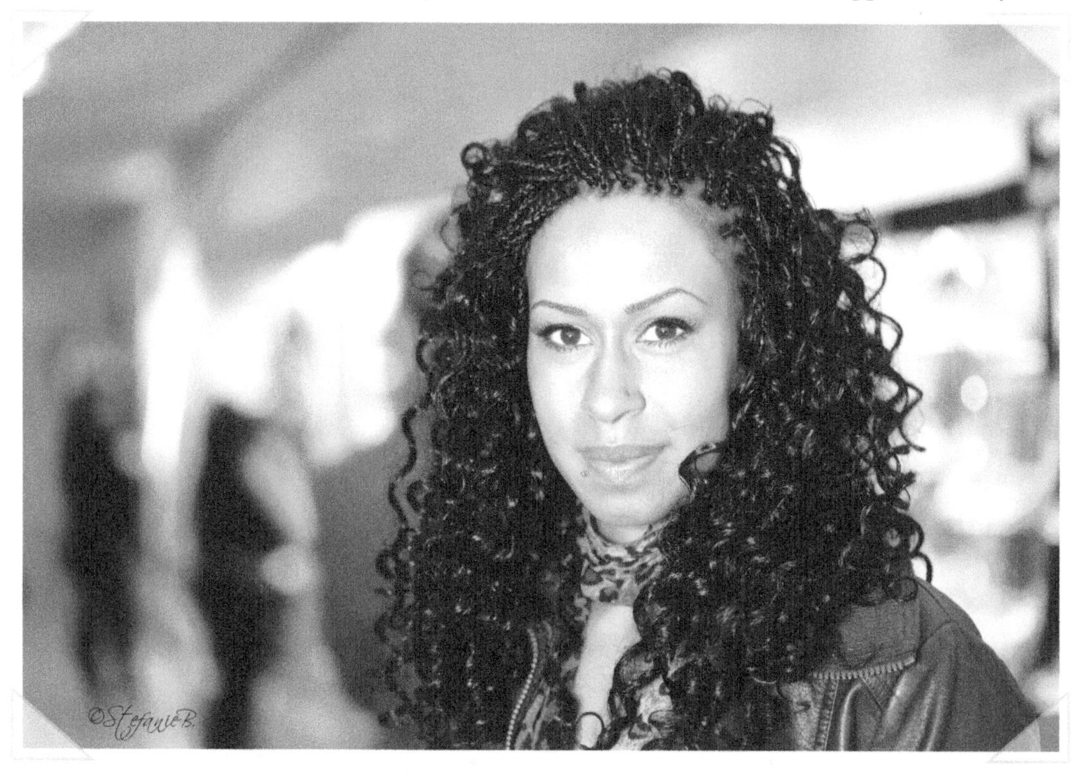

Fig 2.4: Slowly transitioning back to natural gives the mind and body time to prepare for the change.

like you've just had enough of the process, but this is a very valid part of the process for many new transitioners. The truth is, many people attempt to transition and fail many times before they find an approach that sticks! The good thing is, if you relax after abandoning a transition, you're usually going into your relaxer with a much healthier head of hair for having tried to go natural in the first place. It's a win-win!

Transitioning: Five Things To Think About

Transitioning is by far the most popular method of going natural, but it's not all sunshine and roses. Like Big Chopping, transitioning also includes some things you'll need to think about.

1. **Your transitioning hair is neither here nor there.** Transitioning hair is hair that is in limbo—and unfortunately, hair in limbo can struggle. Our hair thrives best when we work with 100 percent of one hair texture. Since the transitioning process requires us to juggle two uniquely different textures, that incompatibility can manifest itself in many ways. Transitioners commonly face problems such as breakage, dryness, excessive tangling and inconsistent styling results.

2. **Because your hair is awkwardly in the middle of two opposing hair types, you don't really get the benefits or look of either hair type.** As a transitioner, your natural styles probably fall flat and are not very full, while your straight styles refuse to lie down and don't look polished. It's just hard to look and feel beautiful with hair that straddles the fence. These challenges can either push forward a transition to natural hair, often far ahead of schedule, or encourage a return to relaxing.

3. **Your transitioning hair may not look healthy.** As you transition and move more and more beyond your standard relaxing time frame, your new growth will begin to play tricks on you. Because the new growth hair nearest your scalp is compact and tends to shrink, it can make your relaxed ends look thinner, scragglier and shorter when they may be perfectly okay. Shedding, tangling and hair breakage, especially where the two textures meet, may also become issues as new growth and relaxed ends compete against one another. When many people see these sorts of changes happening, they often fear that they are doing more damage to their hair by going natural—and many return to relaxing out of fear. The best remedy for these problems, however, is to increase the level of conditioning that you are providing your hair and slowly begin to cut away your relaxed ends. Strategically cutting away these ends will help you in two ways. First, such trims will drastically cut down on any tangling you are experiencing, and second, they will help you get one step closer to your goal of being fully natural.

4. **You'll have to deal with shrinkage!** One of the main reasons that people embark on transitions in the first place is to avoid the short-hair phases of natural hair. Sometimes even the shortest relaxed hair seems long, precious and hard to part with when you are faced with natural hair. Shorter hair draws attention to the face, and for people who aren't quite ready for the limelight, this can feel overwhelming. But, one of the really unique (and ironic) things about natural hair is that, for many of us, no matter how long we transition, our hair will still be short.

How is that, you ask? The answer is, shrinkage!

Although your hair has grown and is longer, the kinks, curls, bends and turns of natural hair will make it appear shorter. (See, Figure 2.3) You can buy a little length by extending your transition by a few weeks or months, but you'll eventually have to come to terms with a shorter-haired you. This characteristic of natural hair means that even waist-length-haired naturals with a high degree

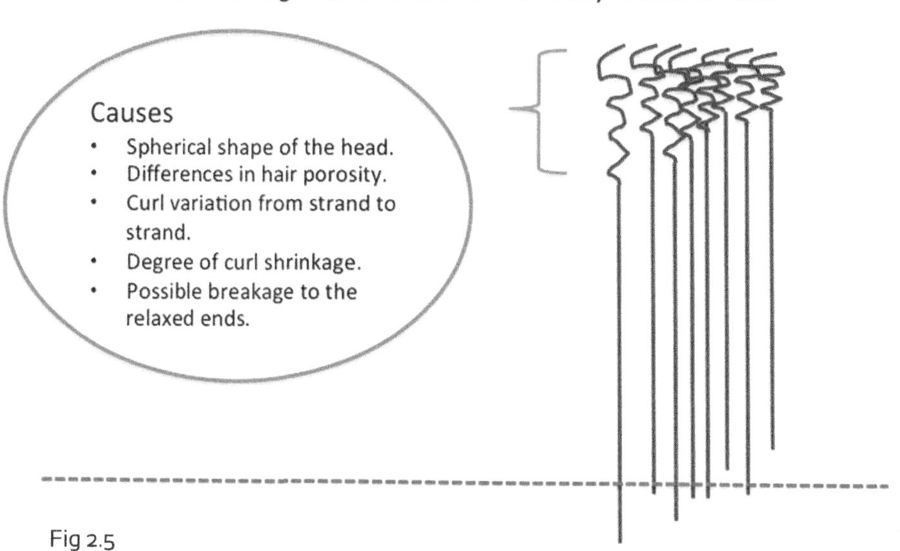

Fig 2.5

of shrinkage can rock short, above-the-shoulder styles one day and much longer tresses the next. Welcome to the amazing world of shrinkage. For the curliest and coiliest naturals, shrinkage is a factor that makes shorter-looking hair part of the deal. But it's not all doom and gloom. Depending on the style you are trying to achieve, shrinkage can also work in your favor.

5. **Your hair may "speak" for you.** Human beings are social creatures, and every aspect of our being speaks to those around us—including our hair. The way we walk, talk, eat and dress all give clues about how we perceive ourselves in the world. Hair, again, is no exception. Natural hair, especially, tends to bring out a wide range of assumptions about the wearer. Of course, what your hair says to one person and what it says to the next may not be an accurate representation of who you really are. Some people may assume your natural hair indicates that you are educated (or uneducated), socially conscious, a rebel, militant, political, wild, fun, earthy and/or carefree. You may or may not be one or all of those things. Of course, relaxed hair also brings certain assumptions and associations with it, too.

Stage 4: The Action Phase

Okay, Let's make it happen!

In Stage 4, we take action and break out the scissors! This stage is complete when the relaxed hair is no more.

It may take a few weeks—or a few years—after your last relaxer, but eventually you will reach a point where you need to *disconnect*. You've held out for as long as you possibly could in the battle between your straight hair and your natural hair, but this is the natural progression of things. Whether it's rampant shedding, breakage or excitement about being fully natural that is the trigger, you will certainly know when *it's time*. The end of transitioning marks the end of preparation in Stage 3 and the beginning of Stage 4: You are now ready for action and your final chop!

Stage 5: The Maintenance Stage

A year down, and I think I'm getting the hang of this!

By the time you've reached the maintenance phase, you've been fully natural with no relaxed hair ends for at least a year. Wearing your natural hair has become habit now, and the chances for relapse back to the relaxed side are significantly lower. This is the stage in which we start to automate the process of being natural.

In the next few chapters, we will really dig in deep and discuss the ins and outs of transitioning.

What Does Natural Mean to You?

Living the natural life can mean so much more than saying goodbye to chemical relaxers. In many circles, you'll find naturals who've given up, added in or rearranged lots of other things to fit into their new model of personal health. Some naturals are comfortable rocking their 'fros with color enhancements, while being natural, for others, means treating their tresses with all-natural, organic hair-care products. Some naturals take it still farther by eating only organic foods and plant-based diets and by delving into other environmentally conscious ways of living. There is no one way to be natural, and your ideas about how to be natural may very well change over time.

What Kind of Natural Are You?

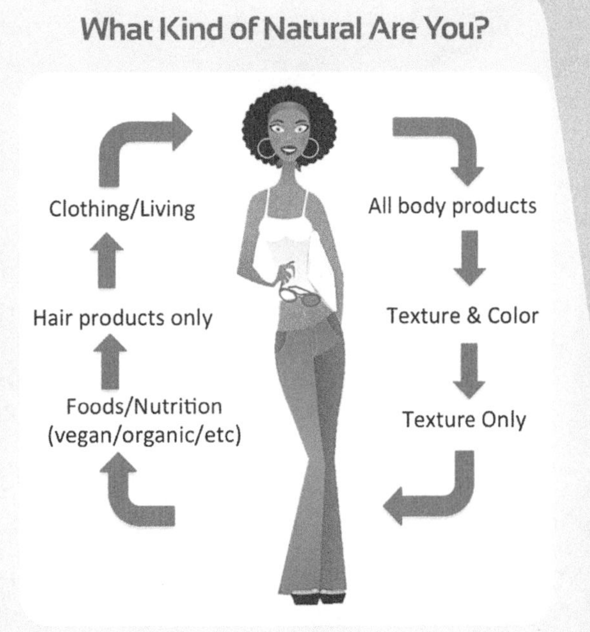

Your Chapter 2 Take-Aways

Many of us experience our journeys back to natural in five stages:

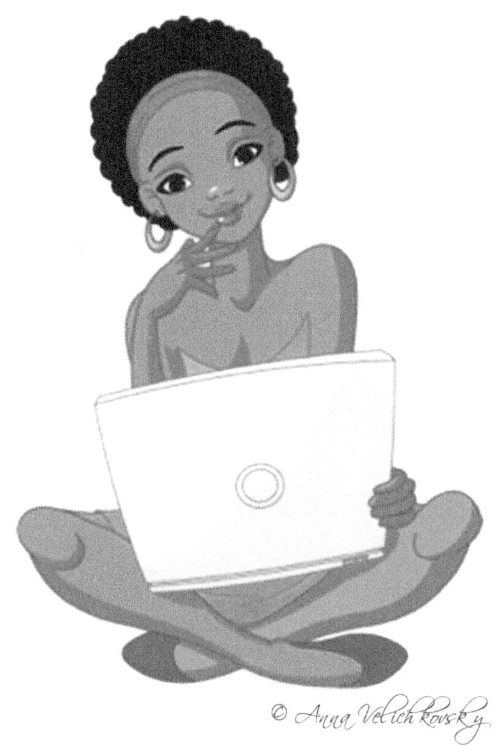
© Anna Velichkovsky

- ✓ Pre-transitioning is a phase in which we are dismissive or show very little interest in natural hair, and may be unaware of the consequences of continuing to relax the hair.
- ✓ Early transitioning is the phase in which we are aware of the consequences of continuing to relax our hair, but we are not quite ready to give up relaxers.
- ✓ Preparation is the stage in which thoughts about being natural meet action! This is the stage in which we either decide to transition or cut straight to the chase and do our Big Chop. Transitioners have an extended preparation phase, while Big Choppers quickly bypass preparation and head straight into the Action phase!
- ✓ Action is the stage during which we perform the Big Chop and have crossed the threshold from relaxed to natural.
- ✓ Maintenance is the stage in which we maintain our change to natural hair.

In the next chapter, we will discuss the two transitions and what they mean for those longing to be natural!

tran•si•tion

tranˈziSHən,-ˈsiSHən/

noun

an event that results in a transformation.

unit 3

Transitioning 101

Chapter 3: The Natural-To-Be

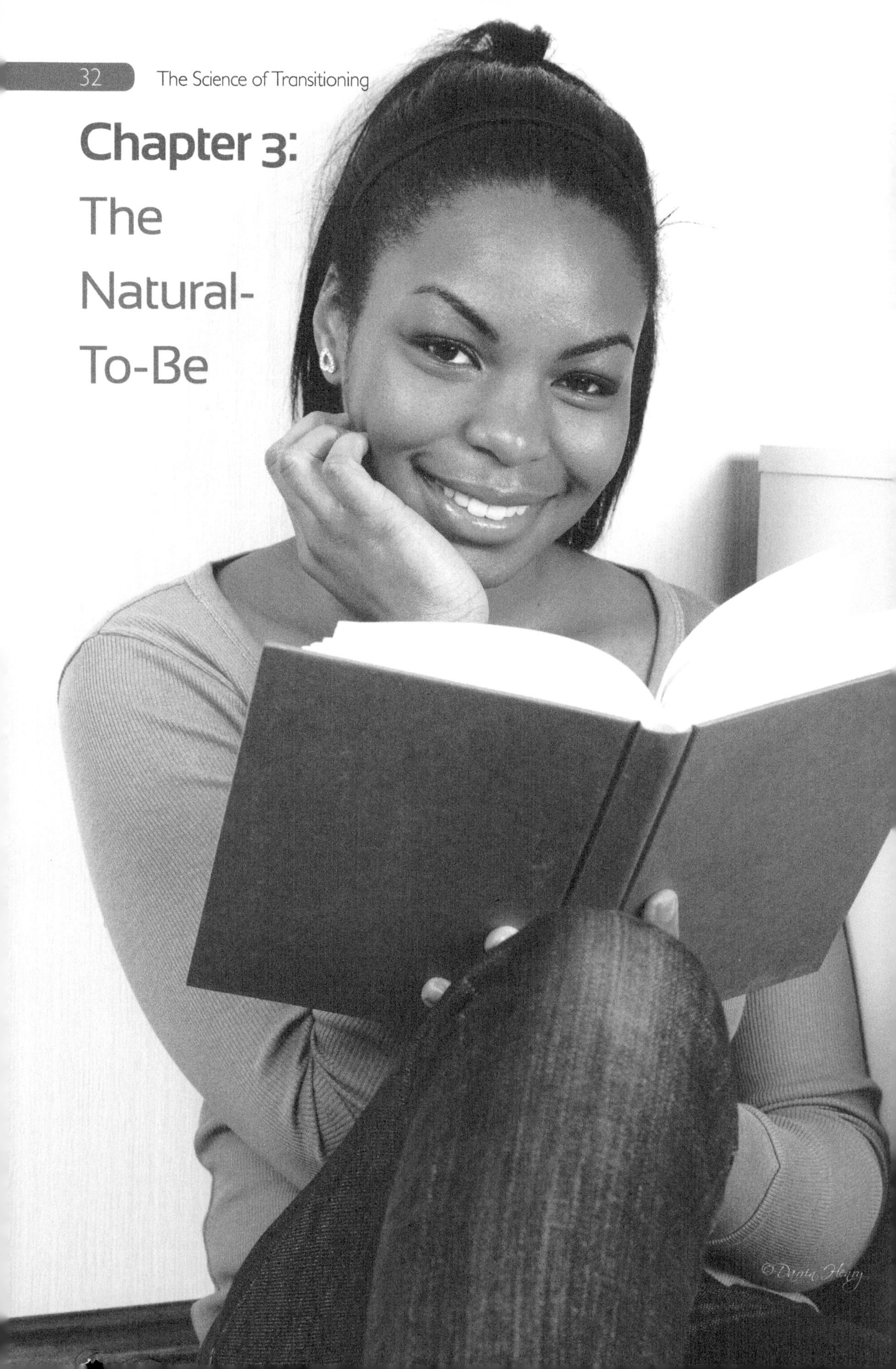

3. Shaping Our Worldview

No hair on earth has the power to stir up emotions and spark discussion quite like ours does. But what brought us here? Why is our hair such a hot topic, and why is changing it such an intense battle for the mind? The short answer is that there is a certain amount of history in our hair. And no matter what your individual reasons for relaxing your hair may have been, it's always important to acknowledge the history of our hair in this world—and the impact of that history on our styling options and choices.

The view that kinky, coily, highly textured hair is unattractive, less desirable and unacceptable is one that has deep origins. Although we are long past the days when any one of us ever walked on slave plantations, we are still seeing the effects of their negative messaging in our beauty discourse. Western media continues to drive home the message that on the scale of desirability, long, straight (usually blond) hair should be prized at the very top, and the kinkiest of coils should be scorned at the very bottom. This negative messaging is so ingrained in our community that many of us haven't seen our hair's natural texture since we were children.

When the first black men and women were forcibly taken from Africa to the Caribbean and North America in the 1500s and 1600s, their captors ensured that more than their hands and feet would be shackled. In order to ensure that the enslaved people's submission would be total, it was also important for their masters to challenge their basic beliefs about themselves, their beauty and their personhood. Hair was wrapped in meaning. African hairstyles gave clues about the wearer's identity, status, rank, religion and age, but these meanings were completely stripped away during enslavement. Many times, the hair of those captured men and women was shaved to dehumanize them and make them into objects ready for sale. The enslaved people's own understanding of beauty ultimately took a back seat to survival when their oppressors imposed their own beauty standards. It was quickly understood that those men and women who happened to look more like their captors (lighter skin and longer, straighter hair) were considered more valuable. Those features ensured their upward mobility and a higher status in society, even after slavery ended. It was pretty simple: If you wanted to be treated well or land a certain job, you had to look a certain way, and that was that.

Even when we celebrated our natural hair and styled it ornately, the "powers that be" did everything that they could to ensure that we "remained in our place." In the late 1700s, Louisiana's Spanish governor, Esteban Miró, developed the *Bando du Buen Gobierno* which was a set of edicts that outlined the guidelines for establishing a successful colony. Interestingly, because he was already suspicious of the free blacks and the "extravagant luxury in their dressing" which he felt was "already is excessive," his edict also included a provision that required women of color to either wear their hair flat, or fully cover their hair with a handkerchief when in public. Specifically women were told that they could not "wear feathers, nor curls in their hair," and that they must comb their hair "flat" or cover it with a handkerchief.

The hair provision was not created because the women's natural hair was seen as unprofessional, ugly or unkempt, but because their hair was seen as too beautiful and too elaborate for their status in society, such that a distinction had to be made. He essentially told them—*You are black women, how dare you dress well and wear your hair decorated, big and curly with pride?* Miró feared that the hair styles that the women were wearing were attracting the attention of white men, and the envy of white women—which upset order in his society. These hair provisions were meant to shame the women of color, and were especially intended to help distinguish lighter-skinned women of color from white women.

But, in an interesting turn of events, the black women of New Orleans turned the edict on its head—literally! The *tignon* (pronounced tee-yoh-n), a headdress of wrapped scarves, was to be worn over the hair in public. The women began to wear the tignons, but styled the headscarves in exquisite and intricate ways. They used colorful fabrics, and added feathers and broaches to the scarves eventually turning what was meant to be a shameful, drab piece of clothing into a beautiful fashion statement that was adopted by white women as well!

Do you know the *power* of your beauty?

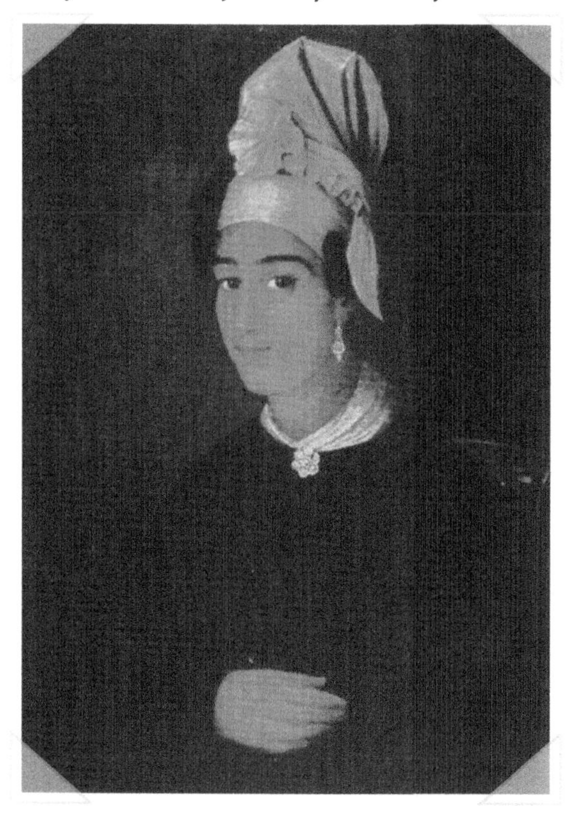

Fig 3.0: Creole woman of color in a headdress, original in the Historic New Orleans Collection at the Cabildo, New Orleans.

3.1 The Language of "Good Hair"

While Miró's edict was put in place to trivialize black beauty and contain the threat of its universal acceptance, others outright denied its very existence. Unfortunately, the idea that European features were superior to others was a message that our people dutifully passed down through the generations—consciously and unconsciously—as a means of survival. The ugly remnants of this history are still with us today, every time someone believes that they *need* a relaxer to be presentable, that their facial features don't fit their natural hair or that they don't have the "right kind" of hair to be natural.

The language surrounding what makes hair "good" and "manageable" today is also influenced by that past. Today's beauty discourse defines good, healthy, manageable hair in very narrow terms because it is controlled mostly by the media and large, multinational product companies that tend to set the rules and parameters of beauty based on what makes European hair look good. Words like *silky, straight, shiny* and *long* come together to create an image of what's considered manageable, desirable hair. The truth is, all of those words are wonderful, but they can be valued as standards for only a few types of hair. If your hair is kinky, coily or curly, your hair by default will always fall short of that "standard" because the standard was never intended to include us. In fact, in many beauty circles, our hair has been held out as the standard of what hair should *not* be! And, of course, companies don't even bother using language that makes sense for our hair because we continue to buy into their current narrow standard in droves.

So, what *should* be the language of beauty for kinky, coily and curly hair? Although none of us is exactly the same, good kinky, coily and curly hair types are served better in the language of beauty by valuing things like *sheen, shape, texture consistency, elasticity* and *volume*. These terms are of greater value and are much more relevant as standards when applied to our hair types. Of course, you'll always have a hard time seeing natural hair as manageable if, instead of *sheen, shape* and *volume*—*silky, straight* and *long* make up your standard and only frame of reference for acceptable hair. The two hair languages work for those for whom they are intended, but their elements are almost completely incompatible. It's not difficult to see why many of us find so much disappointment in our hair when we are constantly holding it to a standard that was never meant for us in the first place.

No More "Problem Hair"

If you take nothing else from this book, I hope that you will understand just how important it is for you to control the language and messaging surrounding your hair. In your journey to natural hair, you will see subtly worded you-are-not-good-enough messages on many products—even on those that are supposed to be celebrating natural hair. Always be aware of cleverly couched marketing language that is meant to disparage and reframe your hair as "problem hair." Curl enhancers, definers and smoothing products tend to be the worst culprits for this kind of fix-your-natural-hair advertising. For more on the topic of language and hair, see "What Happens When You Are Not a Curly Girl?" on page 131.

3.2 Going It Alone?

Most of us think of the transitioning process as a deeply personal journey—and in many ways it is. But unless you live in some remote part of the world with no connection to anyone, it's nearly impossible to transition alone or without affecting the people around you. While the journey to natural hair is certainly a personal one that is all about you—others will also go along with you for the ride! When you start transitioning or are newly natural, you'll find that, believe it or not, some people out there are more deeply invested in your hair than they may initially let on. Some people become very vocal about your hair change, and it's to be expected. It's very likely that when these people first met you, or for as long as they've known you, your hair has always been flat and straight. Going from relaxed hair that lies down flat against your face to hair that stands up and frames your face in a halo is a big change.

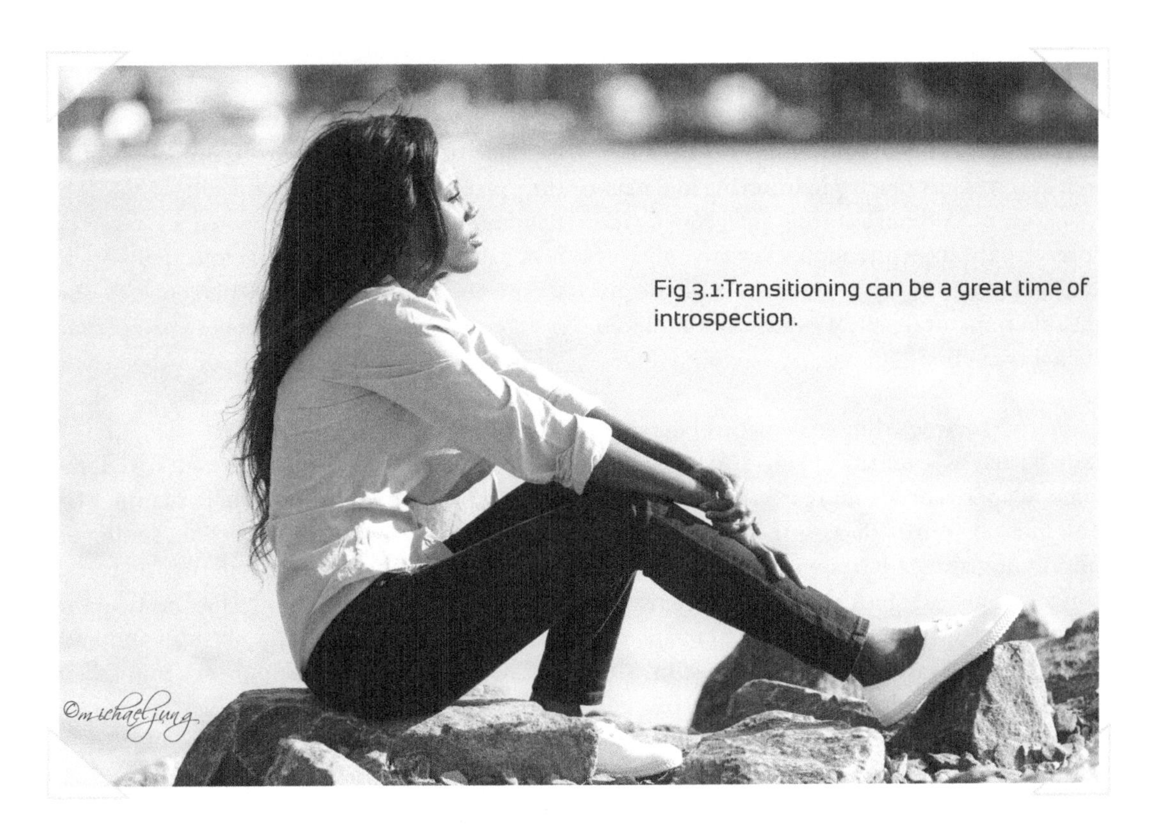

Fig 3.1:Transitioning can be a great time of introspection.

That's what friends are for!

When we asked naturals and transitioners about who had been the most supportive of their hair journeys, one group of people reigned supreme. Their natural-haired friends (80%). Family (73%) and relaxed friends (61%) were a close second and third. The least supportive group? Their hair stylists. (35%)

While we are using our transition to give ourselves time to learn and deal with the change, we can't forget that the people around us will need time to adjust as well. The good news? Fifty-two percent of naturals polled reported that their family members increased their support over time, while only 2 percent reported feeling a decrease in support over time.

3.3 The Two Transitions

When we talk about transitioning, we often discuss it as if it is just one big haircutting and hair-growing event. Although cutting and growing the hair receive the most attention, they are only half of the transitioning story. Before we physically transition to natural hair, we must first undergo a mental transition.

Whether you are deciding to go natural for spiritual reasons, as a means of self-discovery, for fashion purposes or for no reason at all, there's still a mental transition you'll have to make. Transitioning always starts with the mind, well before any physical steps are taken. Where the physical transition focuses on slowly cutting off relaxed hair as new natural hair grows in, the mental transition focuses on slowly cutting off negative thinking as new empowering thoughts come in. The mental transition starts before you do anything to your hair and can continue long after the physical transition is complete. We can see the mental transition at work during the pre-transitioning and early transitioning phases because our thoughts are always the first steps in the natural-hair journey.

We all come to this journey from different places and vantage points. Depending on your background and your specific reasons for transitioning, some of you will need to work harder on the mental part of the transitioning process than others. For those of you who'd like to explore the mental aspects of transitioning, we'll spend quite a bit of time on that in this book. For those of you who are ready to move on to more practical, hands-on transitioning information, you can move ahead to Chapter 4 (page 41), "Your Hair in Transition."

3.4 How Long Will My Transition Last?

The length of any transition depends on the transitioner's specific goals and personal readiness to begin fully working with her natural hair texture. When we asked a group of transitioners in our Super Survey how long they planned to continue their transition, almost 80 percent said that they planned to transition for longer than thirteen months. Interestingly, when we asked current naturals if they were able to actually stick to their transition plans, only 20 percent did. About 5 percent transitioned for longer than planned, while 60 percent transitioned for a shorter time than planned.

Of the transitioning naturals we surveyed, most transitioned for about half their planned time with the average transitioning time lasting only four to nine months. The second largest group included those who transitioned for less than three months, and those who did not transition at all but started their natural journeys immediately with a big chop. Obviously, this was nowhere near the thirteen-plus months many of them may have imagined for themselves as transitioners! The

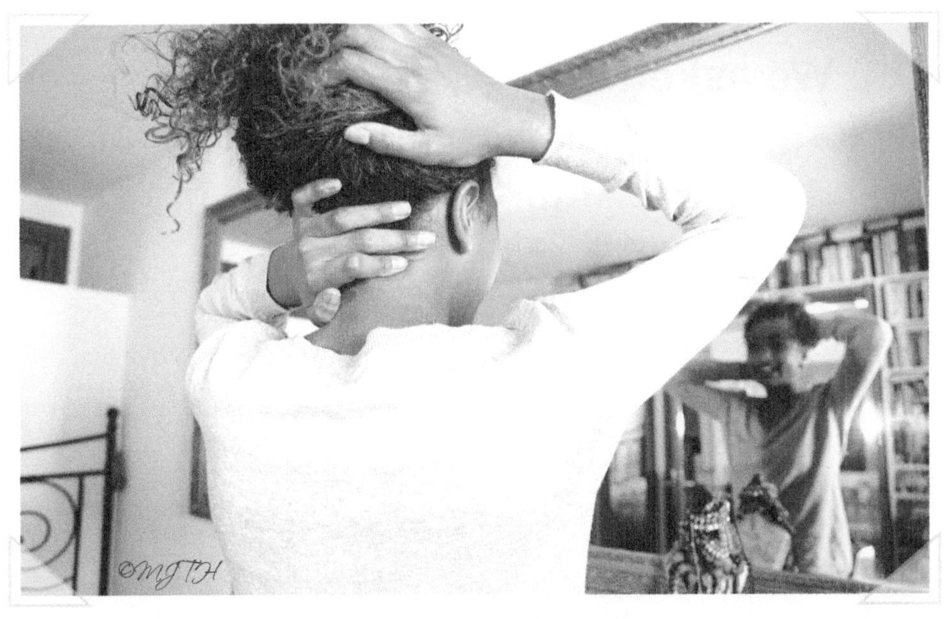

Fig 3.2: The mental transition is all about learning to love and embrace the original, yet new, version of you.

bottom line here is that most transitioners find a reason to chop well ahead of schedule!

Mind over Matter

Remember, there are actually two transitions taking place: physical and mental. The physical transition has a very clear endpoint: It's over once you've removed all of the straight, processed ends. The mental transition is much less concrete, and it is harder to pinpoint exactly when it has happened—and when, if ever, it is complete. You might move through your mental transition quickly and without much thought, or it might be an ongoing process that continues long after the last piece of processed hair is gone. It is not uncommon for the mind to hold the hair captive in the transition, even after the hair is completely natural! We'll discuss the ins and outs of the mental transition

How Long Will My Transition Last?

The amount of time it will take for you to transition depends upon your comfort level with short hair and where you are in your mental transition. If you are ready to go mentally, shorter hair doesn't bother you and you want to part with your relaxed hair sooner rather than later, your transition could technically last less than an hour with a Big Chop.

The Two Transitions to Natural Hair

Physical Transition: slowly cutting off relaxed hair as new natural hair grows in.

Mental Transition: slowly cutting off negative thinking and embracing the original (yet new!) version of you.

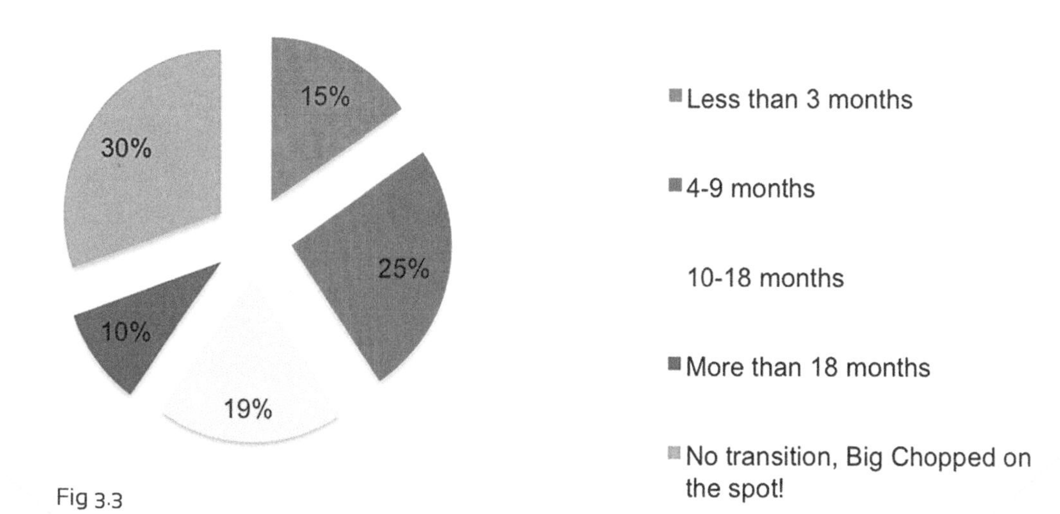
We asked current naturals:
How long was your transition to natural hair?
15%
25%
19%
10%
30%
Less than 3 months
4-9 months
10-18 months
More than 18 months
No transition, Big Chopped on the spot!

Fig 3.3

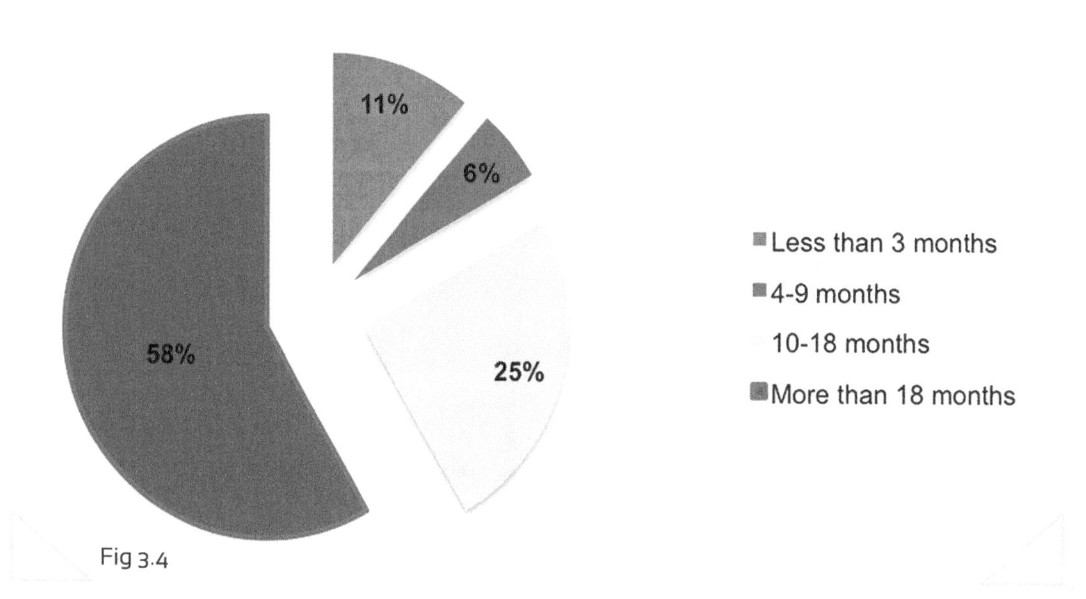
We asked transitioners:
How long DO YOU PLAN to transition to natural hair?
11%
6%
25%
58%
Less than 3 months
4-9 months
10-18 months
More than 18 months

Fig 3.4

in more detail in *Chapter 7, "Your Mind in Transition."*

In the next chapter, we will discuss the physical process of transitioning as well as tips and techniques that you can use to make this period of change worth your while.

Top Five Transitioning Mistakes

1. Treating your new growth like it is relaxed hair and expecting it to behave in a similar fashion.

2. Going through the transitioning process without cutting away the relaxed hair in a timely manner.

3. Allowing the condition of your relaxed hair to determine whether you continue or end your transition (putting the needs of your relaxed hair before those of your natural hair).

4. Not giving serious thought to the mental aspects of the transition.

5. Jumping into the transition without a plan or without understanding the challenges to come.

Your Chapter 3 Take-Aways

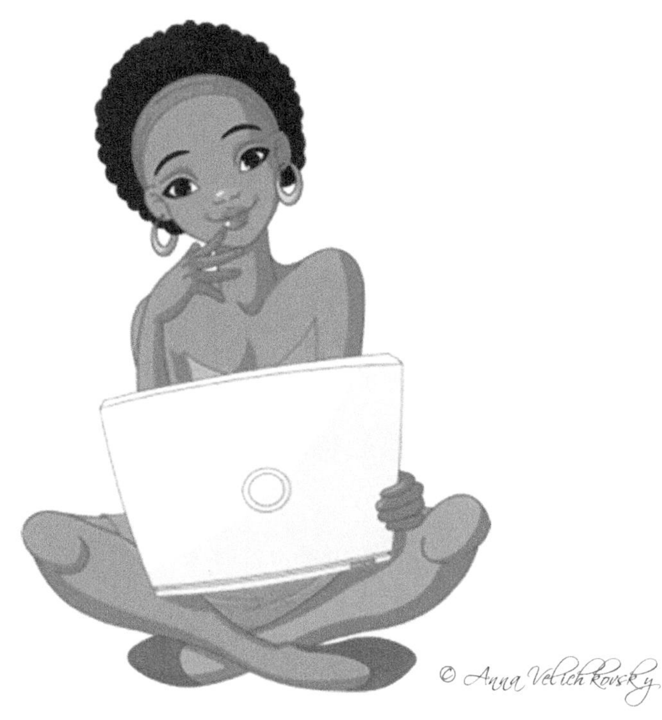

- ✓ There are two transitions that must take place for your journey to natural hair to be successful.
- ✓ The physical transition is slowly cutting off relaxed hair as new natural hair grows in.
- ✓ The mental transition is slowly cutting off negative thinking and embracing the original (yet new!) version of you.
- ✓ Your transition may not last as long as you think! According to our poll, for a variety of reasons, most women who make the journey back to natural do not transition for as long as they originally expected to.
- ✓ The average transition to natural was between four and nine months long.

In the next chapter, we will take you back to basics. What is elasticity? Porosity? The protein/moisture balance? What do they mean for your transitioning hair? Find out in Chapter 4.

Chapter 4: Your Hair in Transition

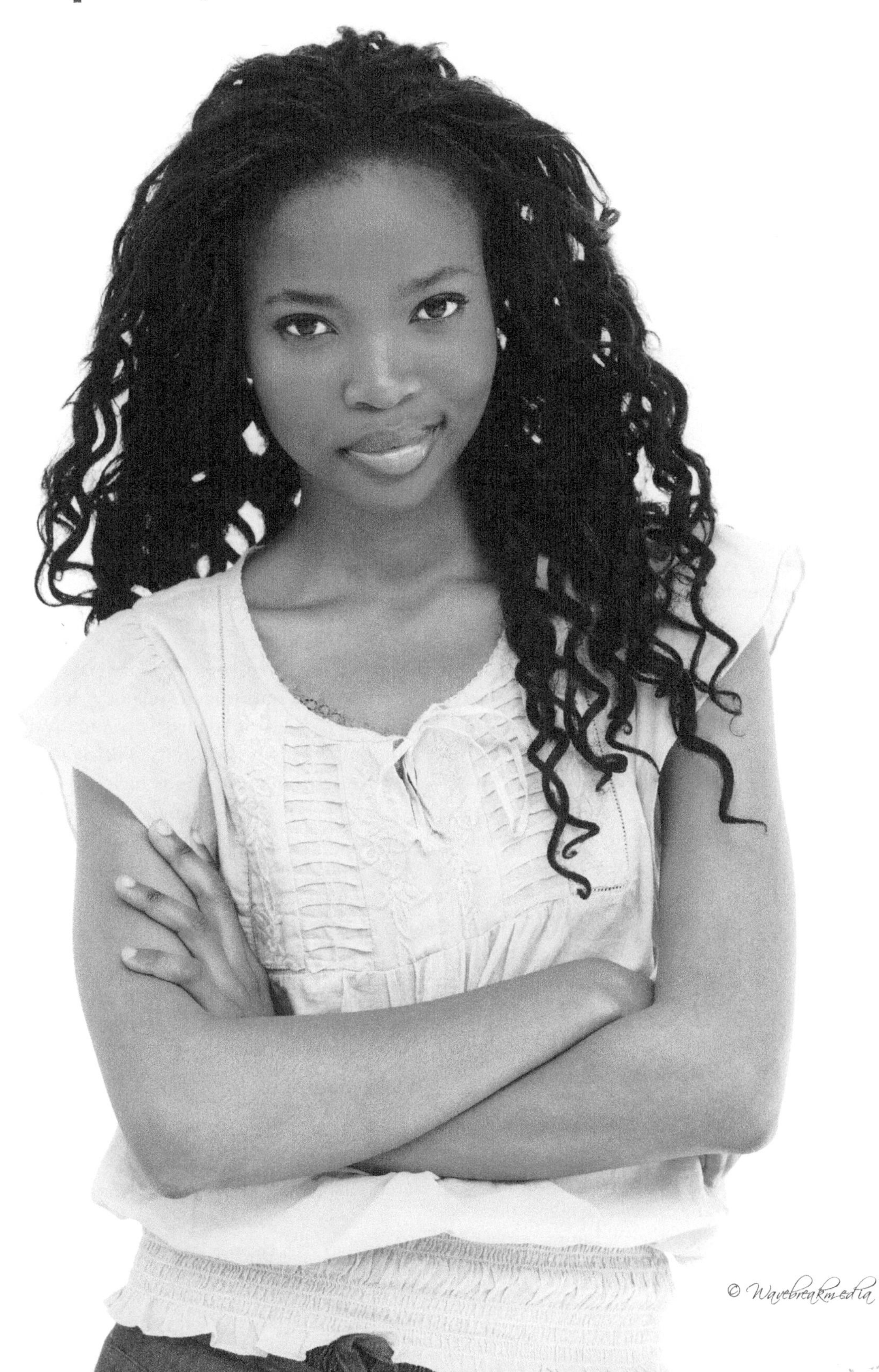

© Wavebreakmedia

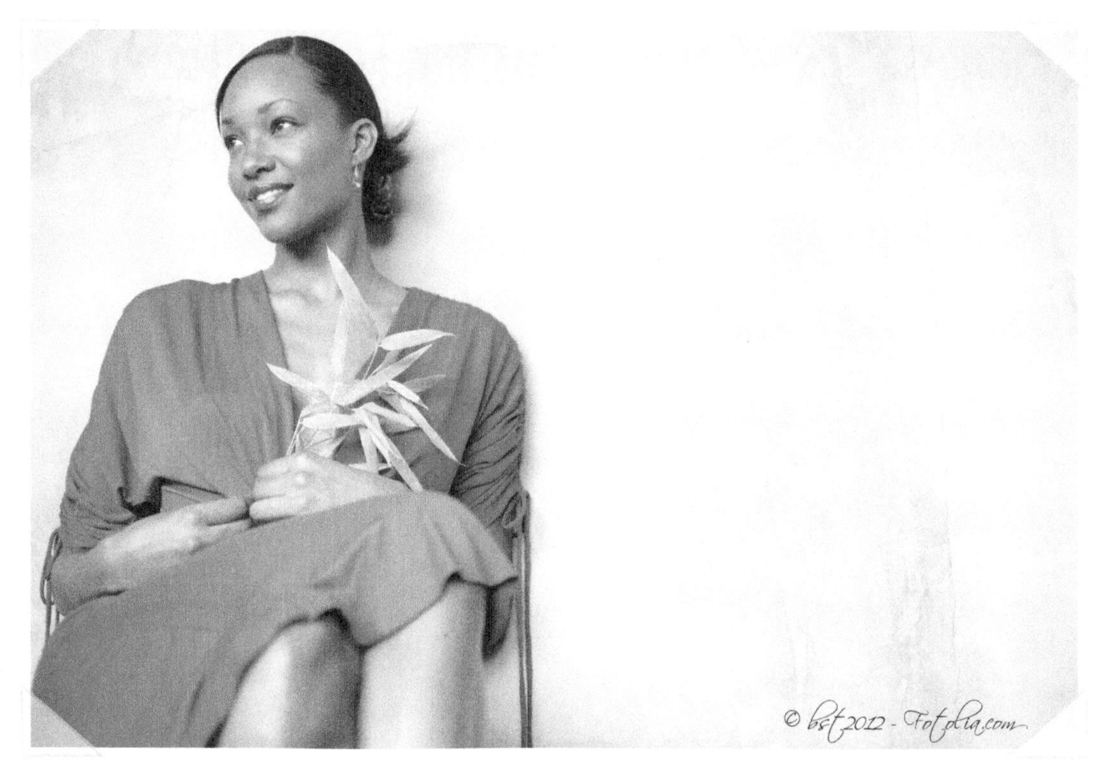

Fig 4.0: How do you begin a transition to natural hair? Easy! Simply allow your hair to grow in without applying chemicals of any kind to alter the texture. You stop getting relaxers!

4. Starting with the Stretch

Up until this point, we've dealt with the mental aspects of the back-to-natural journey. Now, it's time to focus on getting our hair on the same page. We begin our transition with a relaxer stretch. The original *Science of Black Hair* book discusses relaxer stretching, or relaxer deferment, as a technique for improving the quality and thickness of chemically relaxed hair—but relaxer stretching can also be a useful tool for eventually going natural. "Stretching" is simply going without a chemical relaxer for any length of time beyond your normal set relaxing interval. For most people, this means going anything beyond six to nine weeks without a relaxer application.

What separates regular stretchers from transitioners is intent. You are *stretching* when you exceed your regular relaxer interval, but plan to return to relaxing at some point. You are *transitioning* when you exceed your regular relaxer interval with no plan to return to relaxing. It is not uncommon for a basic stretch to eventually develop into a full-blown transition. That is how many natural journeys start, mine included. I regularly stretched my relaxers out to ten weeks, then twelve, then sixteen—until one day I decided just to keep going! Stretching is great practice for going natural.

The Science of Black Hair Super Survey

Survey Says! Of the relaxed women polled in our super survey, nearly **70%** said that they always stretched out their relaxer applications. Another **20%** said that they sometimes stretch their relaxer applications.

Many find stretching their relaxer more than two or three weeks beyond their regular relaxing schedule to be difficult the very first attempt. This is normal. It is always best to set small, attainable goals for the first few stretching attempts. The length of the relaxer stretch is up to you. Whether your relaxer stretch is twelve days, twelve weeks, or twelve months—anything beyond what you are used to is good progress! Successful relaxer stretching takes time and patience, but it gets progressively easier with practice.

4.1 Healthy Hair Care 101: Refresher Class!

Those of you who are familiar with my other hair-care books know that we always cover basic hair and scalp science in every single book. It may not be the most exciting thing, but it is so very important. Your transition is a great time to brush up on and get a grasp of the basic tenets of healthy hair care. For some women, their transition is the first time they've really given their hair care any serious thought. Knowing the basics will go a long way toward ensuring that your transition is a success. Here's your Refresher Class!

Why You Should Always Stretch

Even if you still are not quite sold on going natural, stretching is a practice that is worthwhile in any healthy hair-care regimen. Stretching greatly reduces your exposure to harmful relaxer chemicals that can take their toll on both the hair and scalp over time. Consider this: When your hair is relaxed every six weeks, your scalp and hair are exposed to strong relaxer chemicals up to nine times per year. But, if you stretch your relaxer applications out to ten weeks or more, you will reduce your hair's exposure to as few as five relaxers per year. While reducing exposure isn't the same as no exposure, less exposure is always better. Nearly 70 percent of the relaxed women we polled in our hair survey voted that they regularly stretch their relaxer applications to improve their hair's health, fullness and thickness.

Your Hair & Scalp

Our hair is made up almost entirely of protein. This protein is what gives our hair its strength and resilience. A key part of keeping the hair happy and healthy is protecting this protein structure against attack from day-to-day stressors such as combing, handling and manipulation, heat and, of course, chemical treatments. Our natural hair is hair that has never been through a styling process that chemically breaks down its protein structure. Natural hair is what the cosmetology industry refers to as unprocessed or "virgin" hair.

The Scalp

When you come into this world, your scalp contains as many hair-growing follicles as it will ever have. Most of us have at least 100,000 follicles, but our genes and hair color determine the actual number of strands we have to work with. Underneath the scalp skin is a thriving network of blood vessels and rapidly dividing cells. In fact, of all the cells in the human body, the cells that eventually become our hair are some of the fastest growing. As old cells die and are pushed up by new ones growing in at the bottom of the follicle, the hair strand slowly emerges from the scalp. Cells continue to divide deep in the follicle, die, and get pushed up through the skin. This is the process by which our hair continues to grow, day in and day out.

We like to think of our hair as a living thing—but only a small part of the strand is actually alive. The tiny portion of our hair strand that lies beneath the scalp skin is the only living part of the hair fiber. Everything else is non-living protein. This is why our haircuts, colors and other treatments that take place along the length of the hair strand are relatively painless—and why anything that pulls on the hair from the scalp (such as combing) can be quite painful. It's also why trimming the hair has no impact on the growth rate at the scalp level.

Looking at the Scalp Skin

The scalp is divided into three basic layers. The top layer of scalp skin is called the *epidermis*. This layer is roughly fifty cells thick, and it is the layer we see and work with on a daily basis. It's the layer that flakes when we have dandruff or a dry scalp. This uppermost layer can also be broken down into five more layers: These are the *strata corneum, lucidum, granulosum, spinosum and basale.* For our purposes, the most important of these is the topmost layer—the *stratum corneum*. This skin layer is completely replaced by our bodies about every two weeks.

Just beneath the epidermis is the *dermis*, or middle layer. The dermis contains a network of collagen protein that lends strength and support to the skin. Deepest of all the skin layers is the subcutaneous, or bottom layer. The *subcutaneous* layer is where the scalp's blood vessels, hair follicles and fatty tissue are located. Sweat and oil glands are also located in the subcutaneous layer. The scalp's oil glands produce about an ounce of oil (sebum) every one hundred days to condition and lubricate the hair fiber.

The Curling Starts Here

Our hair's curling and kinking behavior begins right here at the scalp. The shape of our hair follicles ultimately determines the shape of our hair

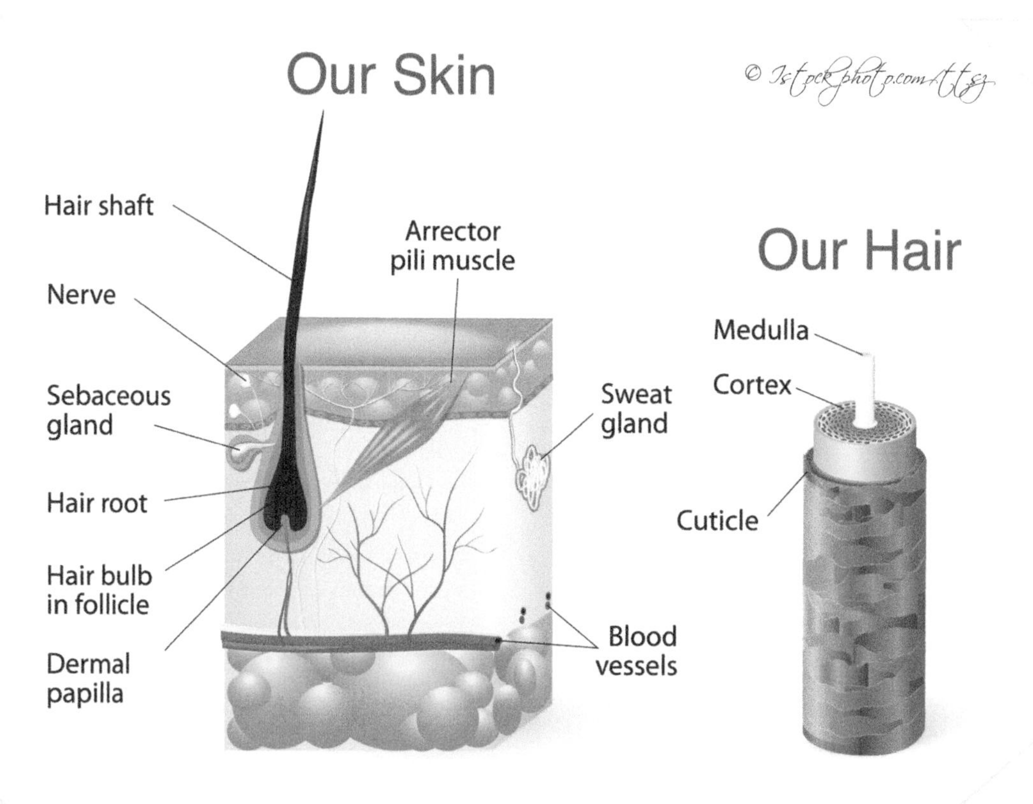

Fig 4.1: Cross section of scalp showing hair growing up from follicle. Illustration of hair's three layers (cuticle, cortex, medulla) at right.

shafts. Curls, kinks and waves come from narrow, oval-shaped hair follicles. The flatter the oval shape, the curlier the hair will be! It helps if you think about follicle shape just like the different icing nozzles that bakers use for decorating cakes . . . or even Play-Doh® shape nozzles. Large, round nozzle openings create simple, straight lines, while oval and crescent shaped nozzles create flat, complex ribbons with lots of character and movement.

The way our hair follicles are positioned in the scalp also plays a role in the shape and curvature of our hair. Follicles that are situated in the scalp at an angle, or in a "hooked" shape will have more kinking and curling than follicles that are completely vertical in the scalp.

The Hair Shaft

Features of the Hair Shaft

A basic hair strand is made up of two (and sometimes three) layers. Let's look at them from the outside going in to the heart of the strand.

Cuticle

The outer layer of the strand, the *cuticle*, is our hair's first line of defense against attack. Think of the cuticle layer as a shield whose job is to ward off wear and tear from the environment and to keep precious moisture contained inside the hair strand. This shield is the layer that determines whether or not our hair actually *looks* healthy. Under a microscope, the cuticle's scales overlap and look like shingles on a roof.

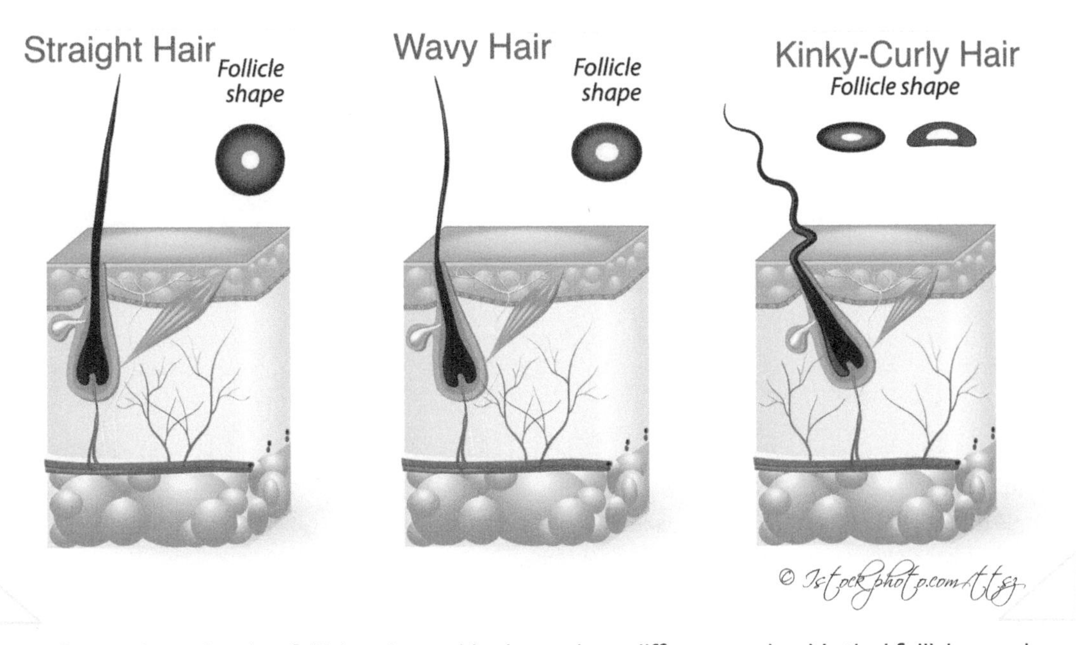

Fig 4.2: Comparison showing follicles situated in the scalp at different angles. Vertical follicles produce straight hairs, while angled follicles produce an explosion of curl.

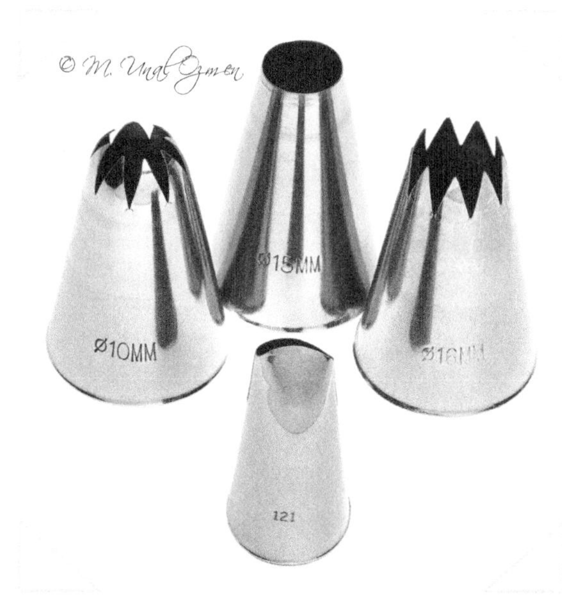

Fig. 4.3: Icing nozzles are the perfect example of how the shape of a tool can influence the shape of the material that is pushed out.

Processes such as permanent coloring and chemical relaxing—even basic things including brushing, washing and styling—slowly weaken and damage these protective scales. Over time, the protective layer begins to chip, split and lift up. When our hair is damaged in this way, it can appear discolored (browner or redder), we may lose length to breakage and the strand may become more prone to tangling with its neighbors. Textured hair is especially vulnerable to this kind of stress and strain. Lifting and chipping happen much more easily, and can occur under much less force, with textured hair than it does for other hair types. Our hair is so delicate that it doesn't take much at all to really damage it.

Cortex

Next to the cuticle, the hair's *cortex* is perhaps the single most important layer of the strand. Fiercely guarded by layers and layers of cuticle, 80 percent to 90 percent of a hair strand's total weight is made up of cortex. For those with fine-to-medium hair strands (strands that are thinner than a typical sewing thread), the cortex is the core of the hair strand. While the cuticle determines whether or not our hair actually looks healthy, our hair gets its basic character—its color, texture, strength and elasticity (stretchiness)—from the cortex. The cortex is the layer within which all chemical treatments (including relaxers) must work in order to achieve their results. Unfortunately, any change to the cortical area weakens the hair considerably.

Medulla

When individual hair strands are very thick, coarse or wiry, they usually have an extra area of hollow space deep inside the cortex. This hollow area is called the *medulla*. Again, the medulla is only found in the thickest hair shafts and may not extend all the way from root to tip along the strand. (Beard hair is coarse and almost always contains a medulla.) To date, scientists have not yet determined the medulla's purpose or its role in hair care so we won't deal with it here.

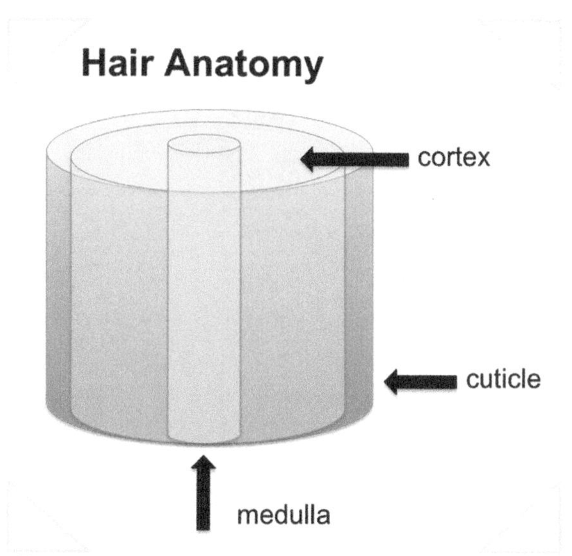

Fig. 4.4: Hair cross section showing three layers: cuticle (outer), cortex (inner) and medulla (innermost).

Anatomy of a Transitioning Strand

A transitioning strand is unique because it contains both relaxed and natural sections along the same strand (see Figure 4.5). At the top of the strand is unprocessed new growth (A), and at the lower end of the strand is relaxed hair (B). Separating these two sections is an invisible boundary known as the *line of demarcation*. The hair strand is quite fragile at this intersection and will break if too much force is exerted on the strand. The new-growth portion of a transitioning strand is the strongest and thickest section of the strand. This hair is robust because it has not had its protective cuticle layers or protein supply diminished by chemical relaxing.

Hard Demarcation Lines

When the incoming new growth and the relaxed portion of the hair strand significantly differ in texture, a *hard demarcation line* is created. The hair that meets at this line is extremely sensitive to breakage and stress because the structural difference between the natural new growth and the chemically altered portion is very stark. Strongly defined demarcation lines can make transitioning a bit more difficult. The practice of relaxing the hair to only 80 percent straightness produces a softer demarcation line and allows individuals to stretch out their chemical relaxers with greater ease (See 4.6). If you are currently relaxed and are considering a transition to natural hair, but aren't quite yet committed, get in the habit of relaxing your tresses to just 80 percent. It will save you later!

Your Hair's Porosity

Porosity refers to how well your hair allows things (mostly water and chemicals) to be absorbed into the fiber. Porosity is also a measure of how well your hair holds onto moisture. Our hair's porosity level can be described as being high, normal or low. Ideally, you want hair with medium porosity—just enough porosity to make moistur-

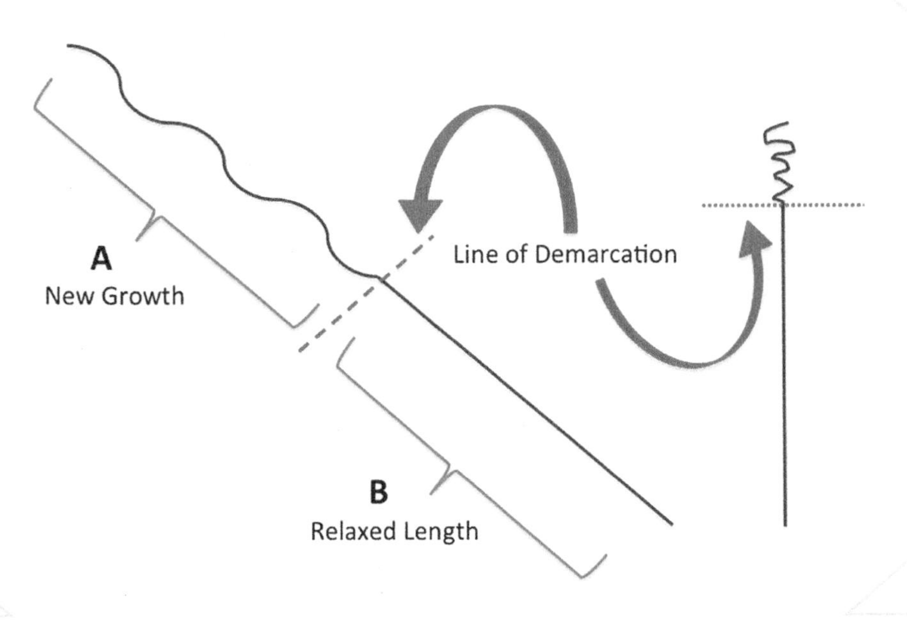

Fig. 4.5: Transitioning strands contain both relaxed and natural sections along the same fiber. The portion nearest the scalp is natural, strong and prone to considerable fiber shrinkage. The portion nearest the ends is relaxed, weaker and not as voluminous. Breakage tends to occur where the two textures meet.

izing easy but low enough to keep moisture in the strand longer. Although some of us are born with naturally higher or lower porosity hair, our hair's ultimate porosity is mostly dependent on the condition of the hair cuticle. Any damage to the hair's cuticle will increase porosity and cause the hair to lose its ability to hold onto the moisture it needs.

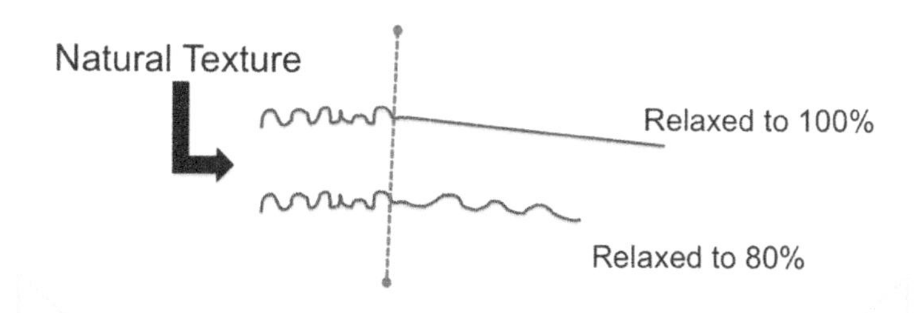

Fig. 4.6: If you are currently relaxing your hair, but considering a transition to natural hair in the future, get in the habit of leaving texture behind with your relaxer applications. This will make the transition to natural hair much easier.

Your hair's porosity may be different on different parts of your head. For example, you may have higher porosity strands around the perimeter of your head because those strands are always exposed to the sun and environment. Strands in the back and center of your head may have lower porosity because they are hidden from the elements by your ponytails and updos.

Your transitioning hair will certainly contain areas of varying porosity. Your natural new growth will have lower overall porosity than your relaxed ends which are highly porous. You will probably see this first-hand when it comes to drying your hair. Your ends will no doubt dry faster than the new growth and hair nearest your scalp simply because it's older and has undergone processing.

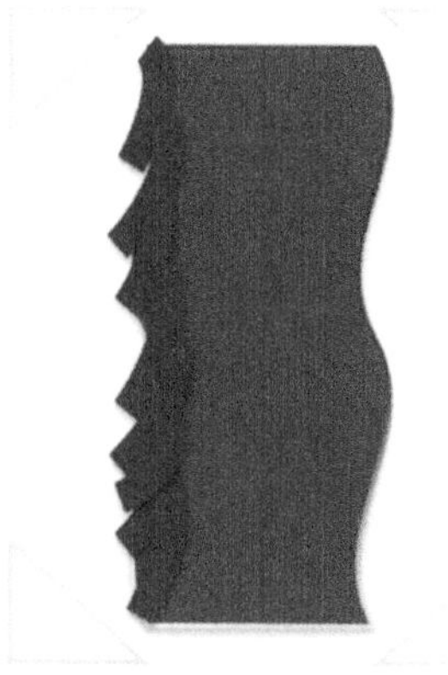

Fig. 4.7:

Normal Porosity

Somewhere in the middle of the porosity extremes lies normal or medium porosity. Hair with normal porosity absorbs moisture into the fiber and is able to hold onto it because the cuticle layers are tight, flat and flexible. Hair with normal porosity is easily moisturized and responds well to chemical processing and heat styling. It also responds best to lighter weight oils like argan oil and jojoba oil.

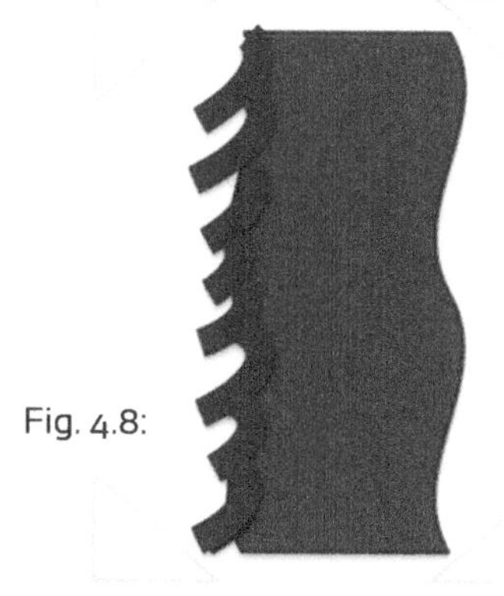

Fig. 4.8:

High Porosity

Most of us have hair that lies somewhere between normal porosity and high porosity. While some people are born with highly porous hair, most arrive at this state because of some kind of damage to the hair's cuticle layers. The usual culprits are excessive heat use, chemical processing and sun exposure.

You may have highly porous hair if:

1. Your hair is relaxed or color-treated.
2. Your wet hair dries very quickly.
3. Your hair soaks up products on contact.
4. Your hair lacks sheen.

High-porosity hair has cuticle layers with scales that are no longer tightly bound or flat. These cuticles' scales are often chipped or ruffled and, in some cases, missing entirely! Because the hair's protective barrier is not as strong, it has a difficult time managing the inward and outward flow of moisture. When it is moisturized, highly porous hair absorbs a great amount of moisture but loses it rather quickly. More often than not, this rapid loss of moisture leaves the hair feeling dry, frizzy and tangly. High-porosity hair needs a good dose of protein restructuring followed by moisturizing deep conditioning to bring it back in line. When it comes to oils, high porosity hair loves heavier weight oils and butters like castor oil and shea butter.

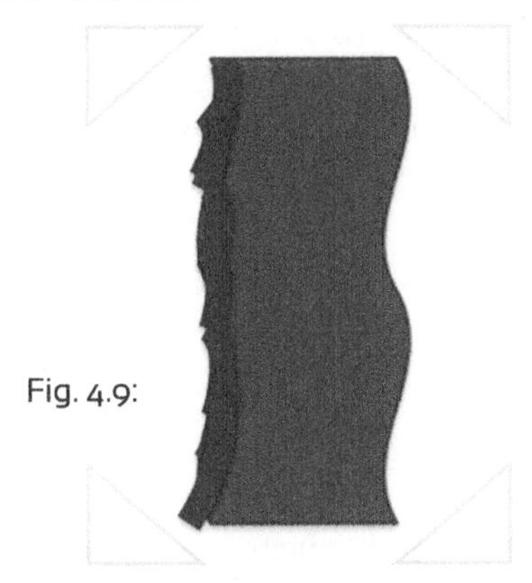

Fig. 4.9:

Low Porosity

If too much porosity is bad, then very little porosity should be ideal, right? Yes and no. Hair with low porosity is generally very healthy hair, with a high degree of sheen. The cuticles are flat, tight and in excellent condition.

Yes, things are great until it comes time to moisturize the hair! Because the cuticle is almost fortress-like, low-porosity hair resists wetting. While this resistance makes low-porosity hair less prone to frizzing than other hair types, it also makes basic moisturizing and conditioning difficult. Products tend to build up on the outside of the strand without really penetrating.

Heat styling can also be harder on low-porosity hair because the strands tend to resist heat manipulation. Because low-porosity hair is also resistant to chemical treatments such as coloring services, stylists will often chemically "soften" a client's low-porosity hair with a high-pH product. The high pH swells the hair and opens up the cuticle, increasing the likelihood of color penetration and ensuring that the color processes predictably and true.

You may have low porosity hair if:

1. Your hair is natural.
2. Your wet hair dries very slowly.
3. Your hair products seem to sit on the outside of the hair, never soaking in.
4. Your hair has lots of sheen.

Compared to relaxed hair, natural hair tends to have lower porosity. If you have low-porosity hair, you may need to use heat via hooded dryers or steamers to help moisture find its way into your hair. Working with lighter, penetrating oil products like coconut oil and avocado oil to seal in your moisturizers will also go a long way toward making your hair feel moisturized rather than coated. Keep moisturizers and oils focused near the ends of your hair, since the ends are the oldest and most in need of protection. Finally, make shampooing a regular part of your healthy hair care regimen. Since low porosity hair tends to accumulate buildup quickly, regular cleansing is important to ensure the fiber isn't overwhelmed with old, lingering product.

Porosity and Hard Water

Hard water can also compound the effects of having hair with low porosity. Hard water is essentially water that has a high mineral content.

This mineral content is usually gained when the water passes over rock formations before reaching your tap. Your water may be hard if your soaps and detergents do not lather well, or if you notice chalky, white buildup around your faucets.

As minerals from the hard water latch onto your hair, they begin to build up over time. This accumulation of minerals on the shaft makes the hair extremely stiff, uncooperative and very dry, regardless of your hair's initial porosity level.

To combat hard water issues in your home, invest in a chelating shampoo. These shampoos are specially formulated to lift hard water deposits from the hair. (*Paul Mitchell Shampoo Three* is a great option.) For a more permanent, yet costlier solution, have your home outfitted with a water softening system.

Porosity, pH and Hair Product Selection

Our hair's porosity levels are influenced by changes in pH. High pH environments increase our hair's porosity, while lower pH environments help reduce porosity. All water-based hair care products have a pH value, so we always have to consider how the pH ranges of our products will impact the fiber. (Oils do not have a pH value.) When we are applying our hair products, we always want to move progressively downward in pH so that the last product we apply has the lowest pH and helps smooth and constrict the cuticle. This downward shift in pH ensures that our hair's cuticle remains in good condition.

Products are generally formulated with this downward pH idea in mind. Shampoos tend to have higher pHs than conditioners, and leave-in conditioners and moisturizers tend to come in at even lower pHs. This downward shift in pH is intentional and helps normalize the pH of our hair toward its healthy, happy acidic range.

When you stick to one product brand for your hair care needs, you are generally safe in terms of having your products formulated with progressively lower pHs. The problem comes when we mix and match product lines. If you are someone who uses many product lines together, be sure to test the pH values of your products to ensure that their pH order is indeed running downward. You can purchase pH testing strips from your local pharmacy, drugstore or Amazon.com.

Porosity at a Glance

Low Porosity

Products penetrate slowly or may never seem to penetrate the hair. The effects of moisturizing products may not be felt at all, or the effects are short-lived.

Normal Porosity

Products penetrate at a moderate rate, and the effects of moisturizing products linger for a while.

High Porosity

Products penetrate very easily, but the effects of moisturizing products are short-lived.

Fig 4.10

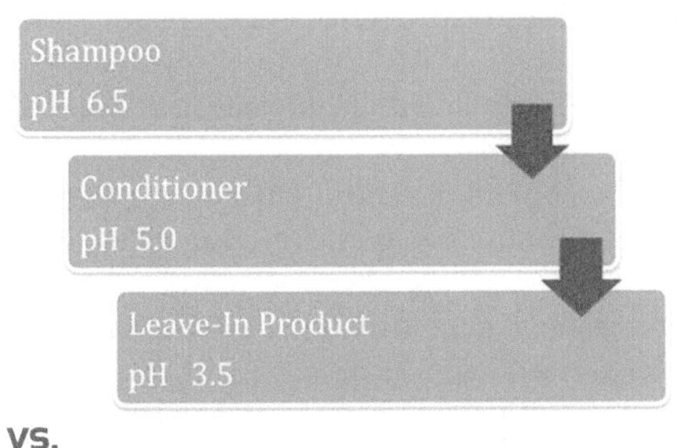

VS.

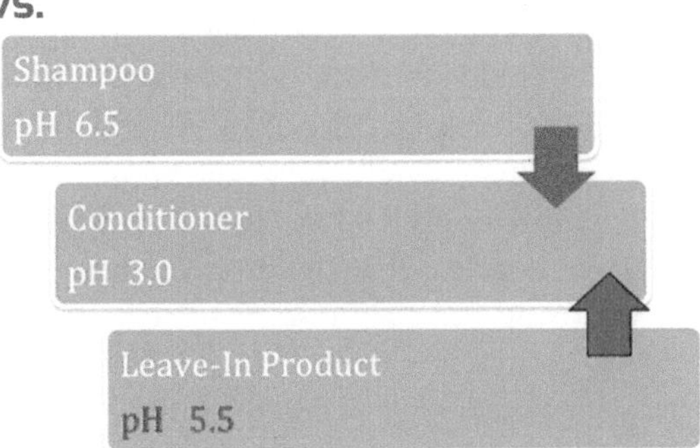

Fig 4.11: The pH values of our products should show a downward trend as we move through our styling routine from start to finish. Swings in pH can negatively impact and affect the way your hair feels.

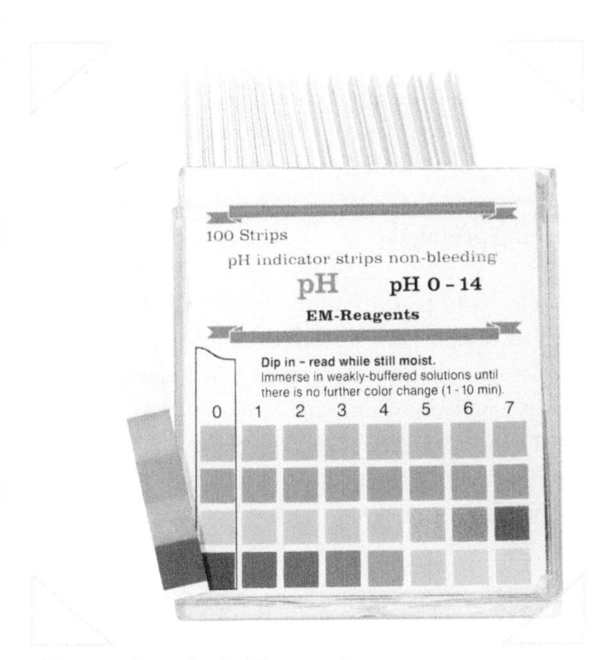

Fig 4.12: Standard pH test strips.

Your Hair's Elasticity

Because our hair strands are elastic, they are able to stretch and then return to their original length when pulled. Elasticity is what gives us great curl definition and bounce. It's also what allows us to pull our hair back into an Afro puff and braid or stretch out our curls and coils with no breakage. Without the proper elasticity, our hair simply breaks.

Our hair's elasticity depends on its moisture content and the soundness of its protein structure. Heat styling, chemical relaxing and the permanent coloring process reduce our hair's elasticity because they attack and deplete both the protein and moisture components of our hair. In order to maintain healthy stretchiness day after day and year after year, our hair must maintain the right balance of moisture and protein. Moisture allows our hair to move through an incredible range of motion without breaking. Protein also supports our strands' range of motion and is what allows it to recover or rebound from the stretch without breaking.

Since your transitioning hair contains both relaxed and natural sections, it will also contain areas of varying elasticity. In its healthy dry state, your natural new growth will have a moderate level of elasticity that allows you to stretch your hair time and time again with very little breakage. Your relaxed ends will tend to have much less elasticity in the dry state and will break with repeated stretching and stress to the fiber. As you

Did You Know?

While dry hair can only stretch to approximately 20 to 30 percent of its original length and still return to normal, wet hair can stretch up to 50 percent beyond its normal length.

progress in your transition and continue to give your hair the moisture it needs, your relaxed ends will likely enter a state where they become "overly elastic." If you take a relaxed strand and stretch it, it will stretch and stretch and then start to thin out just before breaking. This issue with the relaxed ends is caused by protein loss to the fiber.

Protein/Moisture Balancing

Protein and moisture balancing is a key part of any hair-care regimen. If you recall from earlier in this chapter, our hair is made up almost entirely of protein, moisture (water) and binding materials. Our hair's protein is what gives the strand its strength and ruggedness. The moisture component is what gives our hair its flexibility and stretchiness. Together, protein and moisture make our hair both durable and elastic. These elements must be balanced in the hair strand to protect against hair breakage. The hair products we use are usually designed to fulfill either our hair's need for protein or its need for moisture. Using too much of one type of product (products that are too protein-rich when our hair needs moisture, or too moisture-rich when our hair needs protein) will lead to breakage.

Knowing how to identify when your hair needs either moisture or protein is a very important skill for transitioners, especially long-term transitioners who'll be going for several months between relaxer services. Here's the general rule of thumb:

Hair that feels:

- Stretchy, gummy, lightweight, limp or weak needs more protein conditioning.
- Tough, dry, rough, or scratchy needs more moisture conditioning.
- Ambiguous/in-between hair needs more moisture conditioning.

It is easiest to tell whether your hair needs protein or moisture when the hair is wet, but you can also pick up cues from your hair when it's dry. If you are ever unsure about what your hair needs, go with moisture. Giving your hair too much moisture is harder to do than giving it too much protein. This is because moisture is always coming and going from the hair. Hair that was moisturized one minute can easily dry out the next. It's difficult to maintain a surplus of moisture because the water in our hair and skin is always being traded with the environment around us. But protein works differently. When you give your hair protein conditioning, the protein binds to the hair strongly and doesn't go anywhere. Protein only releases its hold on the hair with each cleansing and conditioning session. The effects of too much protein will only wear away after several washings—and until they do, you will probably experience a considerable amount of hair breakage.

Not a 50-50 Balance

Although it is called a balance, the protein/moisture balance for your hair is not a 50-50 balance that dictates you should use protein products half of the time and moisture products the other half. The balance is always heavily moisture-biased because textured hair needs moisture more than anything. A proper protein/moisture balance might include 80 percent moisture-conditioning products and 20 percent protein-conditioning products.

During your transitioning journey, your protein/moisture balance will shift even more toward the moisture side as your natural new growth starts to become the dominant texture. Natural hair that has not had its proteins broken down by the chemical-relaxing process does not need nearly as much protein conditioning to remain in good health as the relaxed hair it is replacing.

As you get deep into your transition, your textures will compete for their different needs. Your

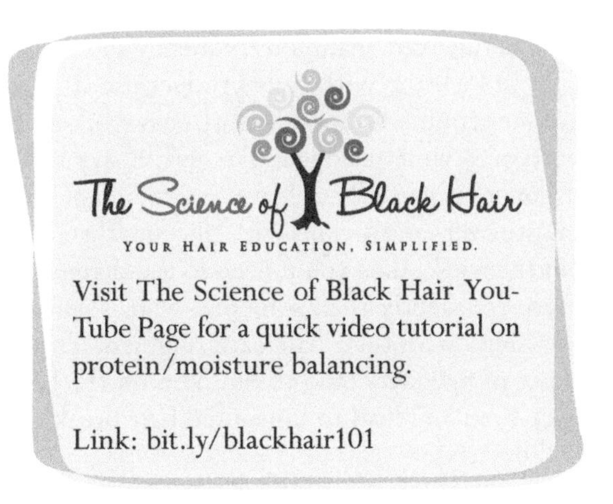

natural hair will want moisture desperately, and at first your relaxed hair will want it too. You'll reach a point where your relaxed length starts to feel limp, weak and stretchy from all the moisture, and it will need more protein to help restore its balance and to prevent breakage. With practice, you will learn how to read your hair very quickly and even predict how it will respond to different things. This level of confidence with your hair does take time, but you will soon have it down!

4.2 Hair Product Basics

How smoothly your transition and newly natural journey go will be a direct reflection of how diligently you keep your hair in a conditioned state. Moisturizing your hair throughout the week is extremely important, but this is also the point in many healthy hair-care regimens where people drop the ball. Many times we think we are moisturizing our hair, but we're really using the wrong products to get the job done. When you are looking for moisturizing shampoos, conditioners, moisturizers and stylers, look for water-based products with water, fatty alcohols, humectants and emollients. (See page 167, the "Hair Product Index" at the end of this book for detailed listings.)

- **Fat (Fatty Alcohols)**

  Fatty alcohols are "hair-friendly" alcohols, unlike the alcohols found in finishing sprays, which are often drying to the hair. Look for common fatty alcohols like cetyl alcohol, cetearyl alcohol, stearyl alcohol and myristyl alcohol in your shampoos, conditioners, leave-ins and water-based moisturizers.

- **Humectants, Emollients and Other Conditioning Agents**

  Humectants are substances that draw moisture from the surrounding air to the hair. Emollients provide a layer of light lubrication to the hair fiber to prevent excess moisture loss. Common humectants, emollients and conditioning agents you'll find in your hair care products are propylene glycol, sodium lactate, sodium PCA, hydantoin, glycerin, polyquaternium, glyceryl stearate, cetrimonium chloride and various types of natural waxes and oils. Many transitioners and new naturals are concerned about the potential health effects of some ingredients. If you are ever worried about the safety profiles of any of the ingredients in your products, check out the Environmental Working Group's website: www.ewg.com/skindeep/.

- **What You Should Try To Skimp On**

  In any moisturizing formula, you should try to stay away from products that contain petrolatum, mineral oil, heavy proteins and other heavy oils. These products will only coat your hair and won't provide much of a moisture benefit. Remember, moisture is water. You cannot moisturize your hair without water being present. You will often hear people say that they use an oil to moisturize their hair, but (since they actually repel water) oils cannot moisturize your hair. Oils can help your hair stay moisturized by coating the hair and preventing water from escaping from the shaft as quickly, but the oils themselves aren't what's moisturizing your hair.

Shampooing Notes

In order to bring the greatest opportunity for moisture into your shampooing phase, you'll want to use sulfate-free shampoos. These shampoos tend to be the gentlest shampoos to use on textured hair. Check out the list of sulfate-free shampoos at the end of this book. (See page 168). Sulfate-free shampoos do not contain:

- sodium lauryl sulfate (SLS)
- sodium laureth sulfate (SLES)
- ammonium lauryl sulfate (ALS)
- ammonium laureth sulfate (ALES)

Many shampoos that are marketed as sulfate-free contain other sulfate-like ingredients or a combination of sulfate-like ingredients that are even more irritating and stripping than the standard sulfates listed above. A key one to avoid is C14-16 Olefin Sulfonate, which is not technically considered a "sulfate" but is extremely similar to basic sodium lauryl sulfate in its potential for irritancy. Of course, whether a shampoo will be harsh and stripping or extra moisturizing and nourishing will depend on its entire formulation and not just one ingredient. There are always exceptions to every rule, but in general, avoiding sulfates will tend to net you more moisture for your hair.

How Often Should I Use Shampoo?

Naturally, your shampoo frequency is up to you—and it may change from time to time depending on your situation. I generally recommend two types of shampoo to include in your regimen: one gentle shampoo for weekly cleansing (every 7-10 days; or every 3-5 days if you are just starting your healthy hair care journey) and one deep cleansing (clarifying) shampoo for use every month. The weekly shampoo is just enough to lift debris without stripping your hair, while the monthly clarifying shampoo is meant to cleanse a bit more deeply and give you a fresher starting point each month.

In general, your shampoo frequency should be kept in lockstep with your product use. If you are someone who uses lots of heavy oils and butters, styling products like gels, heavy conditioners (especially as leave-in products), and moisturizers and serums with silicones throughout the week, then you'll need to use shampoos more frequently than someone who is "product-light" with their hair care regimen. Those types of products tend to build up on the hair over time and lead to unwanted hair breakage and dryness.

Conditioning Notes

We demand a lot from our hair, and the conditioners we select can either make (or break) our healthy hair care regimen. The moisture, "slip" and softness that we get from our conditioners make them a key product in our hair care arsenals. And of course, many transitioners and naturals go through conditioner like there is no tomorrow! While conditioners cannot undo the years of trauma a single hair will experience in its lifetime, a solid conditioner can slow the deterioration process. It is so important to always invest in the best conditioners that you possibly can. This is the place to splurge and it is the part of your regimen that you cannot afford to slack on!

Conditioners work on the surface of the hair to improve its look, feel and texture. They temporarily bond split ends, fill in missing material along the cuticle and add a layer of protection against further assault. As you might have guessed, conditioners also contain a wide range of conditioning ingredients, too. These ingredients are positively charged and absolutely love to stick to our negatively-charged hair strands. (Opposites attract!) The more damage or stress your hair has encountered, the more places the conditioner will want to bind. These ingredients contribute shine, bounce and thickness that will remain long after hair rinsing because they create breathable films on the hair.

Conditioners may be moisture-based or protein-based. Protein conditioners will contain more concentrated amounts of protein to help add structure and strength to the hair, while moisturizing conditioners will be more humectant and emollient-rich. In the first few weeks of any transition, your focus should definitely be on moisturizing conditioners. Where it gets tricky is that many moisturizing deep conditioners also contain some protein. Wheat and silk proteins are the most common gentle proteins in moisturizing deep conditioners. They tend to be extremely gentle and actually enhance the hair's elasticity by helping moisture bind within the cuticle. These formulas are still great moisture-boosting formulas, so don't let the tiny amounts of protein in them concern you.

If we're using lots of conditioner in our regimens, it is also important to clean up after them every once in a while by deep cleaning, or clarifying, the hair. Cleansing the hair with a good clarifying shampoo once a month removes heavy oils, silicones and other styling products that have accumulated over time—and it gives your hair a fresh start! If you are ever experiencing hair breakage that you can't explain, clarifying your hair should be a first step.

Boosting Protein in Your Transitioning Regimen

Chemical processes that access the inner parts of our hair always do damage to the outside of the hair first. Once inside, bonds are broken deep in the hair, leaving you with weaker strands that are always looking for moisture and structure. But chemicals are not the only problem. Heat styling and sun exposure also degrade the hair. Regular protein conditioning will help to keep your hair strong and breakage resistant. Conditioning once or twice per month with a protein-rich conditioner is enough to benefit most people, but always be sure to perform your own wet assessments to determine where you fall. You may find that you only need a heavy protein treatment every other month, or twice a year.

Leave-In & Moisturizer Notes

Leave-in conditioners and moisturizers are combined here because they are both water-based products that use the same ingredient template. This is why leave-ins and moisturizers can be used interchangeably in a healthy hair care regimen. A moisturizer must be a water-based product, so you need one that lists water as its very first ingredient. This top position in the ingredients list indicates that water makes up the bulk of the product formula.

Look for hydrolyzed proteins (ex. hydrolyzed keratin) that are found early on in the product's ingredients list for best results. Hydrolyzed proteins have been engineered to a size that can actually bind to and integrate with the hair in a meaningful way.

These types of moisturizers generally come in the form of light sprays, creams, custards, pastes and puddings. Sprays work well for those with fine hair or braided hair styles, while heavier creams and custards are generally best for those with thicker, coarser hair.

Oil & Butter Notes

The word "oil" is a broad term that includes a wide range of solid and liquid materials including fatty alcohols, triglycerides, butters and oil-soluble silicones. Oils and butters enhance the shine, softness and flexibility of our hair, and they often act as barriers to prevent the escape of moisture from the hair and skin. Lighter-weight essential oils can even offer sensory benefits and healing properties for the user.

What to Look For:

Natural Oils

So what should you look for when buying oils? When you shop for oils, look for ones that are derived from plants, flowers, seeds and fruits. These oils form light, semi-permeable films on the hair to help seal in moisture. Depending on their chemistry, many of these oils quickly wear off from the hair's surface or actively penetrate the hair fiber over time to provide opportunities for re-moisturization of the fiber. Pay attention to where the oil actually falls on its own ingredients list. If your coconut oil has coconut oil listed second from the bottom, it's probably a stretch to even call it coconut oil! The key oil should always be in the top three to five ingredients.

Cold-Pressed Oils

Whenever possible, seek out oils that are cold-pressed. When oils are cold-pressed they retain many more of their natural properties. These oils are made by grinding plants, nuts, seeds, or fruits into a paste. Then the paste is pressed using a tool that causes the oil to separate from the paste. Sometimes the paste is warmed to help it release more oil, but for true cold-pressing, the paste cannot be heated above 115°F. Oils will keep for years if kept in a cool, dry place. Storing oils in dark bottles will also prevent light from breaking them down.

Shop the Grocery Aisle

Sometimes, shopping for your oils in the grocery section is better than picking them up from the hair care aisle. In the grocery aisle, you have access to purer, cold-pressed products and they are often less expensive for larger amounts of oil. Sure, there's no fancy labeling or pretty hair models on the packaging—but you get some of the best oil possible. My coconut oil is food-grade and I always pick up two jars: a jar for the kitchen and a jar for my bathroom!

Moisturizing and Sealing Techniques

Moisturizing is most effective when it is done as a two-step process. The first step to this process is always providing a source of hydration (water) to your hair. The second step is locking in that hydration with a heavier product (oil or butter)—a step also known as "sealing" the hair. Water is the absolute best moisturizer for your hair, but it

Survey Says! We asked our survey participants, *"Which product brands do you consider to be "go-to" brands?* They were allowed to vote for more than one brand, and were also allowed to write in responses if their brands of choice were not included on our original list. Here's what they told us!

1. SheaMoisture 45%
2. Homemade Products 29%
3. ECOSTYLER 24%, Kinky Curly 24%, and TRESemme 24%
4. Organic Root Stimulator (ORS) 23%
5. CANTU 20%
6. Aphogee 17% and Herbal Essences 17%
7. AS I AM 15%
8. Aubrey Organics 13%

Top "write-in" responses:

1. Aussie
2. Giovanni
3. Nexxus
4. Neutrogena Triple Moisture
5. Trader Joe's

needs a little help staying inside the strand. This is where sealing comes in!

Sealing is simply placing a heavier product on top of already hydrated hair, and it is always a temporary state. The goal of applying heavier products after the water source is to simply *slow the evaporation of water* back into the surrounding environment. The longer you can prevent moisture evaporation back into the surrounding air, the longer your hair will feel truly moisturized. Hair that dries out very soon after moisturizing simply does not have a proper moisture barrier in place, or has not been adequately hydrated in the first place.

There are quite a few moisturizing and sealing methods out there, and you'll need to experiment a little to find the one that works best for you and your hair. Some methods work better in specific situations, certain climates and for certain hair types. No matter which moisturizing method you choose, there is one thing that all methods have in common. Water, or a water-based product, should go on the hair before any other product!

We'll take a look at the two most popular moisturizing and sealing methods: the LCO and LOC methods. These sealing methods use acronyms to help you remember when to apply the products you need.

LCO— Liquid + Cream + Oil

L: In the "L" or *liquid* step of the LCO moisturizing and sealing method, a liquid leave-in conditioner product or plain water is applied to the hair first. (Your damp hair immediately after your final wash-day rinse can also be considered your liquid step.)

C: The "C" in LCO refers to a cream-based moisturizing product that is applied after the hair is given the liquid. This cream is a water-based moisturizer that contains water as the very first ingredient. Together with the liquid, this cream helps improve the hair's moisture content by providing an additional source of water and humectants (moisture-attracting ingredients). Since it also contains some oils and emollients, the cream also acts as a light barrier to moisture loss.

O: The "O" in LCO refers to an oil product that is applied to the hair to seal both the liquid and cream products into the hair. In the LCO method, the oil could also be a butter product. The final oil or butter layer acts as a true sealant layer on top of a semi-sealant/semi-moisturizing layer (creamy moisturizer) and a true moisturizing layer (water). In short, the layering is:

Moisture— Semi-Sealant/Semi-Moisturizer— Sealant

The LCO method works best for those with finer strands, and for those whose hair is easily weighed down by products. The hair can even be sealed at the "cream" step for those with the finest tresses. For those people who need a little more sealing power, a hair butter can be used in the place of an oil as an additional layer of protection.

LOC— Liquid + Oil + Cream (or Butter)

L: The liquid step of the LOC moisturizing and sealing method is exactly the same as in the LCO method. Both methods agree on this crucial point—water first! In some variations of the method, "L" just stands for "leave-in conditioner," which may be liquid or otherwise.

O: In the LOC method, oil comes second in line as a direct sealant for liquid moisture.

Did You Know?

Although they coat the hair and repel water, oils and butters cannot lock moisture in the hair forever. Some oils migrate into the hair strand over time (coconut oil), while some simply wear off on their own.

C: The "C" in the LOC method can refer to a water-based moisturizer cream in some variations of the method, or a creamy butter product (non-water-based) in other variations of the method. This third layer is applied to the hair to seal both the liquid and oil into the hair. The cream acts as a moisturizing, semi-sealant layer placed on top of a true sealant layer (oil) and a true moisturizing layer (water). In short, the layering is:

Moisture— Sealant— Semi-Sealant/Semi-Moisturizer

This method works best for those with thicker hair that tolerates oil and butter products very well. It's essentially, a double sealant method. Those with low porosity strands may find the layering a bit much in the LOC method.

Other moisturizing and sealing variations include:
Liquid + Oil
Cream + Oil

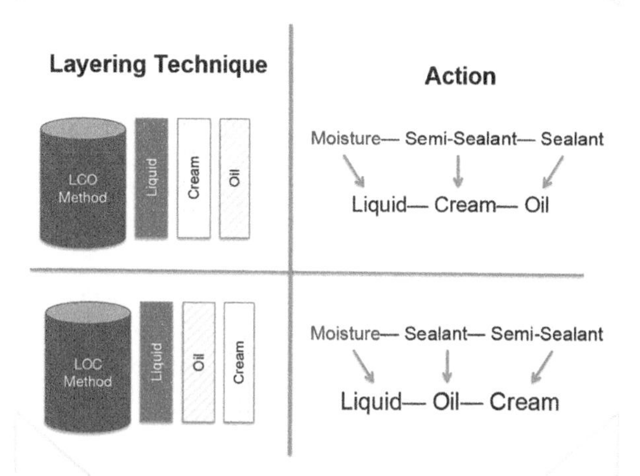

Fig 4.13: Understanding LCO and LOC Moisture & Sealing Methods.

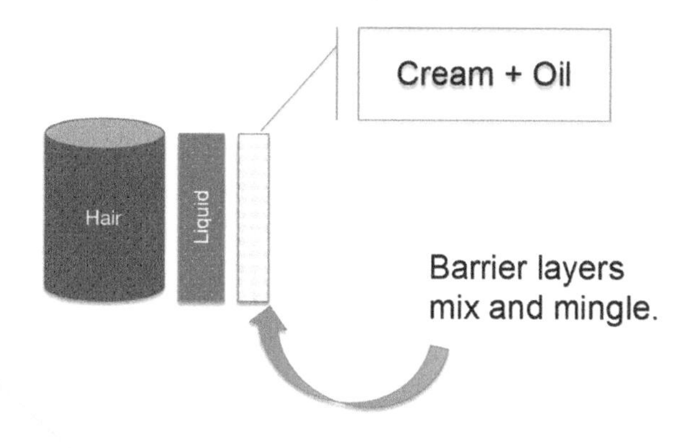

Fig 4.14: In real life, there are no neat, clear lines of layer separation. Creams and oils likely blend together and both work together to slow moisture evaporation. As long as *some kind of barrier is in place*, your hair will stay moisturized longer than when you use water alone.

In the Real World . . .

No matter how you apply your layers, you must keep in mind that this is the real world and there is no such thing as the perfect "layer" or "seal." Unfortunately, there is no way to uniformly apply and distribute the layers and be sure that every hair strand from root to tip receives the same moisture and sealing experience. (This is especially difficult on kinky-curly strands!) Oil and cream layers blend and intermingle in real life—and of course, some strands are missed entirely. But, we try! (See Figure 4.14) The good news is that simply having the combination of layers on the hair after the water will still have the net effect of slowing moisture evaporation. As long as some kind of barrier is in place, your hair will stay moisturized longer than when you use water alone.

Personally, I prefer to use the liquid+ cream+ oil (LCO) or the cream + oil (CO) sealing method for my own hair. I am a fan of layering product so that moisture is packed in closest to the strand where it is useful. Having the more hydration-rich cream layer nearest to

Commonly Avoided Ingredients

When many women begin their natural journeys, they also look for ways to improve the quality of the products they are using to care for their hair. In this section, we will cover a few common ingredients that make most people's "Do Not Buy" list.

Mineral Oil

If you've used any kind of moisturizer in the last twenty years, you've probably come across mineral oil a time or two.

The Problem:

Mineral oil has a softening effect on the hair and skin, but over time, it begins to build up leaving the hair feeling tacky and dry. Those who regularly use water-based moisturizers with mineral oil in them almost always run into problems with maintaining their hair's moisture levels long term. Like many products we use today, mineral oil is distilled from crude oil. The process by which it is made is not earth-friendly in the least, and the oil film that it leaves on the hair can be tricky to remove without using harsh cleansers. In the case of mineral oil, there are far too many great, earth-friendly, plant-based oils that can be used instead.

Parabens

Parabens are a popular, yet controversial group of preservatives that are used in nearly every beauty product from shampoo to toothpaste.

The Problem:

Although parabens are quite effective at keeping products free of microbes, their use is very controversial. Some research has shown that synthetic parabens have the ability to behave like estrogen hormones in the body, triggering "early puberty" in girls and playing a potential role in the development of breast cancer. Trace amounts of parabens have even been found in some breast cancer tumors.

Petrolatum

Petrolatum, and its sister-product mineral oil, is a popular ingredient in many, many hair care products targeted to ethnic consumers.

The Problem:

Petrolatum is a heavy lubricant, so it tends to quickly build up on the hair. At first, petrolatum has a softening effect on the hair, but over time, it begins to build up, leaving the hair feeling tacky and dry. Petrolatum creates a waterproof barrier on the hair that almost completely prevents the user from restoring proper hydration to her strands each day. This inability to get moisture through to the hair creates a chronic dryness problem that ultimately leads to hair breakage. Also, while purified petrolatum is generally considered safe, petrolatum may also be exposed to contaminants during the refining process that cause it to not be as pure.

Silicones

Silicones get a bad reputation in healthy hair care circles—but they actually play an important role in our hair care. Silicones, commonly referred to as "cones" on Internet hair forums, coat the hair shaft in a thin layer of protection that allows the strands to move freely and easily past one another. These products are easily identified by their common word endings: -cone, -conol, -col and -xane.

The Problem:

As with anything that coats or creates a layer on the hair, silicones tend to build up on the hair with regular use.

my liquid layer keeps my hair supple and moisturized. I like to layer my oil on last as a finishing touch for shine and final sealing.

The key things to remember about moisturizing and sealing are:

1. The liquid or water step is where everything counts. It must be first.
2. After your liquid step, experiment to determine which combination of products and layering order works best as a barrier to moisture-loss for you!
3. If your hair feels dry very quickly, reconsider your products or your layering order.
4. If dryness continues to be a problem, revisit your deep conditioning routine. This is where the bulk of your hydration should be coming from.

Your Chapter 4 Take-Aways

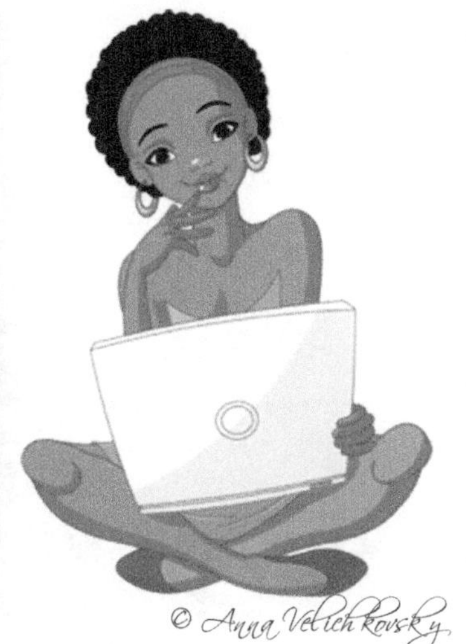

✓ What separates regular "stretchers" from transitioners is intent. You are stretching when you exceed your regular relaxer interval but plan to return to relaxing at some point. You are transitioning when you exceed your regular relaxer interval with no plan to return to relaxing.

✓ A transitioning strand is unique because it contains both relaxed and natural sections along the same strand.

✓ Porosity refers to how well your hair allows things (mostly water and chemicals) to be absorbed into the fiber. It is also a measure of how well your hair holds onto moisture.

✓ Because our hair strands are elastic, they are able to stretch and then return to their original length when pulled. Our hair's elasticity depends on its moisture content.

✓ When it comes to balancing protein and moisture in a healthy hair-care regimen: Hair that feels stretchy, gummy, lightweight, limp or weak: needs more protein conditioning; tough, dry, rough or scratchy: needs more moisture conditioning; ambiguous/in-between hair: needs more moisture conditioning.

✓ It is easiest to tell whether your hair needs protein or moisture when the hair is wet, but you can also pick up cues from your hair when it's dry.

✓ Moisturizing is most effective when it is done as a two-step process. The first step is always providing a source of hydration (water) to your hair. The second step is locking in that hydration with a heavier product (oil or butter).

In the next chapter, we will look at a basic transitioning timeline. How will your hair behave? What can you expect? Find out in Chapter 5!

Chapter 5: The Transitioning Timeline

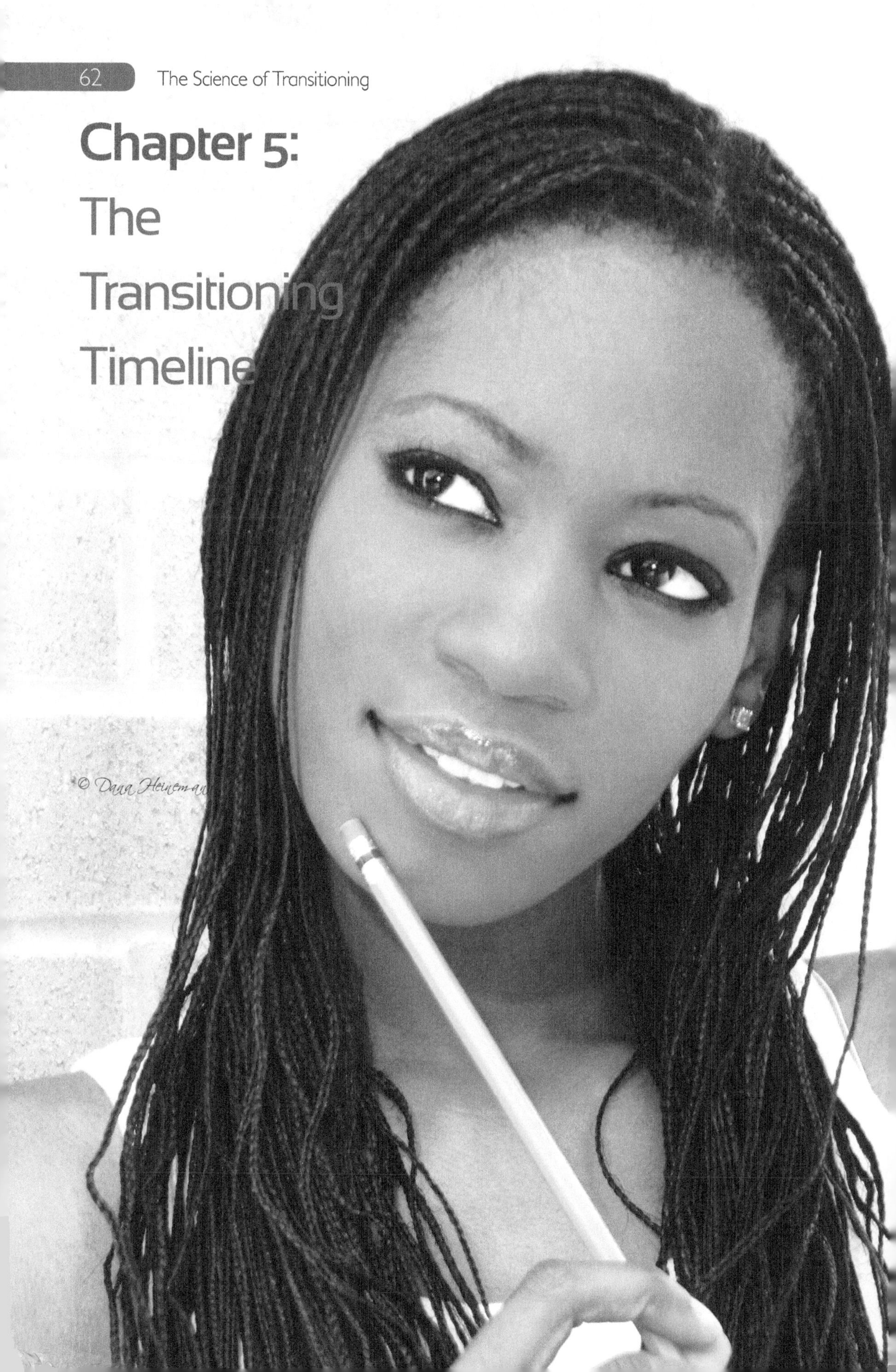

In this section, we will walk you through the stages of a typical hair transition. Keep in mind that this is only a guide, and your own transition may differ drastically from this "textbook" view. This is perfectly okay! No two transitioners or transitions are ever the same. For each section in the timeline, we provide an overview of common concerns and issues (or "What to Expect") and simple things you can do to make the transition easier with "Your Action Items."

When You Feel the Call of Your Relaxer

No matter where you are in your transition, there may come a time when you feel the urge to throw in the towel. This is normal, and you'll need to be ready for it when it happens. Here's a tip: Whenever you feel that urge to relax (usually as you approach your old, regularly scheduled relaxer time . . . or when you're deep into an intense detangling session), put your hair out of sight and out of mind by getting your hair braided, twisted or weaved. These styles will give you a break from your hair drama, buy you time in your transitioning journey and protect your hair in the process. Win-win.

Reward Yourself

Each skipped relaxer application is a victory. A good way to reward yourself for making it through each stretch period is to take the money you would have paid for the relaxer service and save it somewhere. The longer you transition, the more your rewards will add up! Do something positive and fun for yourself—you deserve it!

5. Transitioning: Weeks 0–8

In this stage, you are usually still well within your old relaxer schedule and not much about your regimen has changed. Your transition is still in its infancy, and your confidence is probably at an all-time high! If you're tech savvy, you've probably already got a good list of bloggers and vloggers to read and watch on the web for inspiration.

What To Expect

Since you are still mostly dealing with relaxed hair and very little new growth in the first eight weeks, this stage is probably going to be the easiest part of your transition. You are already pretty good at working with the small amount of new growth that comes in at this stage. Most of the challenges start to arise after the first eight to twelve weeks of your transition.

In the fourth week of transitioning, you will begin to start dealing with an abundance of new hair at the scalp level that simply does not behave like your relaxed hair at the ends. Depending on how fast your hair grows, you may start to see this occur as early as the third week or as late as the sixth week. This new half-inch of hair may feel thicker, harder and sometimes drier than what you're used to. Often, this new growth will not respond to the same products that your relaxed hair seems to love, and the new hair will tend to work against your best your attempts to straighten or flatten it. This would normally be the point when you would reach for the relaxer—but as a new transitioner, your job now is to welcome this new hair and do your very best to nurture it and understand its needs!

Your Action Items

Do Some Spring Cleaning

Once you've had your last relaxer applied and you know for sure that you want to transition,

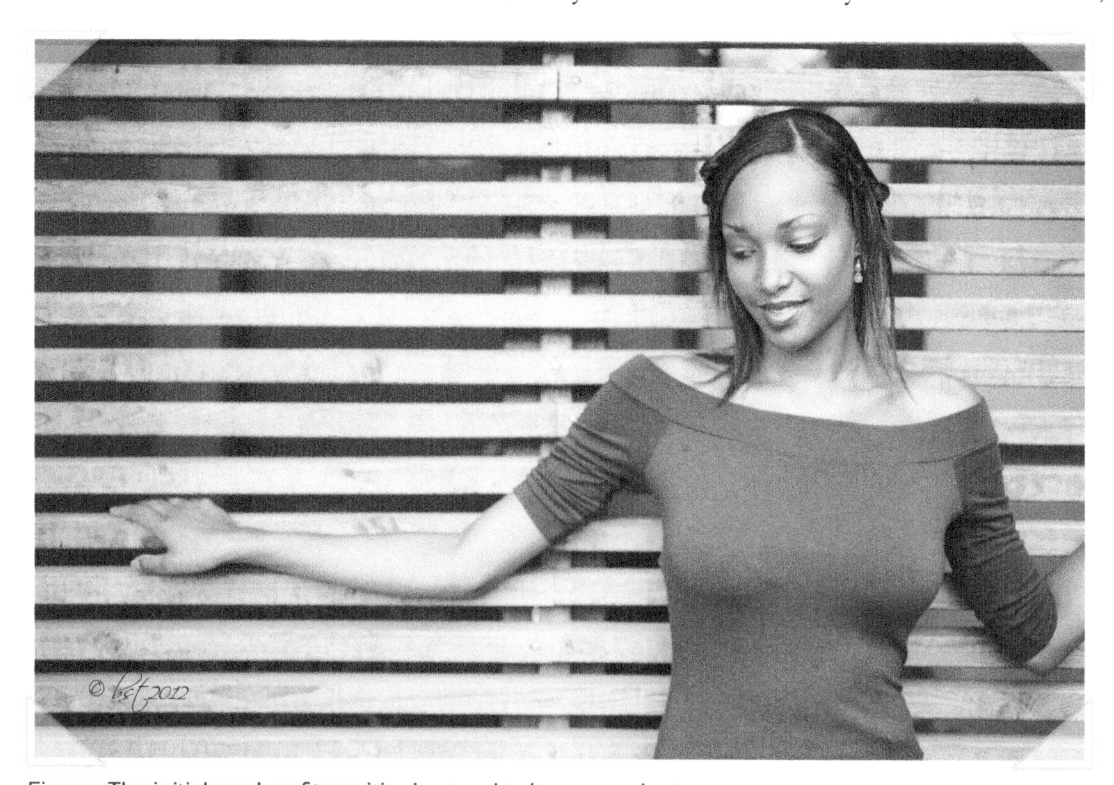

Fig 5.0: The initial weeks of transitioning tend to be our easiest.

Ugly Baby Syndrome

One issue that transitioners may experience during their journey is the old classic: "Ugly Baby Syndrome." When a baby is born, it's a precious miracle, no doubt! But during those first few weeks of life as infants, we're wrinkly, we're scaly and some of us have a face only a mother could love. Our natural new growth faces the same dilemma: It's often judged before it has a chance to grow and show its potential!

For many of us with kinks and coils, that first few centimeters of hair feels strange. Compared to the relaxed hair we are familiar with, our new growth feels incredibly dry, scratchy and rough to the touch. It's this feeling that drives many of us quickly back into the arms of our relaxer on schedule every few weeks or brings an otherwise perfectly smooth transition to a screeching halt. When we try to imagine a full head of this dry, compacted hair, it's no wonder the natural life seems like something hardly worth pursuing. Again, we've judged the baby before we've had time to take her home, feed her, nurture her and love her. Those first few centimeters that are trapped under your relaxed strands are hardly an indicator of what your natural hair is, can do or eventually will be! In the earliest transitional days, we have to, in some ways, *walk by faith and not by sight*. We have to learn to see beyond what is familiar and what is there in front of us.

throw out all relaxer-related items immediately. This may not be a problem for those who have their hair professionally relaxed, but for those of you who do your own relaxers—you've got to get anything that can be a crutch out of the house. Now!

This means no kits, no extra gloves around the house and no other remnants of the life you are leaving behind. Let it go. If it helps, only use hair products from companies that do not also make relaxers. Even seeing the relaxer's name on a shampoo bottle under the cabinet can trigger memories and urges!

Invest in some great moisturizing hair-care lines—there are tons of them out there.

Start with a Good Trim

At the start of a transitioning journey, many people find that a deep trim really jump starts things. A trim is a great way to remove old, bad ends and start off fresh. Trimming also comes in handy as you get into the later stages of your transition. Your hair will grow increasingly tangle-prone as you move through your transition. Uneven ends that are allowed to linger will only lead to a tangling nightmare later on in the transition. A fresh cut will not only give you a fresh start, it will also gently usher you toward the idea of eventually parting completely with the old relaxed hair.

Keep Heat Use to a Minimum

You'll see this action item in each stage of the transitioning journey, because it's just so tempting to fall back on heated styling tools when we are faced with hair that will just not blend in or lie down! The more time that has passed since the last relaxing, the more tempting it becomes to use heat to blend the natural and relaxed hair textures. In fact, many people think that cutting back on the frequency of relaxer use means that they can now use heat more often to style their hair. This is not the case!

Transitioning hair usually requires more heat to keep and maintain styles than hair that has been freshly relaxed. And of course, regularly using this level of heat eventually disrupts the hair's protein structure and curl pattern. Also, since new growth is so close to the scalp, any perspiration at the scalp level will lead to reversion of heat-straightened hair. This can result in the new growth needing to be flatironed on a daily or weekly basis just to keep up with a style. Unfortunately, a routine like this simply trades one detrimental styling aid for another. For more on safer ways to use heat, make your way to *Chapter 10: Supernatural Maintenance Tips & Strategies, page 156 "On Using Heat."*

Let Moisture Work for You.

Hair is most fragile when wet, but the moisture in our hair works as a buffer against heat damage by slowing the rate and distribution of heating. Hair that is adequately moisturized will heat more evenly and safely than dry, brittle hair which heats rapidly. Rapid, uncontrolled heating easily deteriorates the hair fiber. Blow dry your hair on the warmest setting while the hair is dampest, and reduce the blow drying's heat and speed as your hair begins to dry. You want to do the blow drying when your hair's moisture content is the highest, and then adjust the heat downward as the moisture leaves your hair. *Using warm, not hot air, is key.* It'll take longer to dry, but you'll have dry hair that is also quite hydrated in the end.

Seek the Company of Others

You do not have to endure the ups and downs of transitioning alone. Increase your chances of success by finding a strong and motivated transitioning buddy to hold you accountable. Be sure that they are as strongly committed as you are—or even better, more strongly than you are! In life, a stronger person will always influence a person who isn't as strong. The stronger draws the weaker. If your buddy is strong in the wrong direction, you may run into some problems, and it will be difficult to stay the course.

Styling in Weeks 0–8

In the first couple of months of transitioning, detangling and styling will be fairly simple. There is very little new growth to contend with, so there is very little resistance to detangling. During the earliest weeks, you can easily wear the styles you typically wear with your relaxed hair. Smoothed and even straight styles still look great, and roller sets and buns will provide you great protection as you grow out your hair.

Rocking Smooth Styles

A satin hair scarf is a powerful styling tool, particularly during a transition. When applied to damp, moisturized hair, the scarf has the potential to smooth and flatten new growth in just a few minutes. The tighter the scarf is tied and the longer you keep it tied to set the hair, the smoother and flatter the end result will be. At most, a satin scarf needs ten minutes to really set and lay down the hair. Using light styling gels, butters and moisturizing pomades after misting will add shine and control to the smoothed look.

Buns and ponytails work best at the start of a transition, but caution should be exercised as the transition progresses. Slicking and smoothing transitioning hair back into a style can lead to breakage along the edges as new growth attempts to grow

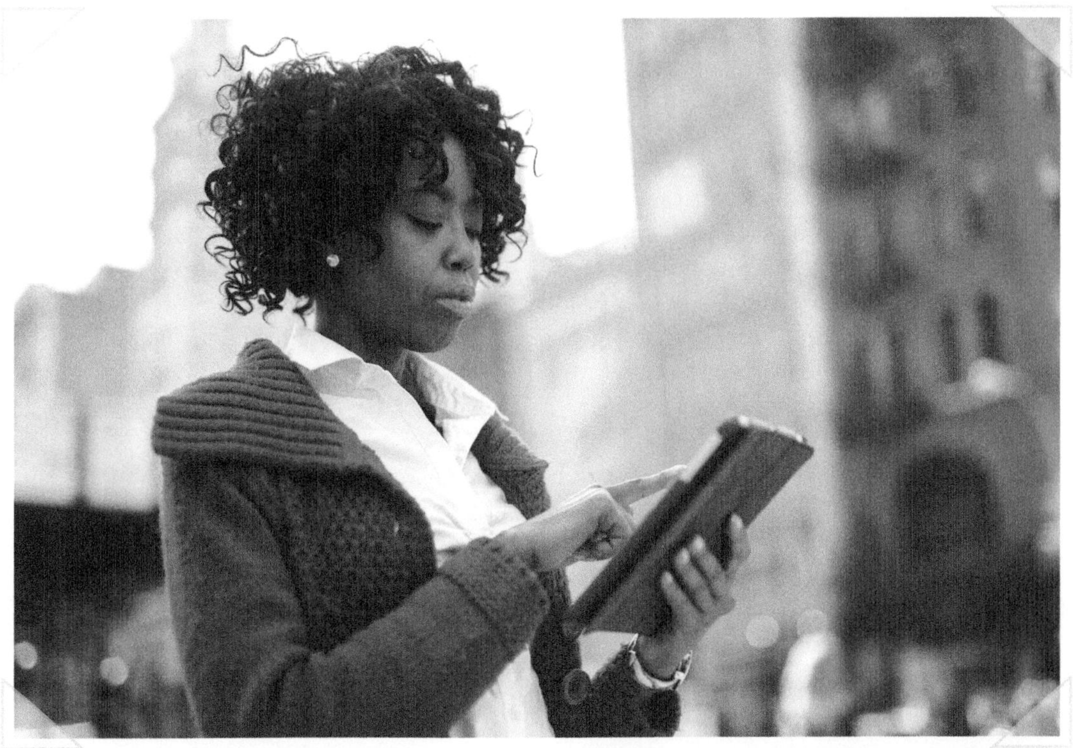

Fig 5.1: There is no shortage of community support within the online natural hair community.

up and out against the pull of the ponytail. Natural hair has its own healthy hair language. (More on this on page 34.) While slicking and smoothing are relatively stress-free for naturally straight and relaxed hair types, it can be stressful to natural-hair types that prefer to grow up rather than down. Trying to work against the nature of natural hair can quickly cause delicate hair edges, where the tension is greatest, to fade. As you get deeper into your transition, your plan should include going the curly route more often than not.

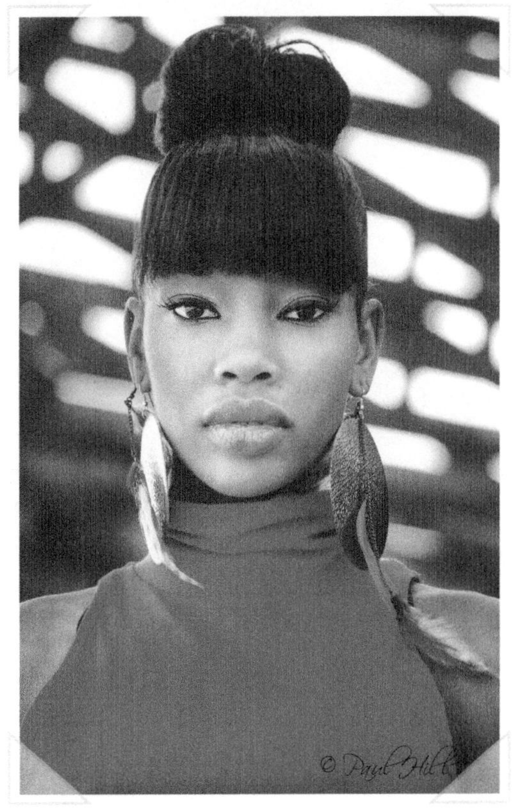

Fig 5.2: With very little new growth present, smooth styles are still an option at this stage.

5.1 Transitioning: Weeks 8–16

As you approach eight to sixteen weeks post-relaxer, your new growth will start to demand some real attention. By now, you will be confronted with the new growth that you'd normally be relaxing at this point. At this stage you probably have one to two inches of natural new growth, and if you haven't turned to braids, wigs or weaves to carry you through, this is the stage

Get Social!

The ability to connect with and follow other transitioners in real time via websites such as www.youtube.com (video) and Instagram or Pinterest (photos) has changed the transitioning game. These online communities are also great resources for learning about new products and techniques to manage your hair during this time. They are also good spots to find a transitioning buddy if you do not have one available to you in your own circle. For styles and techniques, a good video always beats a book!

If you expand your support network by venturing online, here are some good tips to keep in mind:

- Always use discretion when following techniques learned online. Do your research.
- Don't allow yourself to become overwhelmed by the vast amount of conflicting information out there.
- Listen to your own hair, and select a few people who have similar hair types, textures and goals to follow for inspiration.

Now, the last point is very important. It's great to be inspired, but you'll find the most practical information from transitioners who share some special quirks and peculiarities of your hair type. It will save you a lot of heartache and money later!

at which people around you are starting to take notice of your transition.

At this time, you'll need to start addressing your new growth and relaxed length as separate entities for the purposes of your detangling and conditioning efforts.

What To Expect

During weeks 8 to 16, you will need to step up your deep-conditioning efforts. Your cleansing and conditioning schedule will gain more importance because it will become harder and harder to style your hair while it's dry. The more time that passes after your last relaxer, the more you'll find that the only way to really manipulate your hair during this time is when it's wet—or when it has been dampened first. You'll come to rely on wash days to give you your styling flexibility. During this time in your transition, your relaxed length may also start to look very thin and uneven. This is normal.

Getting Over the Straight-Hair Mindset

While many things are the same whether textured hair is relaxed or natural, there are some differ-

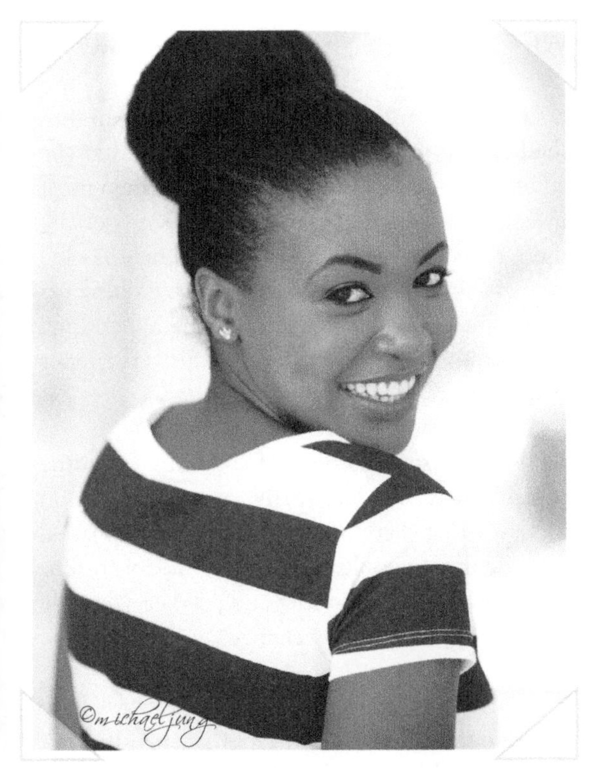

Fig 5.3: Buns and ponytails work best at the very start of a transition, but smoothing them to perfection can put stress on delicate hairlines and edges.

ences between the two versions of your hair that you will need to take into account. Many people have a tough time with transitioning because they still have a straight-hair mindset. One of the major tenets of the straight-hair mindset is that your hair must be smooth, sleek, frizz-free, long and laid down to perfection at all times. Natural hair can be all of those things, too, if you desire—but those traits are not necessarily in naturally kinky, curly, coily hair's character, nor are they in its best interest. Many times, these traits are not achieved without producing some kind of damage in the process. In your natural journey, you'll have to learn how to accept some texture, a bit of frizz, some height, some length shrinkage and some spontaneity.

Another one of the tenets of the straight-haired mindset is the need for daily combing and/or brushing. It has been ingrained in us, for as long as many of us can remember, to comb our hair each and every day as part of basic grooming. But this is something you will need to rethink as a naturalista!

With relaxed hair, gentle daily dry combing and brushing aren't too much of a problem. You can easily go over your hair with a good quality wide-tooth seamless comb each day and experience very little breakage if your hair is in good shape. Finger combing—or using your fingers to style your relaxed hair—is *somewhat* effective but not ideal because it often doesn't leave relaxed hair looking as smooth as it could be.

Your natural hair is quite different. With natural hair you will need to let go of your desire to comb through your hair each day. Daily combing and brushing are just not ideal for most types of natural hair—especially kinky-curly types. Even the gentlest dry combing and brushing often leaves otherwise healthy and strong natural hairs on the floor or in the comb. Why?

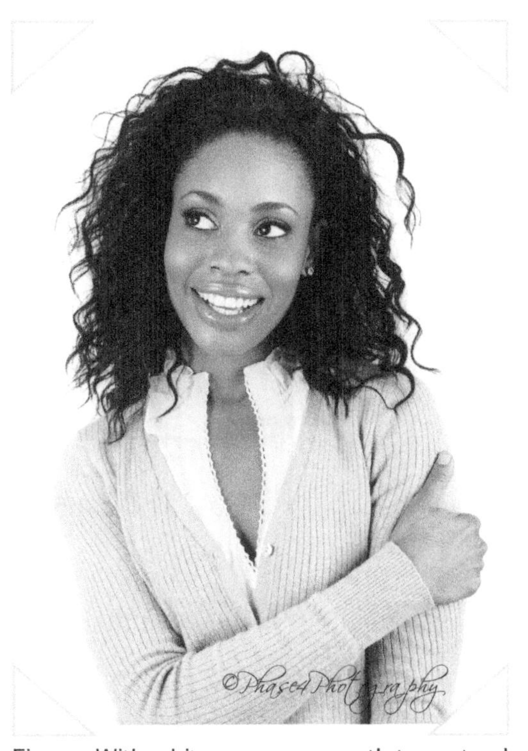

Fig 5.4: With a bit more new growth to contend with, you'll need to be more creative with blending textures in this stage.

Simple. Combing and brushing are about achieving uniform alignment and agreement between neighboring strands of hair. When hair strands naturally run parallel to one another, as straight and loose wavy strands do, achieving alignment is easy with a comb or brush. The act of combing brings these fibers into their natural alignment (or programmed alignment in the case of relaxed strands).

But our transitioning and natural hair strands do not typically align in a parallel manner. The natural sections shrink, coil and clump together unless blown straight. To keep natural and transitioning tresses from breaking, great care must be exercised during the detangling and styling process, and finger styling should be done as much as possible.

So just remember—with textured hair in general (relaxed or natural), keeping combing and brushing manipulation down will always produce a healthier head of hair. It's a matter of mathematics, and the math is simple. The less combing you do, the fewer opportunities you create for breakage to occur. But—and this is a very important but—don't neglect your hair either. Undermanipulation and neglect can create problems during transitioning. Always keep your hair fully detangled to avoid inadvertent matting or the unintentional creation of locs.

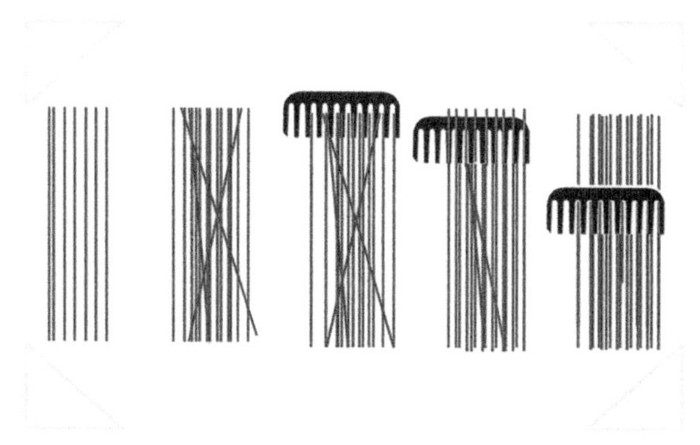

Fig 5.5: Combs are perfect for keeping straight hair aligned properly, it forces kinky-curly hair (which desires nothing more than to shrink, clump and coil) into an alignment that is not naturally ideal.

Why Is My Hair Shedding More Now?

It's not uncommon for transitioners to run into shedding issues just before or sometime after the eight-week-post-relaxer mark—just when most transitioners would normally have been getting their relaxer service. This coincidence has led many to draw the conclusion that stretching relaxers and transitioning actually *cause* shedding. It's a common misconception, and just a reminder that *correlation does not equal causation*.

So what causes this bout of shedding for some transitioners? No one really knows. One good theory is that shedding tends to occur in phases; because most people relax following six-to-ten-week cycles, the shedding and relaxer schedule may simply coincide by chance.

No one likes to lose hair to shedding, but we have to come to terms with the fact that shedding is a natural, healthy and necessary body process. Because it's natural and necessary, it's not something that can be "fixed" or "treated" by adding harsh chemicals to a hair-care routine. Of all the known causes of shedding, however, cutting relaxers (and other chemical processes) from your hair-care routine has never been named as a trigger!

The best approach to shedding is simply to wait it out. Some shedding is normal, and occasionally we all enter periods of heavy shedding as our hormones fluctuate and the seasons change. Assuming that it's not actually hair breakage (shed hairs will always have a white tip on one end), and there are no medical reasons for the shedding, it will eventually subside.

Your Action Items

You'll Need to Dial Down the Heat

When heat is used to blend hair textures during transitioning, hair breakage, and (even worse) irreversible heat damage can result. Many transitioners make the mistake of using more heat on their hair during a transition to blend their textures. Many transitioners reason that since their natural hair seems so tough and they will be cutting off the bad relaxed ends anyway, it's okay to use more heat. This plan, unfortunately, often backfires.

Although natural new growth is quite strong and is fairly heat resistant, it also often suffers considerably with regular heat straightening. New naturals tend to find this out the hard way. Many of them gleefully cut off their relaxed ends, only to be left with lifeless, stringy sections of new natural hair that won't curl or coil at the ends. This, of course, is pretty devastating to new naturals who may have had plans to rock vibrant kinks and curls after the chop. When your Big Chop already resulted in shorter hair than you are used to, losing even more of your hair to damage because you couldn't part with your flatiron during the transition can be difficult. So don't overdo the heat!

Set Up Your Trimming Plan

Since you are postponing the Big Chop with transitioning, you'll need to think about how you plan to do your series of trims to arrive at your final destination. If you trim your hair in line with your hair growth rate, you'll maintain your length throughout the transition. (Keep in mind that natural hair shrinks. You may grow in an inch of natural hair in eight to ten weeks, but cutting that inch from the relaxed ends will make it look shorter.) If you would like to go natural sooner, you can cut at a more aggressive rate.

The commonly suggested time frame for trimming during your transition is about one inch of relaxed hair every six to eight weeks. For those who opt for a longer transition to natural hair, you'll want to trim an inch every three months. For those who'd like a more aggressive rate of transitioning, trimming one inch of your relaxed ends every four to six weeks will get you there.

What I also recommend at this stage is finding a small section of hair that is hidden from view—a section that you will not miss—and go ahead and do a Big Chop on it! (When I personally did this, I used a small section of hair in my nape area. This is very helpful because it allows you to see the real texture of your natural hair and, of course, monitor the growth of your natural hair closely. Remember, relaxed ends make your natural hair look stretched out and lengthier). By keeping a little experimental piece, you can see exactly how your hair responds to products and styling choices—at least in that section. It's a very helpful exercise!

Stay on Top of Moisture & Protein Conditioning

At this stage, you will probably run into your first problems with protein and moisture balancing. Your natural new growth and relaxed ends have very different moisture and protein needs. Relaxed hair needs regular protein conditioning in addition to basic moisturizing conditioning to keep it strong, while your natural hair (your new growth) does not need protein at the same frequent rate. New growth, though, needs constant moisture to keep it elastic and breakage free.

Remember, any time you focus nearly exclusively on moisture, your new growth will love the influx and thrive. But if you keep up the moisture at this high rate and factor in the increased length of time your hair stays damp, eventually your relaxed ends will start to feel weak, extra-stretchy and limp from too much conditioning (think overcooked pasta). If your relaxed length ever begins to feel like this, your hair will need to be strengthened with some protein conditioning in order to prevent breakage. (See page 172 for product suggestions).

When conditioning, you'll need to handle both hair types as two separate entities for best results. If you are bumping up protein, *ensure that only the relaxed length is receiving this treatment*. Your natural hair needs an occasional dose of protein too, but if it receives too much, it will become stiff, dry, tangly and prone to breakage. Be sure to follow your hair's cues to ensure that you are meeting the needs of both hair types.

Consider Preshampooing

If you aren't already doing preshampoo treatments on your hair, now is probably a good time to start. These treatments involve applying an oil or conditioner product to the hair prior to the shampoo stage of the wash regimen. These treatments are great for softening transitioning hair and protecting it throughout the cleansing process. With a preshampoo treatment, you simply:

- Section your hair and apply a lightweight conditioner or oil to each of the sections. Coconut oil is a great oil to use for preshampoo treatments because it both conditions and strengthens the hair. Since water causes the hair to swell, coconut oil is also helpful because it reduces the amount of natural swelling the hair experiences in the presence of water.

- Allow the conditioner or oil to sit on the hair for at least twenty minutes. This softens and detangles the hair, making the cleansing and conditioning process easier later on.

- After you've allowed the preshampoo treatment to sit on the hair, gently detangle each section with your fingers.

- Secure or rebraid sections after detangling to prepare them for cleansing. Cleansing and conditioning your hair in sections is a great way to reduce tangling and breakage.

Get Motivated & Set Clear Goals

Goal setting is an important part of the transitioning process. Write down small, achievable goals, and work toward them one day at a time. Examples of hair goals could be making it to a certain number of weeks without relaxing or learning how to pull off a new style. Cross off each goal as it is completed successfully. Each week post-relaxer is a milestone and a reason for celebration. Visualize your end goal, and continually press toward it. When the transitioning process becomes overwhelming, remind yourself often about your reasons for transitioning to natural hair. Each day will bring new challenges, and some days in the transition will be easier than others. Transitioning may bring out a flood of emotions and in-between moments of excitement and anticipation. It is normal to feel unmotivated, unattractive, discouraged, upset and frustrated as well. When you reach a hair goal, be sure to treat yourself to something nice. You've earned it!

Styling in Weeks 8–16

At this stage of your transition, try to get into the habit of styling your hair in curly styles to match your new growth. This is helpful even early in your transition, when straight styles are still very easy to do. Curly styles prep your mind for shorter hair, and they allow you to better imagine your face framed by texture and curls.

You'll definitely discover that making your straight ends curly is much easier and less damaging to your hair than making your kinky-curly hair straight with a flatiron or blow dryer. The less your relaxed hair and the incoming new growth have to compete with one another texture-wise, the better.

Styles that take advantage of texture such as spiral rod sets, straw sets, braid-outs and twist-outs are the best styling options for transitioning hair.

Beyond ten to twelve weeks post-relaxer, it may be in your best styling interest to place hair in longer-term styles such as braids and weaves to further reduce manipulation. These types of styles give your hair a real break from the day-

Basic PreShampoo Recipes

Preshampoo treatments can be done with one oil or conditioner, or with a mixture of a few products. You can get as creative as your time and schedule allow. Check out these three sample preshampoo recipes from our *Hair Care Rehab* book!

Island Breeze Preshampoo Treatment

Looking for a natural way to boost your hair's moisture levels? Try this simple preshampoo mix before your next wash. It smells great and will help improve moisture levels in your hair.

This Treatment

- Increases moisture levels within the hair.
- Softens hair.
- Improves elasticity.

You'll Need

- 1/2 cup instant conditioner (Suave and VO5 work great, or use your favorite)
- 1/2 can coconut milk (optional)
- 2 tablespoons oil (jojoba or sweet almond oil recommended)
- 2 tablespoons honey

Directions

Combine conditioner, coconut milk, oil and honey, and stir in a microwavable bowl. Warm the mixture in the microwave at ten-second intervals until the treatment reaches the desired warmth.

Thoroughly rinse hair in warm water. Apply concoction to your damp hair in sections. Cover the hair with a plastic cap for twenty to thirty minutes. Rinse, and shampoo the hair as normal.

Avocado Hair Mask

In this recipe, avocados combine with eggs to make a magnificent hair-and-scalp conditioning treatment. Avocado-based treatments are great for hydrating parched hair in the hot summer months.

This Treatment

- Conditions the hair.
- Improves elasticity.
- Hydrates dry, flaky scalps.

You'll Need

- 1 or 2 ripe avocados
- 1 egg yolk
- 1 tablespoon olive oil or almond oil
- 1 tablespoon honey

Directions

Cut the avocado in half, and remove the seed.

Use a spoon to scoop out the avocado pulp and mash it into a creamy paste. Add the egg yolk, honey, and oil, and mix well.

Rinse hair in warm water to lift and remove debris. Section the hair and apply the mask to the lower four inches and the ends of the hair first.

Next, apply the mask higher up the shaft and over the scalp. Cover with a plastic cap for fifteen to twenty minutes. Rinse in cool water.

Cucumber Paradise Conditioning Mask

Cucumbers are packed with water (almost 96 percent) and are an excellent source of vitamins A and C, potassium, sulfur and some B-complex vitamins. Cucumber has been used in the treatment of eczema, psoriasis, and acne because of its soothing properties.

This Treatment

- Conditions the hair.
- Improves elasticity.
- Moisturizes dry, damaged hair.

You'll Need

- 2 peeled cucumbers
- 3 tablespoons honey
- 1 cup aloe vera gel
- 1 tablespoon olive oil or almond oil

Directions

Combine peeled cucumbers, honey, aloe vera gel and oil, and blend into a smooth puree. Apply to the hair for fifteen minutes. Rinse in warm water and proceed to the conditioning stage.

to-day styling challenges of transitioning. Long-term styles are definitely a good rest for your hair, but they don't mean you get to be entirely hands off. Your hair must be treated to moisture and other conditioning treatments, even while protected with weaves or extensions.

5.2 Transitioning: Weeks 16–24

As you may have noticed, your new growth and your relaxed hair have intensified their fight against one another in this stage. Many of your go-to styles are probably not looking as "polished" and "together" as they did earlier in your transition. Between sixteen and twenty-four weeks is a time when you may start questioning whether or not you are capable of continuing your transition—and that's an important question to ask. Many times people assume that natural hair is not for them because their long-term transition has hit some rough spots. But remember, you can't really predict or judge your future experience with your natural hair based on your ability to juggle relaxed and natural hair together!

If your hair is not braided, the people around you are probably starting to notice that something interesting is up with you. They may even begin to comment on your hair if they haven't started already!

What To Expect

During weeks sixteen to twenty-four, you've accumulated a considerable amount of new growth.

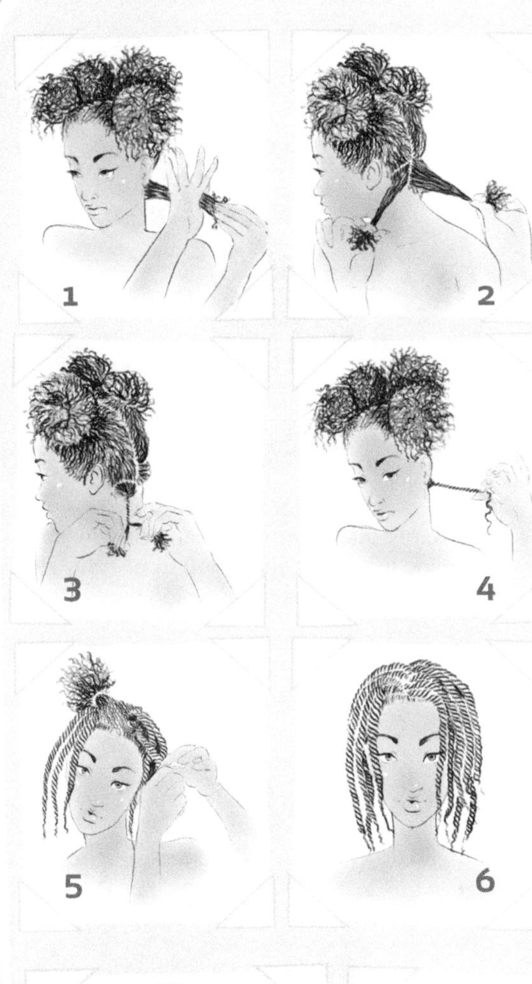

Try It! Twists and Twistout Style

STEP 1. Take a small section of hair, and apply moisturizer/butter along the length.

STEP 2. Divide section of hair in two.

STEP 3. Twist each section over the other.

STEP 4. Twirl the ends.

STEP 5. Continue twisting hair in sections.

STEP 6. Done!

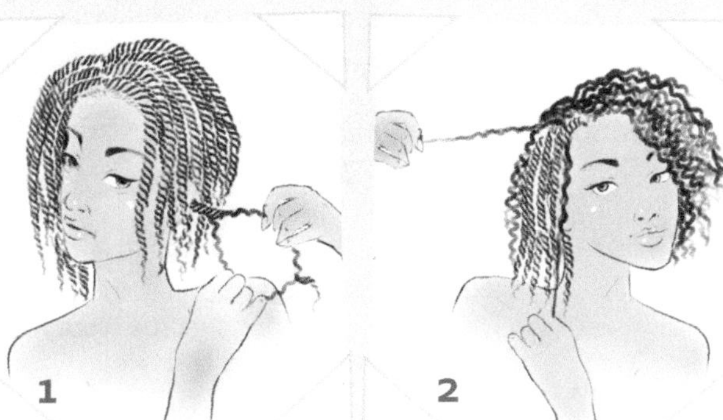

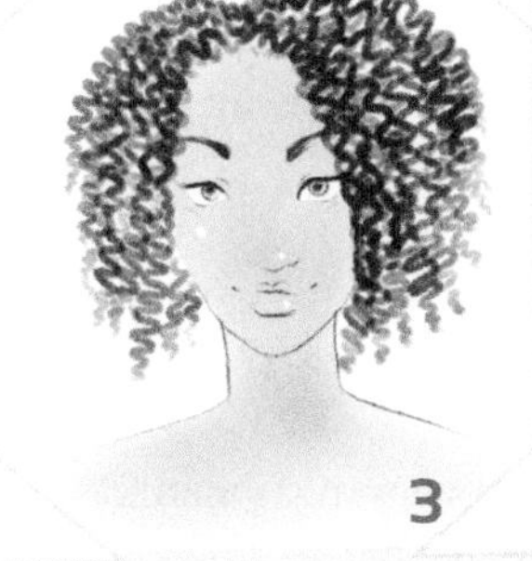

STEP 1 and STEP 2. Unravel twists.

STEP 3. Done!

Ready, Set, Transition!

The best transitioning styles are protective styles such as buns, rod and roller sets, braid-outs, twist-outs, braided styles and sewn-in weaves. Braids, extensions and sewn-in weaves that are carefully done to keep breakage and manipulation low will allow the hair to grow out quickly with little breakage and are great for longer-term transitions.

Headbands are another really helpful tool for transitioners who are heading into the more advanced weeks of a transition. Headbands help to extend the life of most hairstyles you might choose!

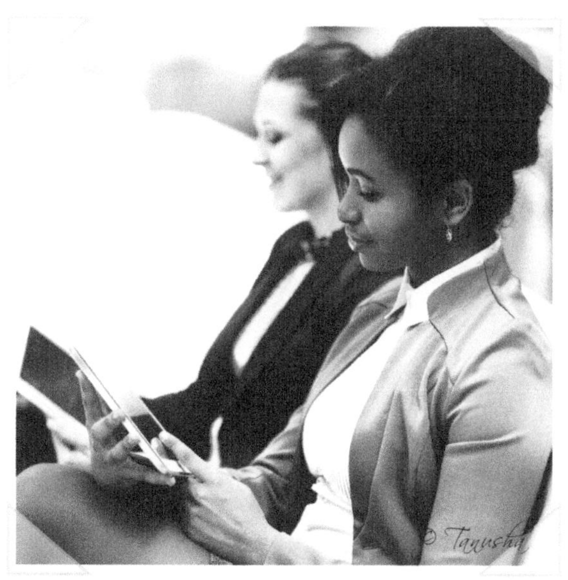

Fig 5.6: At this point in your transition, you are certainly starting to "show"! Your new growth is coming in strong, and trying to blend two textures with straight styles is becoming harder to pull off.

If you have an average hair growth rate of one-half inch per month, you've already grown in two to three inches of new hair. Of course, your three inches may not look like three inches at all due to natural hair's tendency to shrink. For those with slower growth rates, which are not uncommon for many of us, you may have closer to one and one-half to two inches of stretched natural hair at this stage.

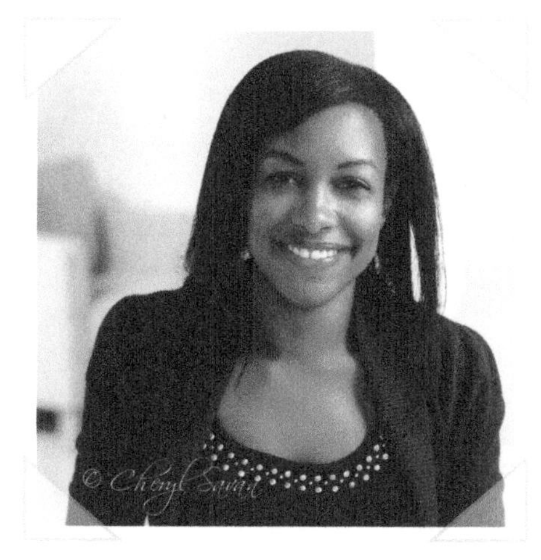

Fig 5.7: As you progress in your transition, your relaxed ends will start to look thinner, although they may be in perfectly good shape. Your natural hair's volume is partly responsible.

Where Is My Hair?

When you've transitioned for several weeks and have considerable new growth present, the ends of your hair will seem thinner and much less healthy than the hair closest to the scalp. You may have started to experience some of this in the previous eight weeks, but for most, this becomes really apparent during this stage. The appearance of thinner ends is especially marked if the hair has been air dried or is naturally fine.

There are a few reasons why your relaxed length is not looking good at the ends, even though it might actually be in good shape. Some of these factors may be working together with others to create your uneven situation.

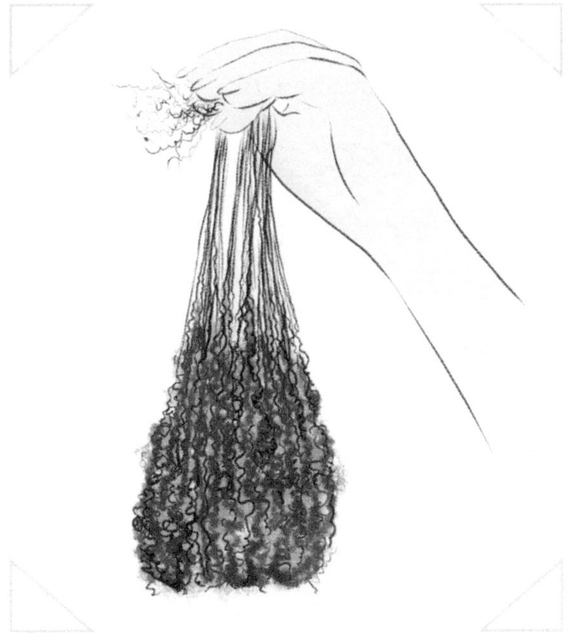

Fig 5.8: Relaxed ends eventually start to appear very thin compared to natural new growth. This is normal.

- **Natural hair is "big" hair.** Even without actual damage to the hair fiber, the ends of relaxed hair appear thin or ratty because the natural hair near the scalp simply has much more volume than the straightened ends at the bottom. The dense network of kinks and coils at the root can draw up tightly and appear much thicker than the straightened ends, even if the amount of hair is the same. Strands of natural hair also tend to be individually thicker than strands of relaxed hair, because the chemical relaxing process attacks and wears down the cuticle. The smoothing stage of the relaxer process also causes strands to stretch out and become thinner—much like pulling on both ends of a rubber band. The longer the transition goes on, the thinner the ends will appear compared to the new growth at the top near the scalp.

- **Differences in hair porosity.** Each hair strand absorbs and retains moisture at a different rate. These strands will stretch when wet and shrink when dry to different lengths, depending upon their own traits and characteristics.

- **Curl variation from strand to strand.** If you are like most people, you have more than one type of curl pattern working on your head. You may have a section that is slightly more kinky than curly or more wavy than curly. You may even have a section that has no defined texture. These varied curl patterns will affect the length of your hair at the ends, even if the straight pieces at the ends are the exact same length. Some curls are simply tighter or looser than the curls immediately around them.

- **Growth rate.** Although our hair strands grow about ½ inch per month, some strands simply grow faster or slower than their neighbors. This may cause your hair to be naturally uneven over time.

- **Spherical shape of the head.** Because our heads are shaped like spheres, our ends will always naturally fall at different points.

- **Possible breakage to the relaxed ends.** This is an inevitable part of any transition. You will experience breakage, even while closely monitoring your protein and moisture levels. Some damage will occur when hairs naturally shed and become entangled in the length of your hair. You have no doubt noticed that it's much easier to maintain a full head of relaxed hair than it is to maintain a head of hair that is equal parts natural and relaxed. One hair type is going to suffer, and it's usually the weaker of the two hair types: the relaxed portion.

Your Action Items

Stay on Top of Moisture & Protein Conditioning

Again, continue monitoring your protein/moisture balance. To keep moisture levels high, try adding conditioner washes (co-washes) in between your regular washings for added moisture.

Uneven-looking hair is common for many transitioners.

Causes

- Spherical shape of the head.
- Differences in hair porosity.
- Curl variation from strand to strand.
- Degree of curl shrinkage.
- Possible breakage to the relaxed ends.

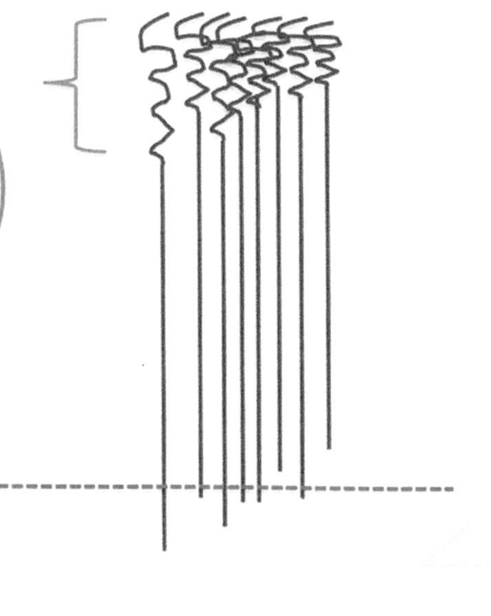

Co-washes are very simple to do. Instead of using your sulfate-free shampoo to cleanse your hair, you'll skip the shampoo and simply use a lightweight conditioner. Your hair will be gently cleansed and conditioned at the same time. Co-washes are quick and will greatly improve your hair's moisture balance until you can get to your regular deep conditionings.

As with most things, too much of a good thing can be bad. Conditioners can build up on the hair over time, especially if your hair has low porosity. You'll want to make sure that you use a shampoo occasionally to deep clean your hair and give it a fresh start. Also remember that conditioner washes cannot take the place of regular deep conditioning. Your hair needs to be regularly deep conditioned to remain breakage-free.

Avoid Perpetual Dampness!

Some transitioners cleanse and condition their hair frequently (i.e., daily or every other day) so that they can manipulate their hair for styling. It is certainly true that transitioning hair is easiest to style and handle when it is damp. However, oftentimes this means spending most days with slightly damp hair that never fully dries. If keeping your hair in a moist state is your strategy for dealing with your strands, you may find that your relaxed ends need more protein than ever to remain breakage-free. Be sure to treat your relaxed ends with the protein they need to stay strong, and continue feeding your new growth the moisture it needs to continue growing in strong as well.

Just Keep Trimming

As we just discussed, your relaxed ends are probably starting to look thinner and more uneven at this time—even with great hair care. This is normal. Stay on top of your gradual trimming schedule by taking off another inch (or more!) of your relaxed length. You'll find that the more even you keep your ends, the less tangling you'll experience on wash day or while styling. The less tangling you have, the less breakage you'll endure.

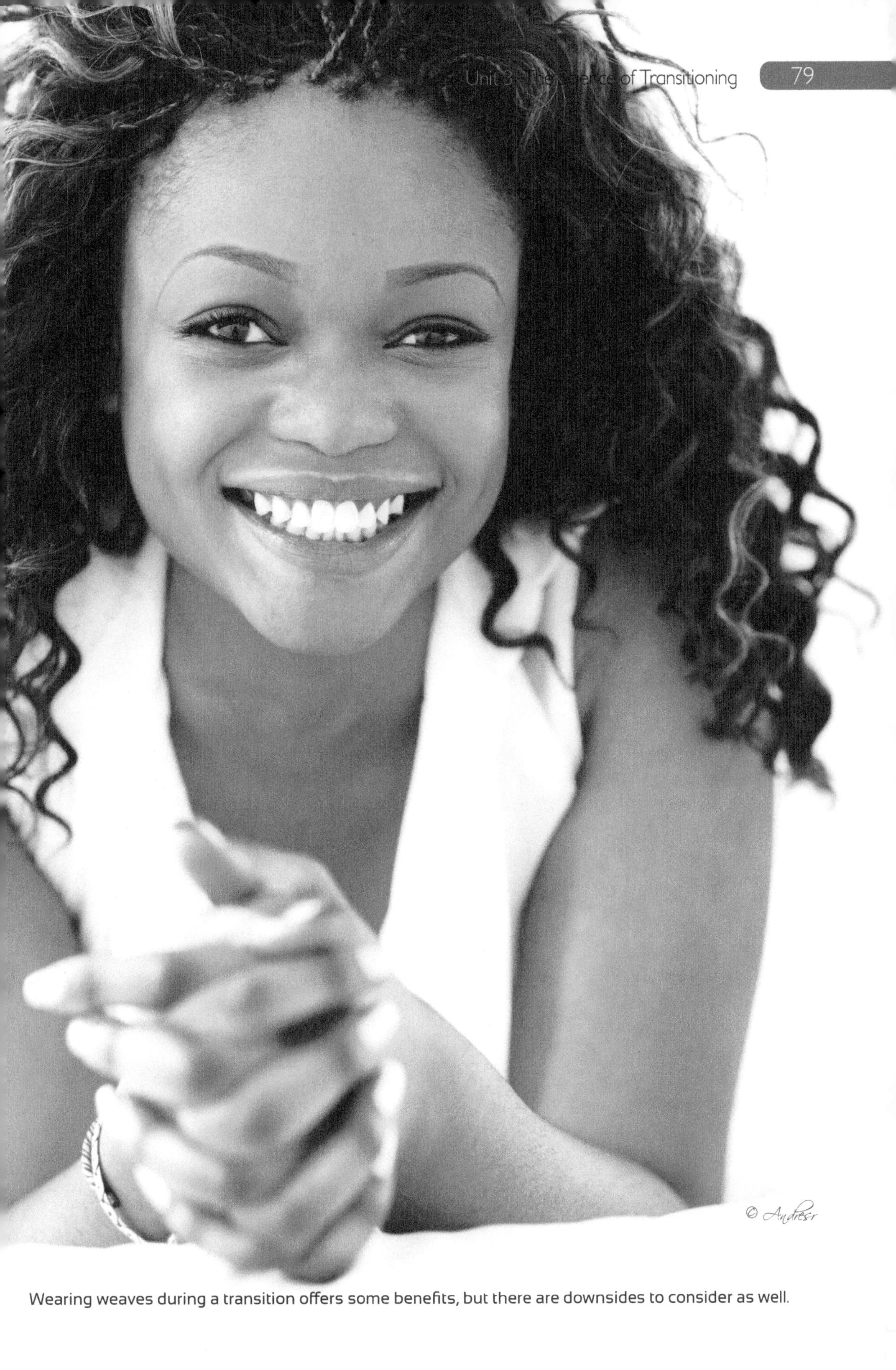

© Andresr

Wearing weaves during a transition offers some benefits, but there are downsides to consider as well.

Styling in Weeks 16–24

At sixteen to twenty-four weeks, your styling challenges will likely start to intensify. Extensions are a very good option for those who have reached this stage of transitioning and plan to continue further. They give your hair a break from the day-to-day styling and manipulation that is required to manage your two hair textures. The more manipulation you perform on your hair, the more tangling and breakage you will experience at this stage in the transitioning process. But there is a catch!

While there are very real benefits to using weaves and extensions on your hair journey, the downside of these styles is that they don't allow you to really work with your hair during a critical point in the learning process: your transition! Working with your hair is just the type of hands-on practical experience you need to survive your first year of being natural—and it's part of the reason why transitioning is so valuable. Transitioning buys you time to learn the ropes. Losing out on this time with your hair may set you up for texture shock when it comes time to do your Big Chop. A vast majority of the *"what do I do with this hair?"* frustration comes from new naturals who sailed through the weeks and months of their transition without having to see, detangle or really style their hair.

If weaves and extensions aren't an option, or if you'd really like to be more with your hair, try braid-outs and twist-outs. (See page 75) If you do not know how to braid or twist flat to the scalp, you can simply do freestanding braids or twists to create the same wavy effect. Add perm rods or rollers to the ends of your braids or twists to secure and curl any straight ends.

You may get to a point where go-to styles like braid-outs and twist-outs don't look good for very long. This is especially true if your new growth and your relaxed ends have a large texture differential. When this happens, spiral rod sets and straw sets (basically curly sets with tighter curls) are also great options for blending the two types of hair during this stage. For those who have the most difficult time blending textures, straw sets are invaluable. As you wear a straw set, it begins to age in a way that mimics kinky-coily natural hair almost perfectly. It's a great style that lasts for weeks and that will help you see yourself as natural even as you transition.

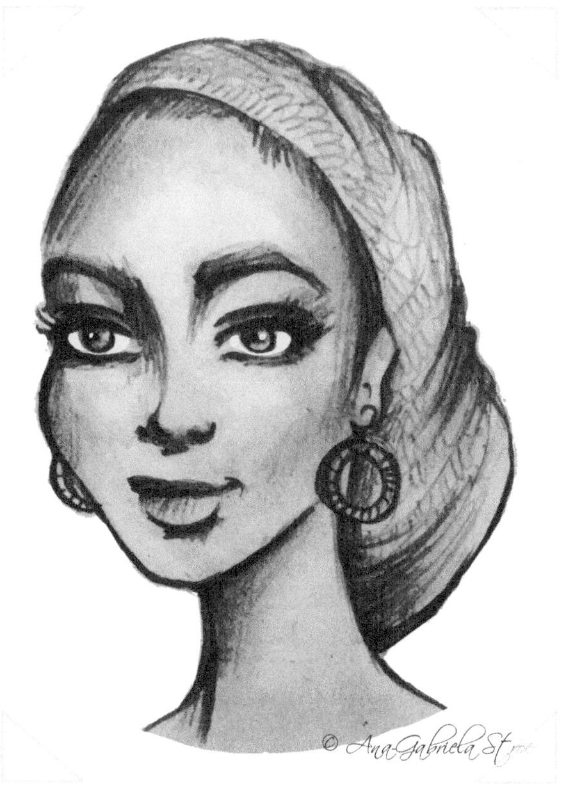

Fig. 5.9: Pinups, headwraps and snoods are other styling options for long-term transitioners who need a quick styling solution.

Remember, depending on your hair type, smoothed styles will only become more difficult to obtain without causing stress and strain to the hair. Those with kinkier, coilier textures will want to reduce the amount of slicked or smoothed styling they incorporate into their regimens at this time. Often, to look good, smoothed and slicked styles require a lot of tension and/or heat, especially at weeks

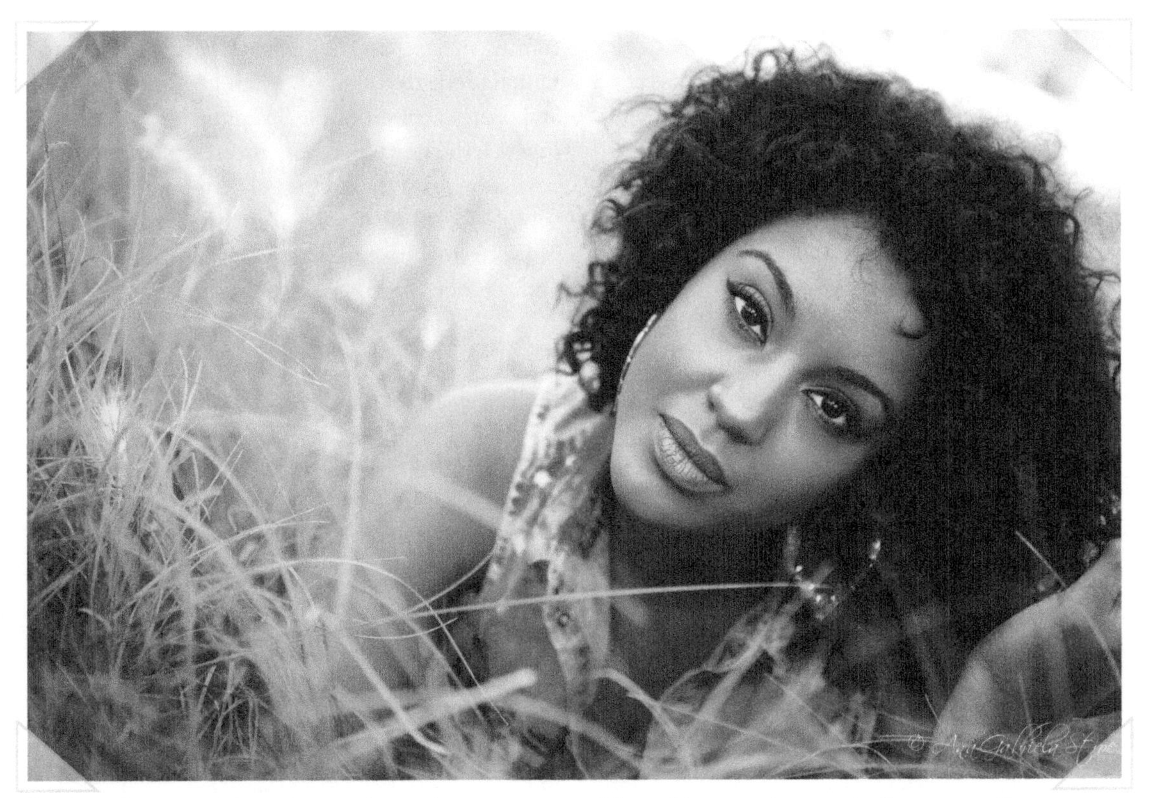

Fig. 5.10: Loose, curly styles are best when you are working with a good amount of new growth.

sixteen to twenty-four of a transition. When there's a large amount of new growth present, the tension needed to pull off the smooth look can undermine the inherently protective nature of the style. Slicking and smoothing just aren't good options, especially if the hair is kept in these types of styles for prolonged periods. Free-form styles that don't place tension on the hair are best.

5.3 Transitioning: 6 Months–1 Year

If you've made it to this point, you've battled through some rough hair terrain, and you are probably working with four to six inches of bona fide natural new growth at your scalp. You may have sections of hair that are entirely natural, either due to some breakage or to your own trimmings along the way.

What To Expect

At this point, count yourself lucky if you aren't facing thinned ends, some intense shedding and possibly breakage. These things are a normal part of letting go even with the very best hair care! You'll really begin to notice these changes if your hair is not in extensions, a weave or another braided style. If you've gone up to a year without a relaxer and you've been trimming on schedule as suggested, your new growth may be gaining length on your relaxed ends at this point. At five to six inches in length, your incoming natural hair is certainly making its presence felt!

Action Items

Keep Trimming

Yes, you've guessed it! At this point, you may want to become a bit more aggressive with your

Fig. 5.11: You've been in it for the long haul! You have considerable new growth and it is quickly assuming its place as your dominant texture.

trimming schedule. You are almost ready to be fully natural and are likely only a few inches of relaxed hair away from your goal.

Stay on Top of Moisture & Protein Conditioning

Again, it's vitally important to monitor your hair's moisture and protein balance. This is absolutely key to fighting breakage during any long-term transition. Keeping the correct balance does tend to get a bit tricky as you make it into the advanced stages of transitioning—but it's still very doable!

Breakage is one of the most common complaints among those who transition for extended periods of time. Most hair breakage during a transition occurs as a result of too much hair manipulation and an imbalance of protein and moisture in the hair. New growth tends to crave moisture conditioning more than the chemically relaxed length, which tends to waver between needing moisture and protein conditioning. Weekly deep conditionings are the key to keeping moisture balanced for both new growth and the relaxed length. Stay on top of—and ahead of—your breakage by keeping your new growth happy with lots of moisture and the occasional dose of protein.

If you are not already conditioner washing, consider adding co- washes between your regular washings for added moisture. These will greatly improve your hair's moisture balance.

As we've stressed in the previous transitioning weeks, heat use should be minimized as much as possible to prevent damage to natural tresses. Using heat to blend natural and relaxed textures during a transition can have a permanent effect on natural hair, causing it to lose its precious curl pattern. You've come way too far to lose all of your new natural hair to breakage now. You probably also noticed, from any previous straightenings that you've done, that your hair does not look all that great straightened anyway. Heat-straightened transitioning hair quickly swells and reverts, making it a waste of your time and efforts!

Styling at 6 Months & Beyond

If your hair is not in a braided or weaved style in this phase of your transition, damp hair styling now will begin to show its true worth. Water softens the texture of natural new growth and allows it to be arranged and smoothed into a style with less breakage.

Rocking curly styles during this time will offer a welcome break from day-to-day styling manipulation and also prepare you to envision yourself with hair that closely frames and hugs your face.

If you are experimenting with braids, twists and sewn-in weaves at this time, be sure to wear these styles for no more than four to six weeks, with two-week break periods between installations. If

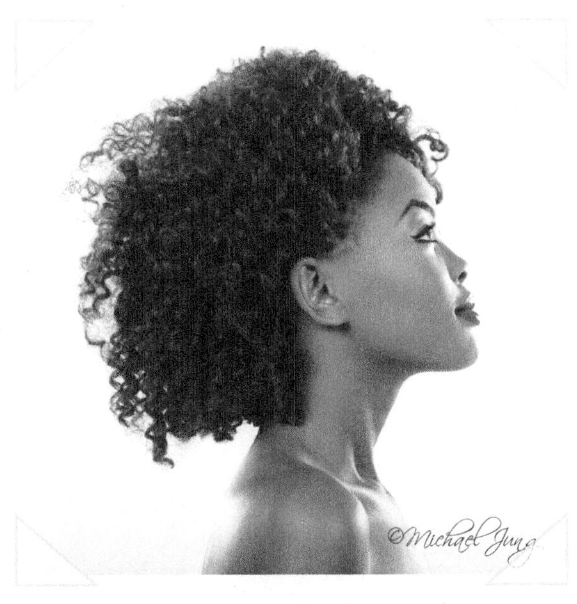

Fig. 5.12: Braids that mimic a natural texture are great for putting you in a natural frame of mind.

your hair is kinky-curly, kinky twists are a great option because they allow you to see what your natural hair's own twists—as opposed to sleeker, Senegalese twists—will look like. Staying on top of your trimming schedule as you alternate in and out of these longer-term styles will ensure that you are fully natural in no time.

5.4 Transitioning: 12 Months & Beyond

If you've reached this point in your journey, many of the practices and techniques from previous months will still apply to you. In Chapter 3, we discussed the fact that while many transitioners see themselves in a long-term transition, many more end up returning to fully natural much sooner than they'd planned. If you recall, many of the transitioners we polled stated that they planned to transition for as long as eighteen months. In practice, most transitioners never quite make it beyond a year (that is, unless they are wearing a longer-term hairstyle such as braids or a sewn-in weave to carry them through the planned transition period). The truth is, most transitioners who wear their hair "out" during their transitions quickly find during the later weeks that a choice to disconnect will have to be made sooner rather than later.

What To Expect

If you've gone a year or more without a relaxer and you've been trimming every six to eight weeks as suggested, your new growth may be longer and more substantial than your relaxed ends at this point. At five to six inches or more in length, your new natural hair is certainly the dominant texture!

Your natural growth is now commanding more attention and is no longer as willing to cooperate with your styling wishes. This incoming new growth is so much stronger than the relaxed length at the ends of your hair that you'll eventually start to see the problems with your relaxed ends really intensify. Relaxed hair and

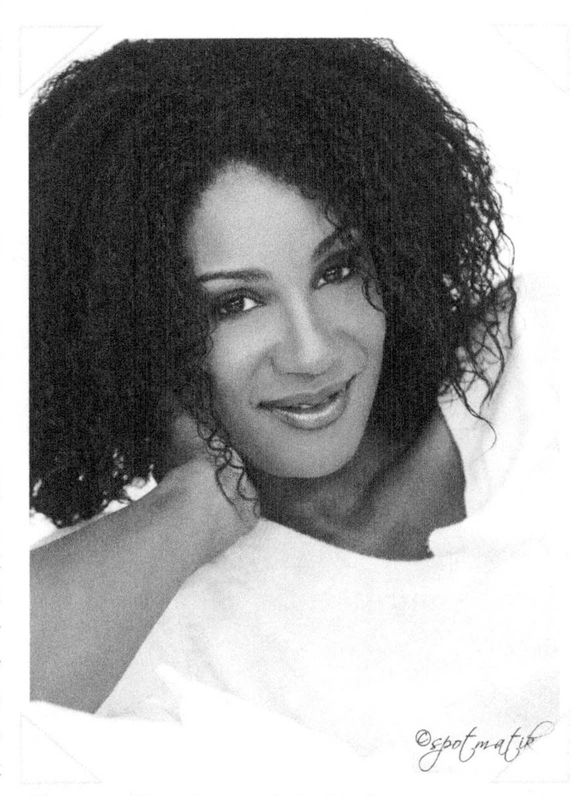

Fig. 5.13: If you've made it this far, you are nearly completely natural!

incoming natural growth are just not compatible, and it's extremely difficult to maintain the two textures together on the same head with success for long periods of time. Since relaxed and natural hair types have differing needs, customizing your hair-care treatments to each hair texture also will become more and more important as you progress through your transition.

Your Action Items

Keep Styling Manipulation Down

More than anything, overmanipulation of the hair during a transition can lead to breakage and excessive tangling. Keep rocking those long-term-wear styles such as braids, protective weaves, simple curly sets or buns to keep down manipulation from combing during your transition.

Keep trimming!

Work toward bringing your transition to a close by continuing to trim your hair at a pace that is comfortable for you.

Do Some Thinking about Your Journey

The Big Chop can be a scary prospect for any transitioner. Take the time to think about your reasons for holding out in transition. Are there hair goals that you are trying to reach, or is it something else that keeps you from bringing your transition to a successful close? What's holding you back from parting with your relaxed ends? If it's just plain fear or anxiety, acknowledge it—and think back to your original reasons for wanting to transition to natural hair. Don't let fear stand in the way of achieving a worthy goal for yourself.

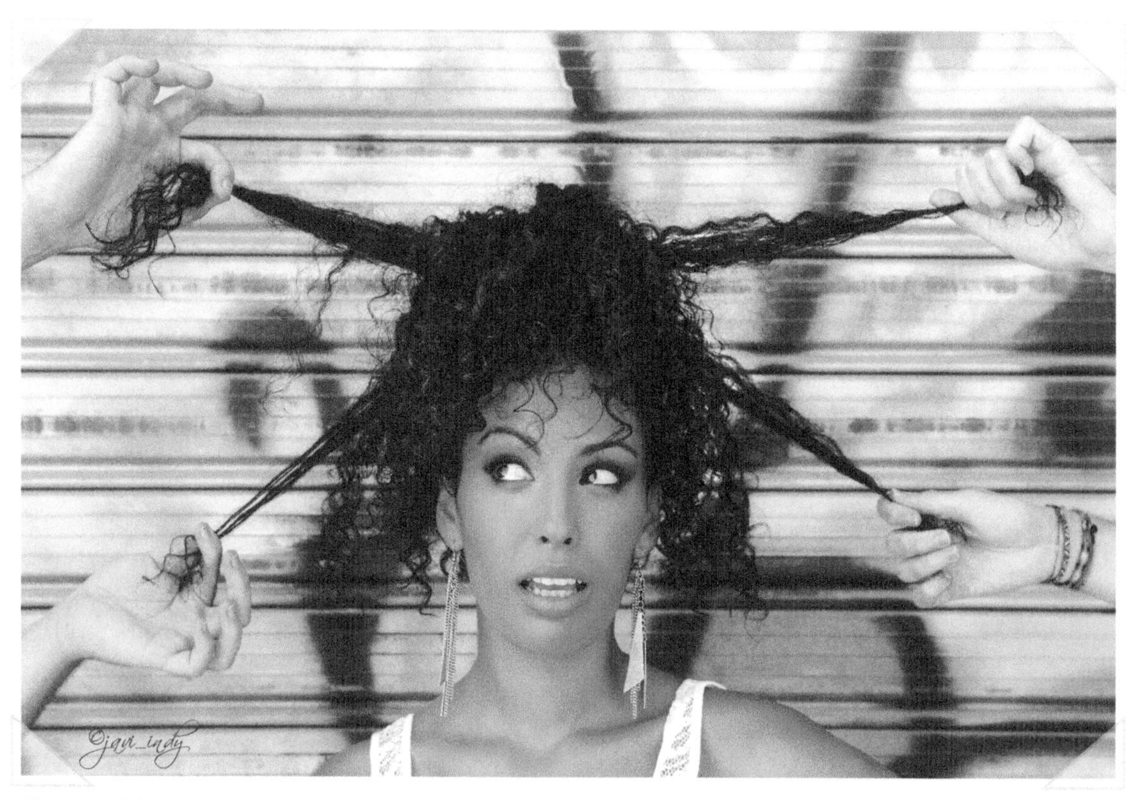

Fig. 5.14: Always take time to consider your reasons for holding out in your transition.

Styling at 12 Months & Beyond

A year into your transition, you can really begin to see where your natural hair ends and your relaxed hair begins. What remains of the relaxed ends at this point is a stringy, uneven mass of hair that is something of a challenge to style and detangle. At this stage, you may start experimenting with "wash-and-go" styles that take advantage of your incoming texture and curl pattern. Since you have considerable new growth at this point, your wash-and-gos probably look very good! If you still have a lot of relaxed ends remaining, you should simply braid, twist or roll up those ends to help them blend better with the rest of your natural hair.

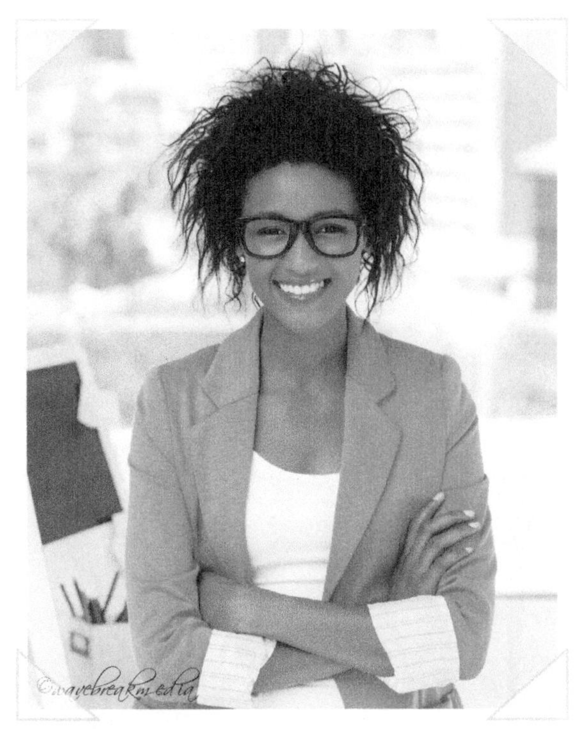

Fig. 5.15: This long-term transitioner has relaxed ends that are ready to go. You can see the outline of her beautiful, thick Afro underneath the relaxed ends. Many of us continue to hold on to thinning relaxed ends for a variety of reasons.

Your Chapter 5 Take-Aways

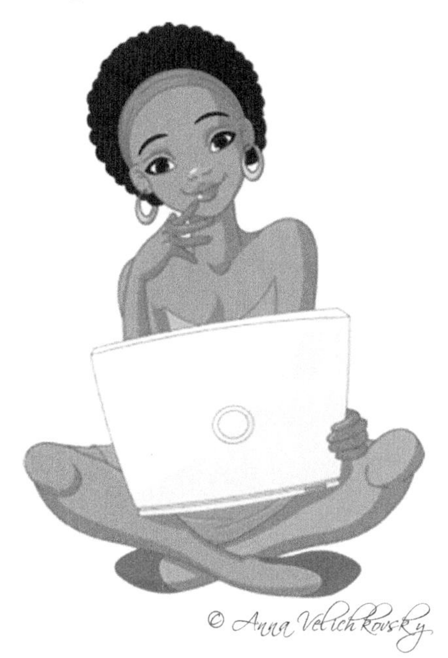

- ✓ Monitor your protein/moisture balance to keep breakage under control. Your new growth thrives with lots of regular moisture, and does not require much protein conditioning. However, your relaxed ends need regular doses of protein with moisture to keep from faltering.
- ✓ Avoid the temptation to dial up the heat during your transition. Styling transitioning hair to match your relaxed texture is hard on the hair. For best results, style your relaxed ends to match your new growth as closely as possible.
- ✓ Trim your relaxed ends on a regular basis to keep your transition moving along.
- ✓ If you are experimenting with braids, twists and sewn-in weaves, be sure to wear these styles for no more than four to six weeks, with two-week break periods between installations.

In the next chapter, we will discuss the ins and outs of caring for transitioning hair. How should your regimen look? Which are the best detangling and trimming methods? Find out in Chapter 6.

Chapter 6: Special Transitioning Topics

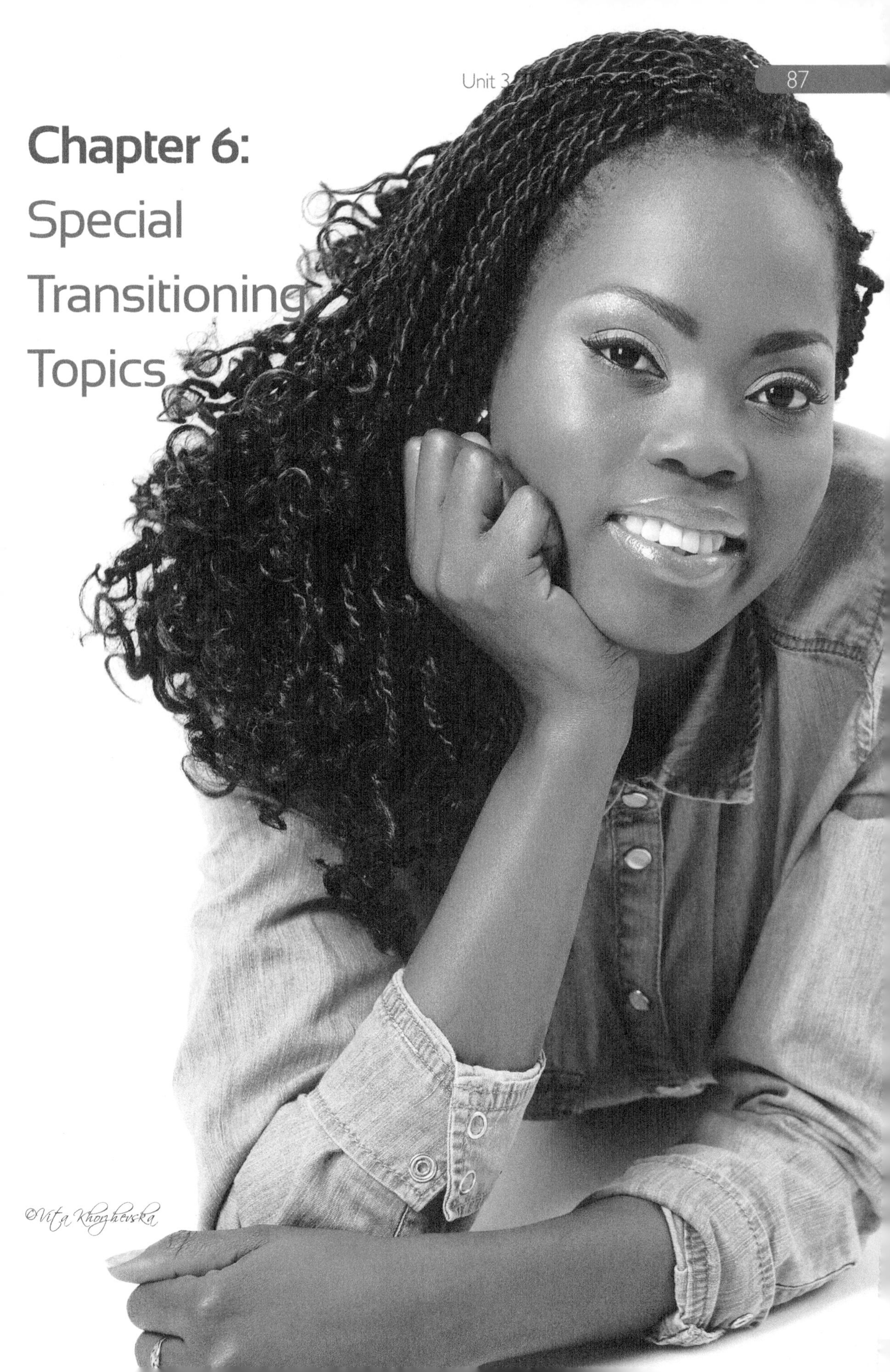

6. Sample Transitioning Regimen

Before we get started, it's important to point out that since there is not just one type of natural hair, there is not just one type of hair-care regimen or technique that works universally for everyone. What you'll need to do is borrow different strategies and techniques from other successful regimens to customize one of your very own that works for your hair's needs.

No matter what type of hair you have, all hair needs some basic things: moisture, protein and a low-manipulation, low-heat environment. How much moisture and protein your hair needs—and how much manipulation and heat use your hair can tolerate—will all depend on the unique characteristics of your hair. Individual variation is the thing that makes hair care both fun and frustrating. Experimentation is required! You have to fumble and fail a bit to know exactly what is going to work for you. Always listen to what your hair is telling you. Remember, this is your journey, and you are in the driver's seat. Tweaks and adjustments are 100-percent encouraged.

A basic healthy hair-care regimen will have both moisture weeks and protein weeks. Moisture weeks should occur about two to three weeks out of the month, with one or two weeks set aside for protein conditioning. A simple schedule would look something like the sample calendar below:

In the sample regimen, deep conditionings are done weekly and are scheduled on Saturdays. After every two moisture weeks, there's a protein week to follow. During the protein week, you will simply add in a protein conditioner or reconstructor of your choice, and then follow it with a moisturizing conditioner. You will use a moisturizing conditioner every single week.

Remember, the regimens and techniques provided here are just simple guidelines and should not override what your hair is telling you to do—or what you know works very well for you. For example, if your calendar is saying that it is your protein week and your hair is feeling very, very dry, that's a definite sign that your hair needs more moisture, not more protein. Individual tweaks may very well make a recommended regimen work better for you!

Monday	Tuesday	Wednesday	Thursday	Friday	Saturday	Sunday
Week 1 Moisture	→	→	→	→	Deep Condition	
Week 2 Moisture	→	→	→	→	Deep Condition	
Week 3 Protein	→	→	→	→	Deep Condition w/ Protein	
Week 4 Moisture	→	→	→	→	Deep Condition	
Week 5 Moisture	→	→	→	→	Deep Condition	
Week 6 Protein	→	→	→	→	Deep Condition w/ Protein	

Moisture Week Regimen

During your moisture weeks, you will focus on providing daily moisture for your hair and doing your moisturizing deep conditioning. Although the sample regimen suggests that you deep condition once per week, you should feel free to cleanse and condition your hair midweek if necessary. You have the freedom to customize the sample to fit your own lifestyle and needs.

Daily Moisturizing Regimen (Morning & Evening)

Apply a water-based moisturizing product to your hair once or twice daily as needed. Follow the moisturizer with an oil to help seal in your moisture and preserve your hair's conditioned state. Focus your moisturizing efforts at the ends of your hair. You may refer back to page 56, Moisturizing and Sealing Techniques for more information. Also see page 167, the "Hair Product Index" at the end of this book for a detailed listing of daily moisture products.

On Wash Day

1. Choose a sulfate-free shampoo from the shampoo list.

2. Divide your hair into four to six sections, and loosely braid or twist those sections to the ends.

3. Keeping the braids intact, thoroughly saturate your hair with warm running water for five minutes to remove any topical debris on the strands and scalp.

4. Apply your moisturizing shampoo, and gently work it into your hair with the pads of your fingers.

5. Rinse the shampoo thoroughly.

6. Apply a moisturizing deep conditioner from the conditioner list.

7. Cover your hair with a plastic cap.

8. Sit under a warm dryer for twenty minutes. If you are short on time, try for at least ten minutes. When it comes to deep conditioning, your under-the-dryer times may vary, depending upon your personal schedule and the condition of your hair. A good rule of thumb is to condition the hair until it begins to soften. Depending on your hair type and condition, this may happen as soon as ten minutes after application of the conditioning product or not until thirty or even forty-five minutes have passed. Using heat will always speed up your conditioning.

9. Rinse out the conditioner with cool water.* Proceed with leave-in conditioner and your preferred styling methods.

Protein Week Regimen

After a few weeks on a moisture regimen, you'll need to get a boost of protein into your regimen. During your protein weeks, you will focus on providing daily moisture for your hair and doing your protein deep conditioning at week's end. You will perform your daily moisture regimen as usual; the only difference is that you will add in the protein conditioner at the end of the week during protein weeks. If at any time during your scheduled protein week your hair feels dry or brittle, **skip the protein week conditioning** and treat your hair to more moisture. Do not resume your protein weeks until your hair's moisture balance is corrected or you begin to feel your hair go limp and almost gummy to the touch when wet.

---

* If your hair has low porosity (see "Your Hair's Porosity," page 47), you may find that rinsing in cool water makes your hair feel hard or takes away from your hair's moisturized feel. If this is your experience, simply skip the cool-water rinse and use tepid water instead.

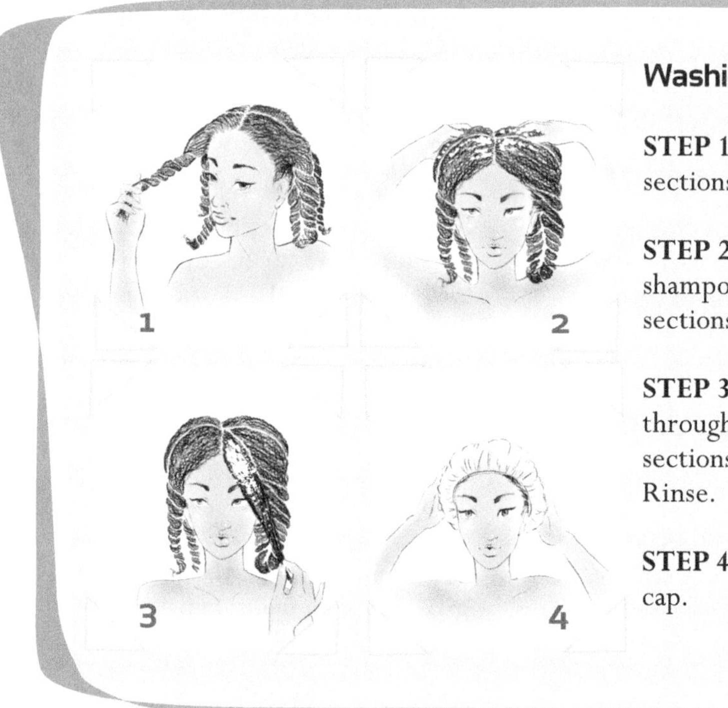

Washing & Conditioning

STEP 1. Separate hair into sections.

STEP 2. Apply and massage shampoo into scalp, keeping sections intact. Rinse.

STEP 3. Work conditioner through the hair in small sections from root to tip. Rinse.

STEP 4. Cover with plastic cap.

Again, you have the freedom to customize the sample regimen to fit your own lifestyle and needs. It's important to understand your hair's protein/moisture balance and adjust your conditioning weeks to suit its needs.

Daily Protein Regimen (Morning & Evening)

You will simply follow your standard moisturizing week process of applying a water-based moisturizing product to your hair once or twice daily as needed. You may also select a protein-rich moisturizer if your hair needs an extra protein-infused moisture boost—but always follow your hair's cues. If your hair ever begins to feel stiff during your protein week, revert back to giving your hair moisture. Continuing down the protein path will only result in unnecessary hair breakage.

On Wash Day

1. Follow Steps 1–5 from the Moisture Week Wash Day Regimen on page 89.
2. Apply a protein-rich conditioner or reconstructor from the conditioner list, and concentrate the product on the ends of your hair and any relaxed length. Follow the directions on the product label, and rinse out.
3. Apply a moisturizing conditioner to restore softness to the hair and aid with detangling.
4. Allow the moisturizing conditioner to remain on the hair for at least ten minutes.
5. Rinse the conditioner with cool water. Proceed with leave-in conditioner and your preferred styling methods.
6. During your Protein Week, continue to follow your daily moisture regimen. Pay attention to how your hair is feeling, especially the relaxed ends, add a protein-based moisturizer or leave-in to your daily routine. As you get deeper into your transition, you may need to increase the frequency of your Protein Weeks.

Customize Hair Care to Each Texture

As your transition progresses and the natural texture becomes dominant, customizing the product regimen to the two types of hair—natural and processed—may become necessary. Each hair type has its unique needs and challenges. For example, natural new growth tolerates frequent hydrating and conditioning better than relaxed hair. Similarly, the regular protein treatments that relaxed hair thrives on may prove to be too much for natural new growth over time. Remaining attentive to your hair's needs as the texture changes is very important for preserving your hair's health.

6.1 Detangling Your Transitioning Hair

Transitioning strands are especially prone to tangling because the strands do not maintain parallel alignment from root to tip (See Figure 5.5). Since our curly/coily strands have the tendency to intertwine with one another and connect with neighboring strands, more combing force is needed to realign these hairs. For these reasons, combing and brushing through transitioning hair (especially dry hair) should be minimized as much as possible. Get in the habit of using your fingers first to do much of your detangling work, then if a deeper detangle is necessary, work your way down with progressively smaller combs.

With textured hair—relaxed, natural or transitioning—using a divide-and-conquer approach to handling the hair is absolutely essential. Separating your hair into four to six sections is easier on the hair and allows for better hair management than tackling the hair as a unit. If things get too difficult during detangling, split those larger sections into smaller, workable sections. (See "Detangling Your Natural Hair," page 134 for an illustrated view.)

Avoid dry detangling whenever possible. The sections you work with should be damp or saturated with either conditioner or oil, especially if you will be using a tool other than your fingers for detangling. Moistening the hair always increases its flexibility, so that it can be manipulated over a greater range of motion without incurring breakage. Dry detangling will always result in more hair on the floor and in your comb. Use your fingers whenever you plan to detangle your hair in its dry state.

Once your new growth starts to become significant, usually at about six to eight weeks post-relaxer, try this method for detangling your hair on wash day:

1. Start with your hair separated into four sections. (Six or more sections may be necessary if your hair is very thick or if you are several months into your transition.)

2. Apply a moisturizer or other conditioning product to the hair to soften it and prepare it for detangling.

3. Use your fingers to carefully remove any large tangles from each section.

4. Follow the finger detangling with a large-tooth seamless comb to detangle. There are two ways that you can safely detangle hair with significant new growth.

    Method 1: You can start from the bottom of the relaxed ends and work all the way back up to the scalp, or

    Method 2: (Recommended) Isolate the new growth and relaxed ends, and treat them as two separate sections. In this method, you would:

    - Start from the bottom of the relaxed ends and work up to your hair's line of demarcation (where the relaxed hair and new growth meet).

- Support the line of demarcation by holding it to prevent unnecessary pulling and tension on this delicate point.
- Continue to support the line of demarcation as you carefully detangle the new growth. Use your comb to gently "tap" into the new growth layers.
- Once the new growth has been loosened and detangled, work back downward through the line of demarcation with your detangling. Be extra gentle here. The relaxed ends should already be detangled and will easily fall into place.

5. Twist the detangled section out of the way, and move on to the next section.

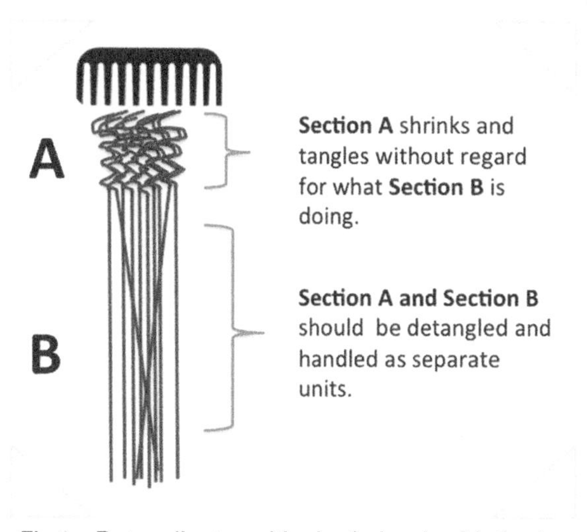

Fig 6.1: Detangling transitioning hair using Method 2.

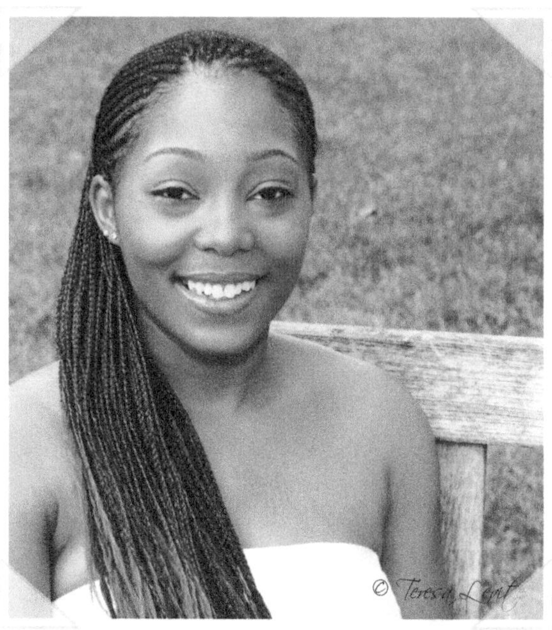

Fig 6.2: Braids and extensions are a great way to give your hair a break during your transition.

6.2 Caring for Braids & Extensions

Braids, extensions and weaves are cornerstones of transitional styling. In fact, nearly 40 percent of the transitioners we polled in our hair survey reported that they have used these styles to make it through their transitions. These are some of the best protective styles because they are extremely low maintenance, require no heat and can be worn for weeks at a time. When you are battling with two textures that want nothing to do with each other, breaking out somebody else's hair can help you forget the drama of your own!

These styles, however, aren't perfect. Weaves and braids are great styling options that give our own hair lengthy breaks from manipulation and styling, but misuse of these styles in a hair-care regimen can result in hair loss, breakage and thinning in affected areas. Braided styles and weaves should be worn for no more than four to six weeks at a time with two-week break periods in between installations.

Tips for Braids, Weaves & Extensions

Take a Good Look at Your Hair

Before you put in the first braid or lay the first track, you must make sure that your hair is in good condition. If your hair is breaking or thinning, you need to treat that condition BEFORE you install your extensions. Remember, damaged hair going into the style is always going to be damaged hair coming out of the style. Literally. Once your hair is in braids or a weave, it's difficult to give it the treatment that it really deserves. Take a few days while your hair is out of your weave, braids or extensions to condition and rebuild your hair first, then move into your protective style. This will save you a lot of heartache when it comes time to take your style down.

If you don't stay on top of your conditioning situation, those four to six weeks without proper treatment will simply manifest as breakage. Add in the natural shedding that will need to take place after your hair has spent weeks in confinement, and you are going to have a lot of lost hair on your hands, no pun intended! Who wants to see their hard work circling down the drain and blanketing the floors? Don't let it happen to you!

Keeping Them Protective

To get the most protection out of the hair-braiding process for sew-ins, cornrows and twisted and braided extensions, follow these steps before arriving at your braider's shop:

- Thoroughly shampoo and deep condition your hair with a gentle, sulfate-free moisturizing shampoo.
- Carefully detangle hair with a large-tooth comb.
- Moisturize the hair with a water-based moisturizer, and seal the hair with a healthy oil of your choice.
- Gently blow out the roots with a blow dryer on the COOL setting. (This will cut down on breakage, since some braiders are hard on the hair and will rake through delicate tresses from root to tip with a rattail comb.)
- Be sure that all tangles have been removed by gently going through your hair with a comb.
- Carefully moisturize and oil the hair again for protection during the braiding process.

Braiders should work with clean, conditioned, moisturized and oil-sealed hair only.

Once seated in the braider's chair, you should always remain involved in the process to avoid leaving the shop with a damaging style that is too tight and works against your healthy hair goals. Make sure, especially, that the braider does not pull the hair too tightly around the edges. The hair on the hairline and edges is very delicate and cannot take high loads of tension for extended periods of time, especially near the line of demarcation.

Support the beginning of each braid or twist initially by placing an index finger at the start of the row or braid while the braider is advancing down the line. As you anchor the braid with your finger, gently introduce a counterforce toward your forehead (in the opposite direction of the braider's progress). Introducing an oppositional tension to counter the braider's tugging motion will reduce braiding tension along the hairline. This counterbalancing method prevents the braider from applying too much braiding tension or force in one direction as she or he collects more hair and moves down the row or braid.

Once your braids are installed, take note of your hair's condition. If you notice any of the following symptoms, your braids are too tight:

- small red or white bumps forming along partings, and at the hairline and edges.
- an extra-shiny look to partings and exposed areas of your scalp.
- white-tipped hairs sticking up from your braid where it starts at the hair line.
- excessively dry, flaking skin along parts, particularly at the frontal hairline.

Braided and twisted styles may loosen over time as the hair begins to grow out, but some strands are simply pulled out from excessive tension placed on the follicle. Unfortunately, this damage cannot be repaired and can mean permanent hair loss in the future.

Fig 6.3: Small microbraids are a great option for surviving a longterm transition, but be sure to monitor your hairline for signs of tension and stress.

Healthier Cornrows

The best types of cornrows for growing black hair are "advanced" cornrows (also known as Ghana cornrows, banana cornrows or step-up cornrows). Advanced cornrows generally start small and incorporate additional pieces of weave hair as the cornrow advances along its line. Because they grow larger only as the line advances, this type of cornrow is less likely to put stress on growing hairlines. The same "too-tight" warning signs apply for all cornrows, braids and weaves.

Keep an Eye on Size
For individual braided extensions (box braids) and twists, make sure that the parted sections are in line with the size of the braid. Do not overload small parted sections with large, heavy braids. The parted section is your base for the braid. Placing a large braid on top of a small section of your real hair will increase your hair's breakage potential as it struggles to support the weight of the braid. For cornrows, a similar principle applies.

Shampooing, Conditioning & Moisturizing Braids & Weaves

Just like hair worn in other protective styles, hair worn in braids and weaves still needs to cleansed and moisturized on a regular basis. To maintain your hair's health and to get the most out of these protective styles, it's very important to keep up your shampooing and conditioning routine (with some adjustments) while your hair is braided or protected with a weave hairstyle. Being completely hands-off is not a good thing! Strive for cleansing every ten days or so, but not less than once per month. Moisturizing should occur on a daily basis.

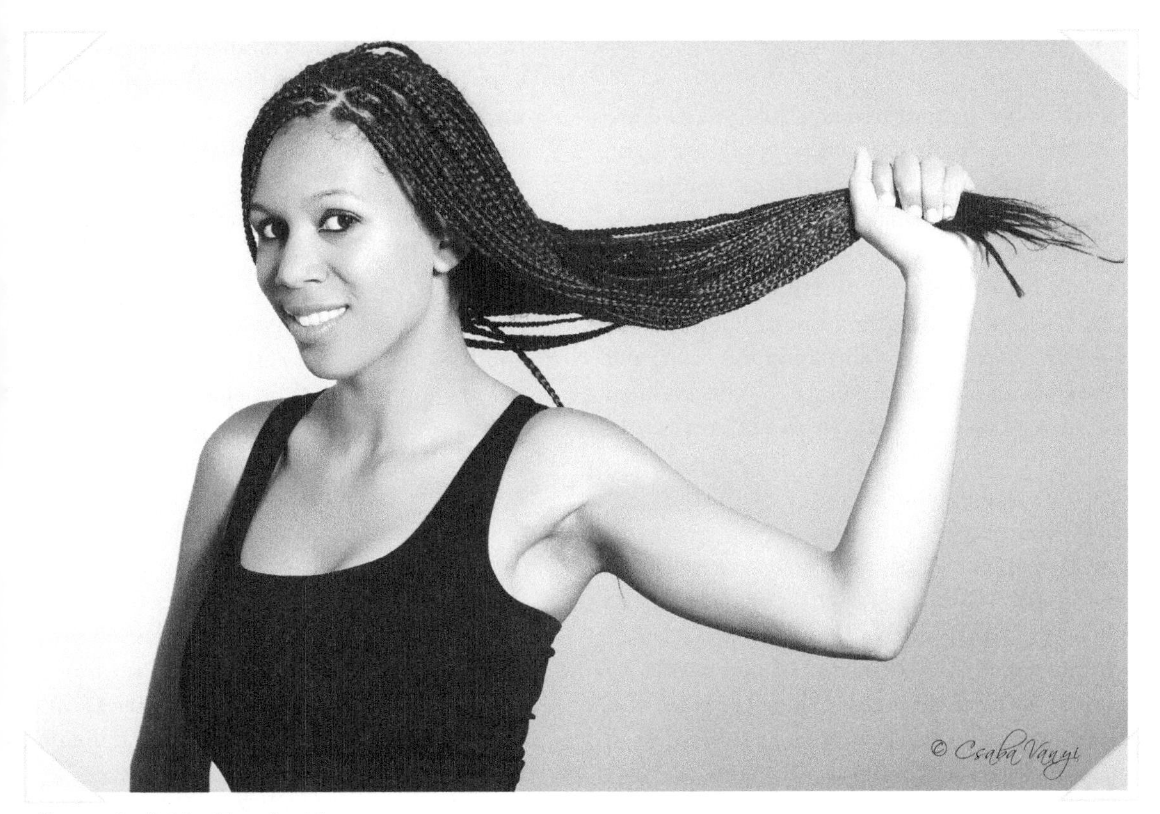

Fig 6.4: Individual box braids.

Tweaking Your Hair Products

When you are transitioning your hair with the help of these confined styles, it is extremely important to remember both the moisture and protein needs of the hair—just as you would if the hair were out and loose. Alternating your products will ensure that your hair gets the treatment it needs from week to week.

Diluting your products will help your moisture-based and protein-based hair products actually get through to your hair. Using a squeeze, spray or applicator bottle is a great way to ensure precise product placement between tracks, along cornrow lines and along the length of braid extensions. Because of their mist and drip action, these tools allow products to reach the hair a lot better than thicker creams and oils. Conditioner, however, is especially likely to build up if it is not diluted properly and rinsed well. To prevent buildup, simply transfer several capfuls of your shampoo or conditioner to squeeze bottles or applicator bottles and add enough water to make a full bottle. Shake up your mixture, and you're done.

For water-based moisturizers, liquid products are best. You can simply use various braid sprays and leave-in conditioning sprays to meet your hair's moisture and protein needs. To save time, energy and product, focus the application of the product on your actual hair near the top portion of the braid—and not along the braided length. Your real hair's ends need conditioning the most, and these ends very likely are going to be concentrated near the first one-third of your extension's length.

To ensure that the moisture stays with your hair, always follow your moisturizing product with a heavier oil or butter. This final seal will keep your braids, twists and other styles moisturized much longer than simply applying a moisturizer and moving on. Moisturizers may be sealed with an oil or butter by smoothing the oil product into the palms of your hands to create a thin film and then gently pressing down on the braids or twists with your hands.

Other Tips

- **Protect it.** A stocking cap placed over extensions at night, especially cornrowed styles, can help prevent frizzing and extend the life of your style.

- **Work your way down.** Always move your fingers downward along the braids and lines when cleansing or moisturizing to avoid roughing the hair.

- **Keep it dry.** Always make sure that you fully dry your hair under wigs, weaves and braids once you have rinsed or washed it. Damp hair is a recipe for odors, mildew and bacterial growth.

- **Expect some shedding.** Our hair sheds around the clock as a natural response to living. When your hair is confined by a braid or weave, the shed hair falls from the scalp but is trapped in the braid and is unable to fall completely. The shed hair must wait until the style is taken down before it is freed. If your hair has not been properly maintained under a weave or braids, it may begin to suffer from extreme breakage and matting when the style is removed because the natural shedding compounds tangling.

- **Lay it to rest.** Remember, our hair needs regular rest periods between braid and weave applications. These rest periods allow us the opportunity to thoroughly examine the condition of our hair and apply the correct moisture and protein treatments to keep it growing without breakage. Rest periods between weaves or braided styles should be two to four weeks in duration, and wear periods for these styles should be no longer than eight to twelve weeks at a stretch. Today's weave hair often looks good and holds up much longer than twelve weeks; nevertheless, after this amount of time in the style, our hair requires attention and basic maintenance to prevent excessive tangling and matting.

6.3 Trimming Transitioning Hair

Trimming transitioning hair can be both intimidating and tricky, but it's a necessary part of any transition to natural hair. Because our transitioning hair is naturally springy, coily and fluffy at the roots, in many ways, trimming transitioning hair can seem like cutting a moving target!

How Often Should Transitioners Trim?

The hardest thing for most transitioners to deal with is the fact that they will have to part with some of their hair. How often you trim your hair depends on your own goals and of course, your fondness for shears! Everyone is different, and there is no one trim schedule that works for everyone and every situation. You have to find what you're comfortable with and try to stick to that plan as best you can. Doing small trims every six to eight weeks will keep your tangling under control, keep your transitioning hair looking its best, and progress you toward your goal of natural hair in good time.

You may also need to add in some maintenance trims if you notice any of the following things starting to happen:

- **Split Ends.** If you're seeing lots of split and damaged-looking ends, these are perhaps the most obvious signs of a problem. Split ends are a big deal, and they must be kept under control if a transitioner is to keep her sanity during the detangling process on wash day! Split ends will always find a way to tangle and catch on neighboring strands. You don't want that!

- **Thin Ends.** You may have uneven, jagged and thin-looking ends. Interestingly, damage isn't the only reason for this! As you move through your journey, your hair will naturally start to look thin—even if your ends are actually in good shape (see page 76). Although your ends may be in impeccable condition, the fact that they are not even makes them very prone to tangling, matting and excessive friction between neighboring strands. Another good reason to trim any ends that look like this, even when they are healthy, is that they may be detracting from the overall beauty and look of your hair. Healthy though they may be, jagged, whisper-thin ends just don't look as good as a full and even hemline.

- **Hair Breakage.** You may also be seeing lots of hair breakage. Sometimes when we hold on to ends for longer than we should, those ends will simply do the honors for us! If you notice an increase in broken strands—or just an increase in tangling in general (usually from those strands getting caught in other strands while trying to fall)—it's time to break out the scissors.

Get the Proper Tools

Before you start trimming your hair, always make sure that you have the right tools in place to get the job done. If you haven't done so already, now is a great time to invest in a good pair of hair shears. (See Figs. 8.3 A and B) These shears should be dedicated hair shears and should never cut anything else in your house—not paper, not threads and definitely not store tags from new clothes! Using these shears to cut anything other than hair will dull the blades quickly. Dull blades do not make even cuts but simply push the hair around within the blades before you cut. This damages the freshly cut ends of your hair, even as you remove old damage!

Trim Wet or Dry?

In general, trims done on textured hair types should be done when the hair is dry and (preferably) in the style that is typically worn. However, when you are trimming transitioning hair, you may occasionally need to break from the traditional advice to trim only when dry—especially when you are doing your Big Chop! Dampening your hair will allow you to properly distinguish between your natural new growth and your relaxed ends when you are trimming.

NOTE: Using heat first to straighten transitioning hair before trimming can negatively impact the long-term health of your hair. Not only does heat straightening shorten the lifespan of your relaxed ends, but it can also put your new growth in jeopardy. Use heat on your transitioning hair with caution.

Basic Trimming

1. Separate your hair into four to six sections.
2. Split your first section in half, and then in half again. This gives each section four mini sections.
3. Gently detangle a mini section, and slide it between your index and middle finger. Smooth your fingers down the length of the hair, and stop about one inch above the place where you would like to trim. Use your sense of touch to guide you. You can generally feel a texture change between the healthier part of the strand and the part that needs to go. It may go from softer to wirier or rattier.
4. Use your fingers to firmly hold the hair in place, and slowly trim just above the problem, working straight across.
5. Repeat this process for all other sections of hair.

(See page 135 on "Trimming Your Natural Hair" for additional information and an illustrated view)

Twist/Braid Method of Trimming

1. Section off one square inch or less of hair .
2. Loosely twist or braid the hair from root to tip.
3. Slide fingers down the length of the twist, and trim areas where hair is thin or ratty.
4. Pin completed twist, and move on to another section.
5. Repeat this process for all other sections of hair.

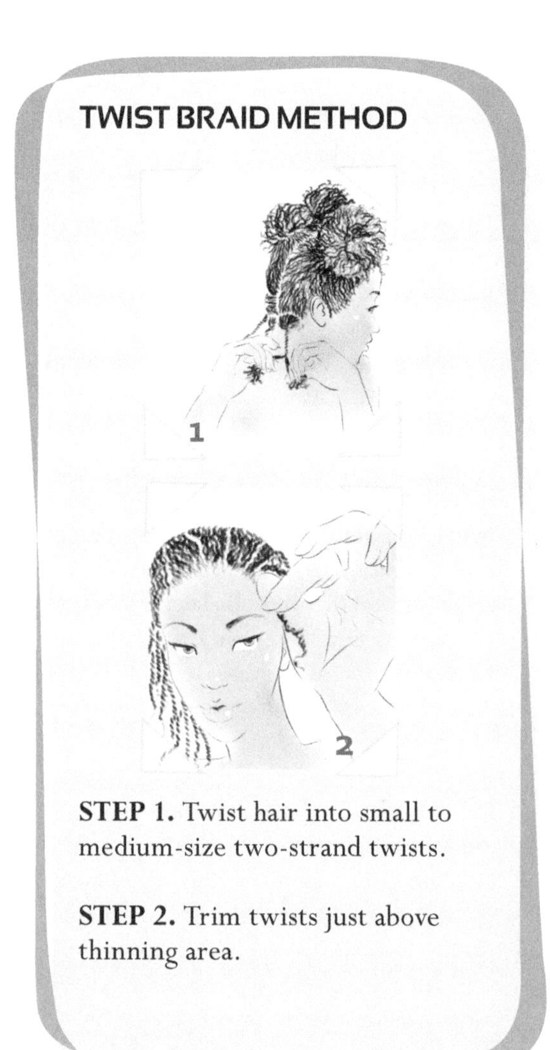

STEP 1. Twist hair into small to medium-size two-strand twists.

STEP 2. Trim twists just above thinning area.

Your Chapter 6 Take-Aways

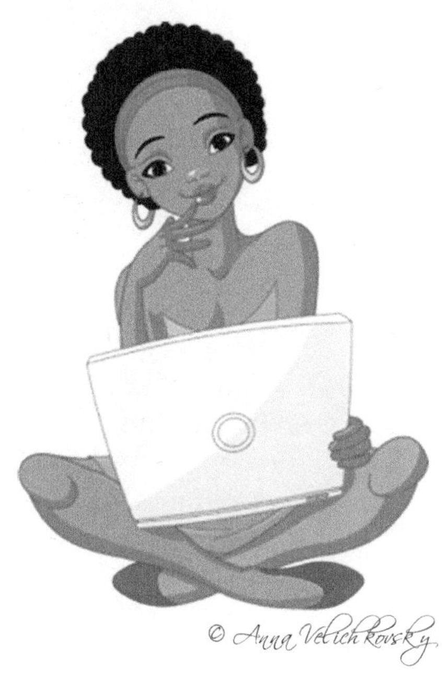

- ✓ There is not one type of natural hair or one type of hair-care regimen or technique that works universally for everyone. You'll need to borrow strategies and techniques from other successful regimens to customize one of your very own that works for your hair's needs.
- ✓ Avoid *dry* detangling whenever possible. The sections you work with should be damp or saturated with either conditioner or oil, especially if you will be using a tool other than your fingers for detangling.
- ✓ Braids, extensions and weaves are some of the best protective styles because they are extremely low maintenance, require no heat and can be worn for weeks at a time.
- ✓ Doing small trims every six to eight weeks will keep your tangling under control, keep your transitioning hair looking its best and progress you toward your goal of natural hair in good time.

In the next chapter, we will dig a little deeper into the mental transition that we briefly touched on in Chapter 3. This chapter will help you understand why the mental transition is so necessary and how you can manage its ups and downs!

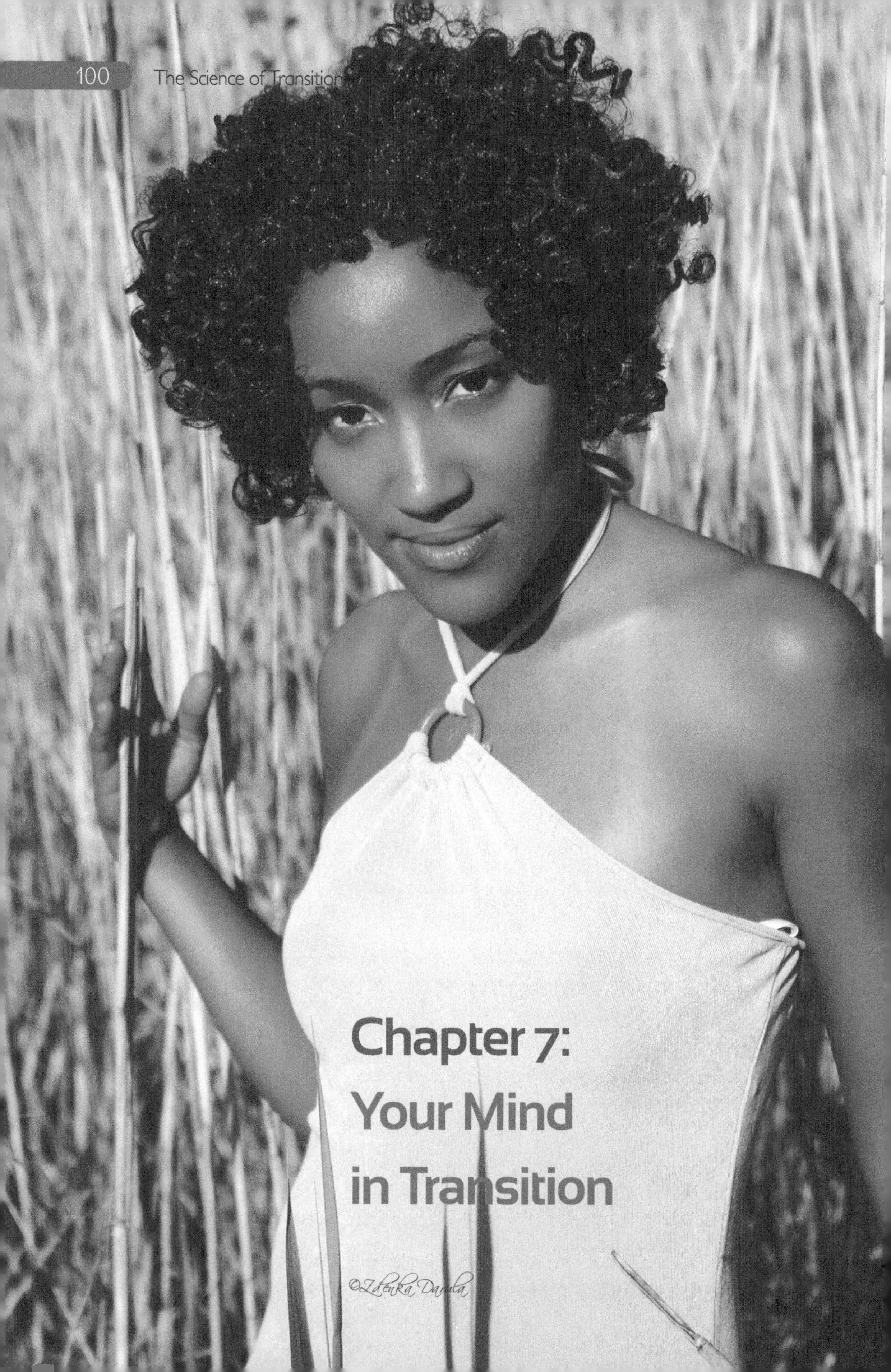

Chapter 7: Your Mind in Transition

Whether your goal is to lose weight, change careers, leave a draining relationship behind or accomplish some other goal, change always begins with the mind. Transitioning is no different. It also requires an alignment between the *mental you* and the *physical you* in order to hold.

The you who is *physically transitioning* will always want to follow the lead of the you who is *mentally transitioning*. When the two transitions are not in lockstep, there is always going to be friction and instability. If you leap forward with physical changes before your mental self is ready, you'll soon find yourself back at square one, freshly relaxed. Time spent in the physical transitioning process is helpful because it buys time for the mental transition to take place. The physical transition gives the mind the necessary time to adapt and get on board with the coming changes. Very often our time in transition shows us that we have some negative thinking to undo. The mental transition is so important that we'll spend quite a bit of time on the topic in this book.

7. The Emotional Rollercoaster

Earlier in this book, we compared transitioning to ending a long-term relationship. Closing a chapter on any relationship is difficult, but it's especially difficult when the relationship is one that the majority of people around you expect you to stay in for better or worse, till death do you part! Although more and more women are choosing to wear their natural hair today, in many places wearing natural hair is still simply not the norm. People may not understand why you want to end a perfectly good relationship to enter into a new and uncertain one.

Needless to say, transitioning can bring up a wide variety of emotions and feelings, and many new naturals ride an emotional rollercoaster. As a person in transition, sometimes you'll feel fierce, and at other times you'll feel like wearing a bag over your head. You might even go from feeling beautiful and invincible one day to feeling ugly and defeated the next. These feelings are completely normal and are a part of the growing process for you on your journey. Don't run from your negative emotions. Be honest with yourself. Confront them. Try to understand where these feelings are coming from. As you begin to get used to your changing hair, the negativity will eventually give way to both creativity and positivity if you keep an open mind. We will look at some challenges that you may encounter during your mental transition and try to understand where some of these challenges come from.

Three Great Tips for Mastering the Mental Game

Here are some tips for making the mental transition:

1. **Know Your Reasons for Making the Transition.**
   We all have different reasons for transitioning. What are yours? Being able to answer this question is critical and will help you stick out your transition, even when times get tough. Is it to reduce your exposure to harmful chemicals? Or to jump on a fashion trend? Are you trying to get in touch with the original you, or are you transitioning out of necessity due to damage from relaxers? A combination? While all reasons are valid, they need to be enough to overpower your desire to relax your hair again.

The reasons that provide the most value and staying power in a transition are the ones that really cause you to dig deep and make changes in yourself and in your attitude. For example, if improving your personal health or setting an example for your daughter are some of your top reasons for transitioning to natural hair, re-relaxing puts you in a more problematic moral position than someone whose reason is just to "try something new." In short, the stakes are higher for you to succeed at transitioning if your reasons really have an impact on you.

Why Am I Doing This?

There are so many reasons for wanting to transition from relaxed to natural hair—all of them equally valid. What are your reasons? Here are some reasons our Science of Black Hair Facebook fans gave!

- Reduce exposure to chemicals.
- To try something new.
- Curiosity.
- It's a challenge.
- It's healthier.
- It's the original me.
- To set an example.
- To prove to myself that it's possible.
- Necessity.
- Just to do it.
- To benefit from better length retention so that I can achieve my longer hair goals.

2. **Know What Relaxers Really Do & Put Them in Perspective.** Remind yourself that relaxers are made up of highly corrosive chemicals that have no place on or near your scalp. And let's be honest: If you are like many women, you've already been burned a time or two. Ask yourself, *Is this the price I'm willing to pay for beauty?*

If straight hair is still an option you'd like to keep on the table, there are safer, healthier alternatives to help you arrive at your straight-hair goals. Using a blow dryer, flatiron, or "wrapping" a roller set are just a few temporary options. But keep in mind that in order to remain in optimal health, naturally kinky, coily and curly hair wants to be left to its natural ways. Going from curly to straight will always introduce stress to the hair—whether the methods are permanent (with relaxers) or temporary (with heat). Temporary methods, of course, are generally less traumatic for the hair.

3. **Make Your Environment Supportive.** If you are someone who frequents salons, look for a salon home that specializes in natural hair or that has a diverse clientele including naturalistas. If patrons of your current salon relax or wear weaves religiously, feeling motivated during your styling session can be difficult. Surrounding yourself with like-haired people will inspire your own styling creativity and get you accustomed to seeing "done" hair that isn't always stick straight, weaved or heat fried. Exposure to the possibilities and potential of natural hair in a salon setting really helps you to develop an appreciation for the versatility of highly textured, kinky-coily hair.

7.1 What To Do When There Is No Support

If you've been a longtime smoker and one day you just tell everyone, *Guys—I'm done with cigarettes. I'm quitting*, you can expect almost unanimous support from family, friends and even strangers. Everyone is happy that you are letting go of such a terrible habit. As human beings, it is natural for us to rally around the ones we love when they turn away from something in their lives that is causing harm. It's just in us to cheer on the ones we love when they make positive changes.

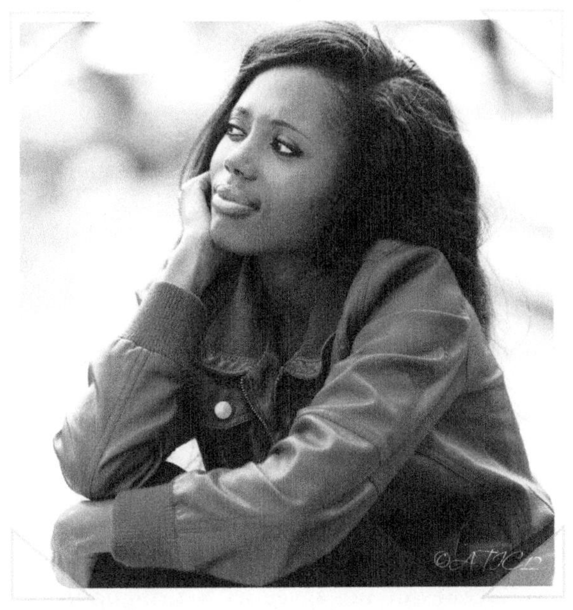

Fig 7.1: While some of you will receive complete support from your circle of friends and family during your transition, many others will face a longer road ahead.

But somehow, the story changes and friends and family members can drop the ball when the threat we are abandoning is the threat of chemical relaxers. Of course, we would never attempt to place chemical relaxing on the same level with smoking as a possible life-or-death issue, but these chemicals do still pose a real hazard to both the hair and skin. Despite the fact that transitioning is very much a step in a healthful direction, it's a possibility that taking this positive step can set you up for unfair scrutiny and even ridicule.

When we choose to go natural, often we are making the difficult choice to leave behind everything we know and start on a new path. Many times, we are on our own—the very first in our immediate circles to go on this journey. The newness of our experience may cause us to feel more vulnerable and sensitive to other people's words and actions than normal. During this time, we may feel like we need more validation and support from the people around us. While many people find the support they need at home during their time of transition, others may find that support surprisingly lacking or completely absent.

While friends, coworkers and peers may be easy to ignore, close friends and family pose a special challenge. Whether your usual support system is outspoken and vocal about their dislike for your change or uncomfortably quiet and neutral about your change, feeling excited about your hair journey can be difficult when your family is not on board with you.

So, what do you do when your support system is unsupportive?

The first thing to keep in mind is that just because certain friends and family are not on board with your decision to go natural does not mean that your goal is not a worthwhile pursuit. The fact that you thought enough to embark on this journey in the first place shows that it is worth something to you. Also, keep in mind that it is normal to face resistance from others, especially if they fear you are doing something worthwhile!

Are They Really Unsupportive?

Lack of support from family and friends is one of the biggest challenges that a new transitioner or new natural will face. Many newbies are surprised to find that the same people who were most supportive of their other life goals do not share the same enthusiasm about their new decision to go natural. Sometimes, however, what

The Science of Black Hair Super Survey

Survey Says! The majority of women we polled in our hair survey (80%) voted that they would continue on with their transition even if a spouse/partner or significant other disapproved.

Natural Support

If you are not getting the support you need, branch out! Attend natural-hair meet-ups in your area, or connect in a big way online!

Going natural is one of those things that really pushes the inner you to shine. The process will, if nothing else, decrease your reliance on others for validation. This is a good thing. Going natural is an amazing opportunity for you to practice being more self-reliant and independent. Going natural is so much more than just switching from one hairstyle to another. The journey can truly become one of personal, inner growth—if you allow it.

we may think of as a real lack of support may not be what it seems.

Sometimes support is as simple as giving someone space, offering a listening ear when they are emotionally full or providing a shoulder to cry on. While outright discouragement and intentionally hurtful words are easily seen as unsupportive, it is also easy to write off such things as silence or someone's apparent lack of interest as unsupportive, too. Although these things can be hurtful, consider that they may not be signs of someone being intentionally unsupportive. Some "unsupportive" friends and family aren't aware that you need them at a time like this, or they may be unsure of how to support you. Sometimes unsupportive comments come from friends and family because they are genuinely concerned about what you'll face as a result of wearing your hair natural and want to "protect" you. Some close friends and family members may just be really bad at expressing themselves. Or maybe they are insecure or unsure of their own beauty and are projecting their fears onto you.

Tell Them How You Really Feel

When you aren't getting the support you need for your transition or life as a new natural, sometimes a heart-to-heart chat with those you love is in order. Let them know how your decision to be natural affects you and is important to you. If something is known to be important to you, then for people who love and are concerned about you, that something will naturally carry more weight with them—even if they do not agree with it. Be up front about the kind of support that you need during your transition, and think very carefully about whether or not particular individuals really have the capacity to give that support. Does your friend or loved one have the time, the right resources, the skills, the experience? For example, your stylist may have been the go-to girl for your relaxed-hair roller sets and other straight styles, but does she have the necessary skills and experience to see a full-scale transition and Big Chop through to the end?

The Truly Unsupportive

Sometimes friends and family can be hard on us. If this is true in your case, you'll have to tread carefully. Take in constructive feedback, and toss out unconstructive feedback. To the extent that you can, remove negative people from your life—or at least limit your contact with them. Many times people who discourage your decision to go natural are simply reflecting their own fears and social conditioning about natural hair and beauty in general. Their fears often can be laid to rest with information and by simply exposing them to natural hair.

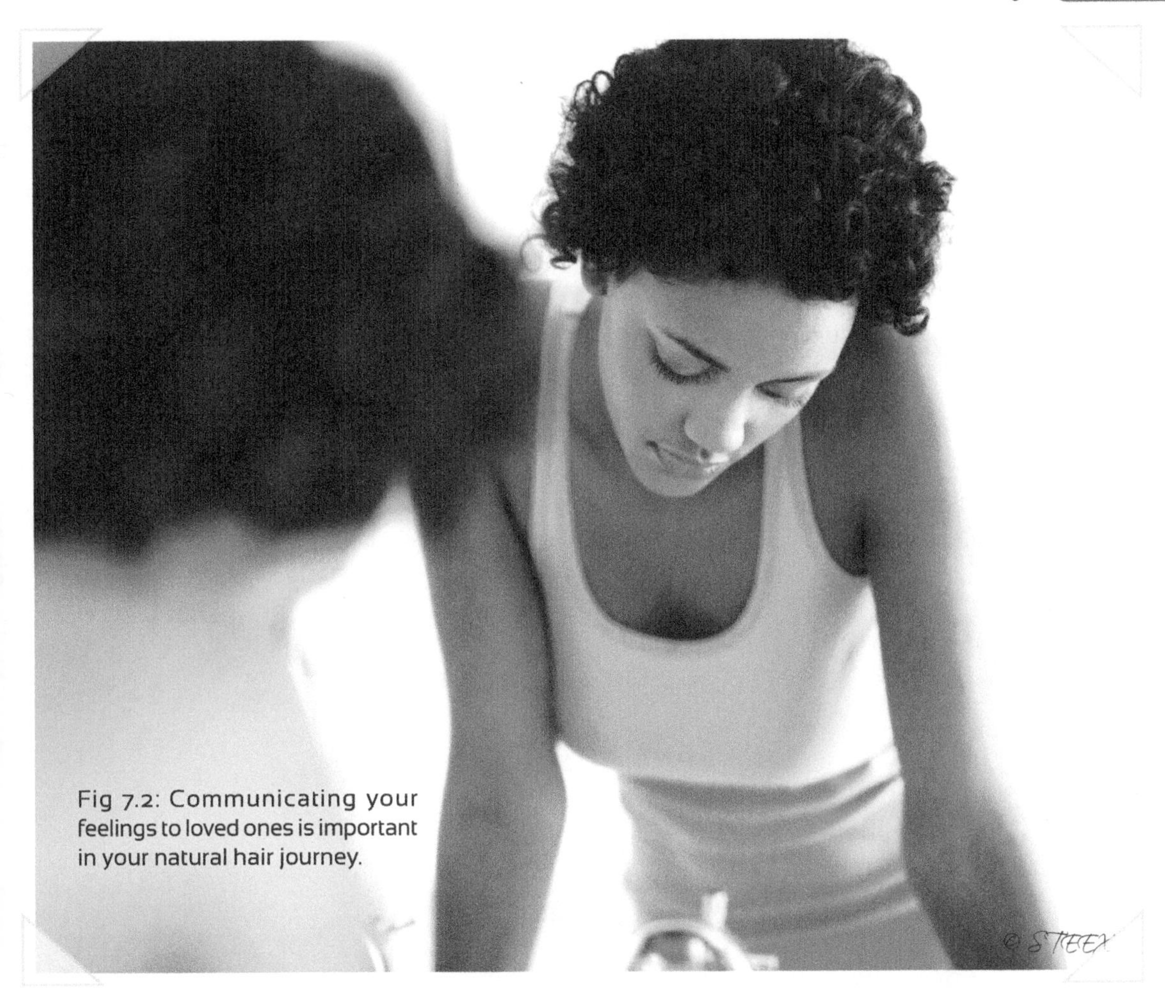

Fig 7.2: Communicating your feelings to loved ones is important in your natural hair journey.

Keep Pushing Ahead Toward Your Goal

Don't lose sight of your goals by trying to calm and cater to everyone else's objections, insecurities and fears. Remember, you do not need anyone's approval to be the best and healthiest you that can be. At times, you may find you need to tune others out to protect your own vulnerable spirit and confidence. Turn the tables by using their lack of support to bolster your determination to succeed. Don't forget that sometimes you may be the light that someone else needs to see in order to take that first step in her own transition. Once they see your transition done, and done well, you may be surprised by how many people will hold up your example as their inspiration.

Finally, remember, while it is ideal (and would be really nice), it may not be possible for every single friend and family member to have your back on this decision right away. Just as it took time for you to fall in love with the idea of wearing your hair in its natural state, it will take those who are closest to you some time, too. Remember your supporters, like you, are people with their own lives, goals, views and ideas. Sometimes when you are dealing with a lack of support, you have to give yourself more of what you wish you could get from others. If you aren't feeling the love and support you need from certain friends and family members, this means you will need to commit to providing that love for yourself.

7.2 Dealing with Other Naturals

The sudden need to be vocal about your hair doesn't always come from those who don't like or have natural hair. Sometimes other new naturals and seasoned veterans who've been natural for years may give you strife over your hair decisions, particularly the speed and manner in which you reclaim your natural hair and how you style it.

Just Cut It Off!

When transitioners complain about tangles and breakage and all of the other things that tend to accompany transitioning, it's easy for some well-intentioned naturals to tell them (often in love but, occasionally, in disgust) to simply "just cut it off!" Now, this advice at face value, is usually quite valid because just cutting it off *will* solve most of the physical problems with tangles and breakage you may get from trying to reconcile two incompatible hair states. But this answer can be insensitive to the process that some transitioners need to go through to ensure that they are able to mentally stay the course. When transitioners chop before they are ready, it may affect their chances of staying the course.

It is important to understand that transitioning is more than just hanging on to hopeless hair. It's more than just straddling the fence in a sea of indecisiveness and cowardice. It's not a sign of weakness, either. For some in-betweeners, it's a smart, strategic decision that will solidify their resolve going forward. For some, it's an honest recognition that, *Hey, I'm still working on my alignment*—or that *I'm really not quite ready for a drastic change . . . yet.*

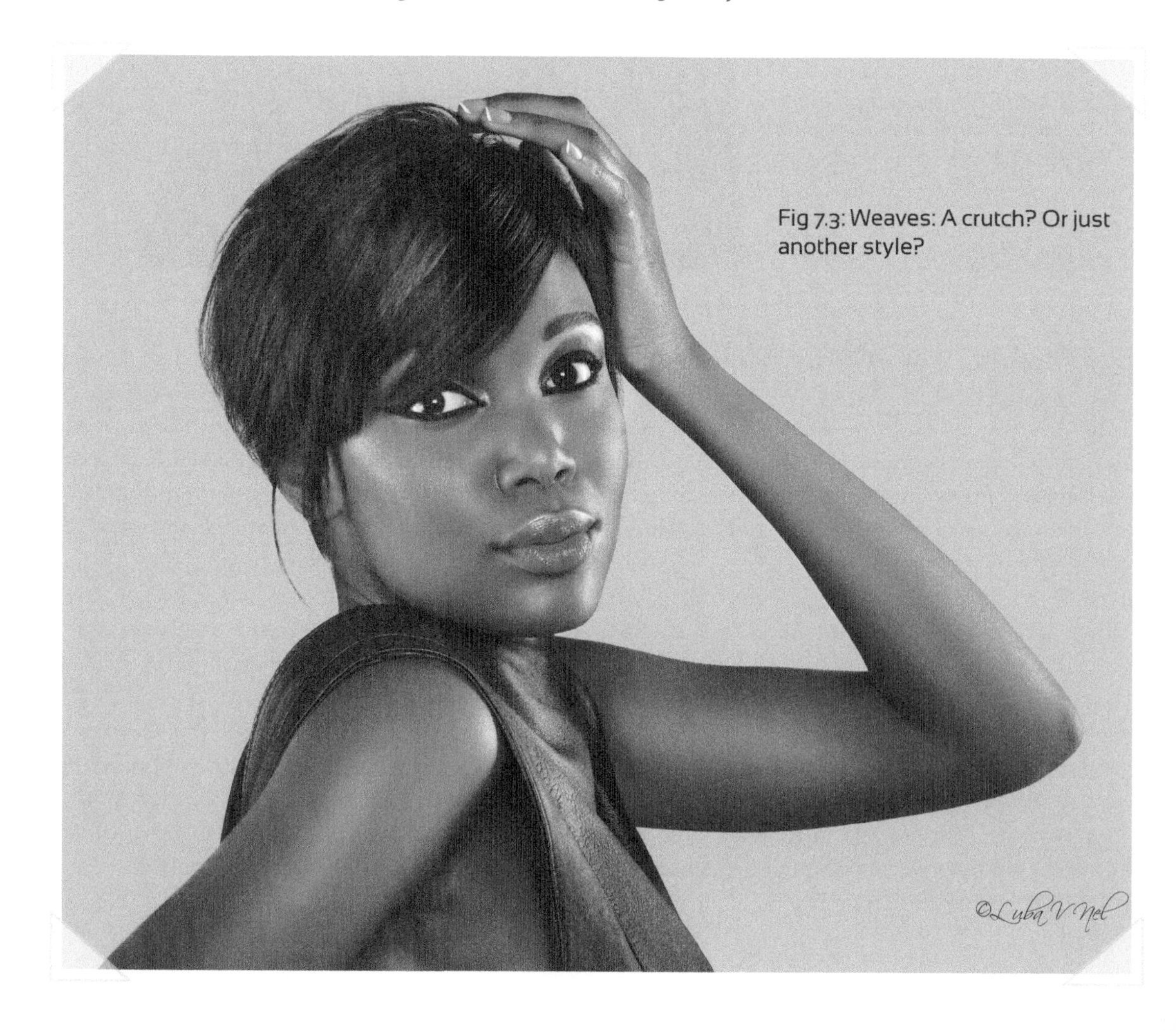

Fig 7.3: Weaves: A crutch? Or just another style?

Why Are You Hiding under That Weave?

Another issue that often comes up, for those who've already completed the transition and are now newly natural, is the issue of styling. For many new naturals, styling shorter hair is a challenge. Often these new naturals will seek out alternatives to wearing their shorter hair, such as wearing extensions or weaves. Other new naturals as well as some seasoned naturals may view this reluctance to wear their natural hair out as a sign that the new natural does not really want to accept her hair—or as a sign that she is not yet willing to learn how to care for natural hair.

In some cases, these assumptions may be true. Remember, just because someone physically has natural hair does not mean they aren't still in transition. Some new naturals who wear weaves and extensions right away may have chopped before they were truly ready. Because they rushed, they may not be in complete love with their new hair just yet, and may still be in the throes of a mental transition—which is a necessary part of the total transitioning process. Some may still be questioning their decision to be natural. Some may be struggling to understand and like their texture, and still others could be going through some things in their lives that mean caring for hair needs to take a backseat for a while.

Of course, not sporting natural hair right out of the gate could also mean that the new natural is still in experimentation mode. She may absolutely love and be committed to her natural hair but is looking for a styling break, in need of a quick styling change or trying out a protective style that will allow her natural hair to grow out a bit more first.

Your Journey, Your Way

Whether you are taking the lengthy route to natural hair, relying on extensions because you aren't sure about your hair, or riding out the shortest stages with your new hair by turning to a weave, no one should make you feel bad for going through your own journey and your own process the way that works best for you. It's impossible to ever know someone else's reasons for adopting a particular styling choice—and really, it's no one else's business to know! We must always remember to embrace one another and teach one another in love. No two paths are the same or more valid than the other, nor must they strive to be.

7.3 Natural Hair in the Workplace

A very valid concern that many transitioners and new naturals face is how their hair will be perceived in the workplace. Even though we are seeing more natural hair in the professional world, there are still those out there who think that natural hair is inappropriate. Add to this the growing number of hair-related lawsuits and protests popping up left and right, and it's no wonder many people are worried. For many, the idea of big, uninhibited, carefree ringlets and cottony coils pushes the boundary of what is acceptable for work. It is one thing when coworkers feel this way and quite another when the people who hold the keys to your advancement (bosses, managers and supervisors) in that environment are the problem.

Take Advantage of Our Hair's Versatility

You can make natural hair's versatility work for you in the workplace. Natural hair offers a menu of styling options that are appropriate for any work environment. If you work in a highly creative space where personal expression is encouraged, your natural hair can be worn in ways that inspire and command attention. If you work in a traditional corporate environment, the same hair can be styled in subtle, subdued ways that still whisper chic sophistication. With natural hair, you really can have it both ways!

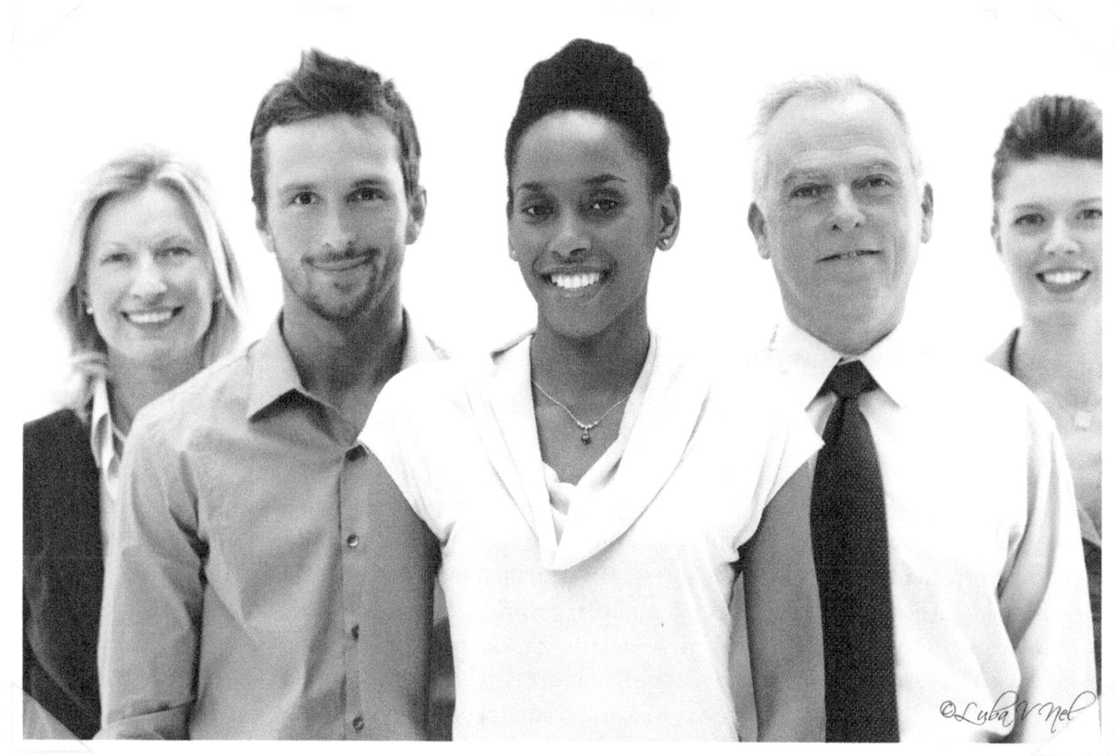

Fig 7.4: Natural hair is professional and can be styled to suit any workplace.

Check Yourself

A good thing to remember is that much of the negativity we expect to experience is simply us projecting our own fears about being natural. That's normal, and it's okay! It's like preparing to be on stage—you imagine everything that could possibly go wrong, and because you gave energy to those thoughts, they often materialize in just the way you feared! If you give too much weight and energy to other people's thoughts, you'll find it hard to do anything in life—going natural or otherwise.

Essence magazine ran an online poll asking women if wearing their natural hair had affected their success in the workplace in a negative manner. About 13 percent responded that they *knew it did* affect their success because they'd experienced it directly. Fifty-six percent responded that they *thought it did*, although they'd never experienced it personally. These poll results are far from scientific, but underscore the point that what we think is going to happen may not be in line with what is actually going to happen out there. Only a small percentage of those responding to the poll

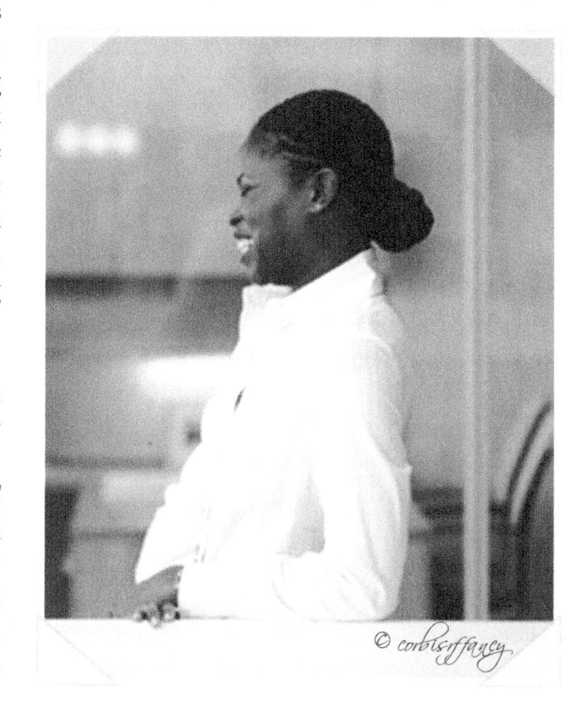

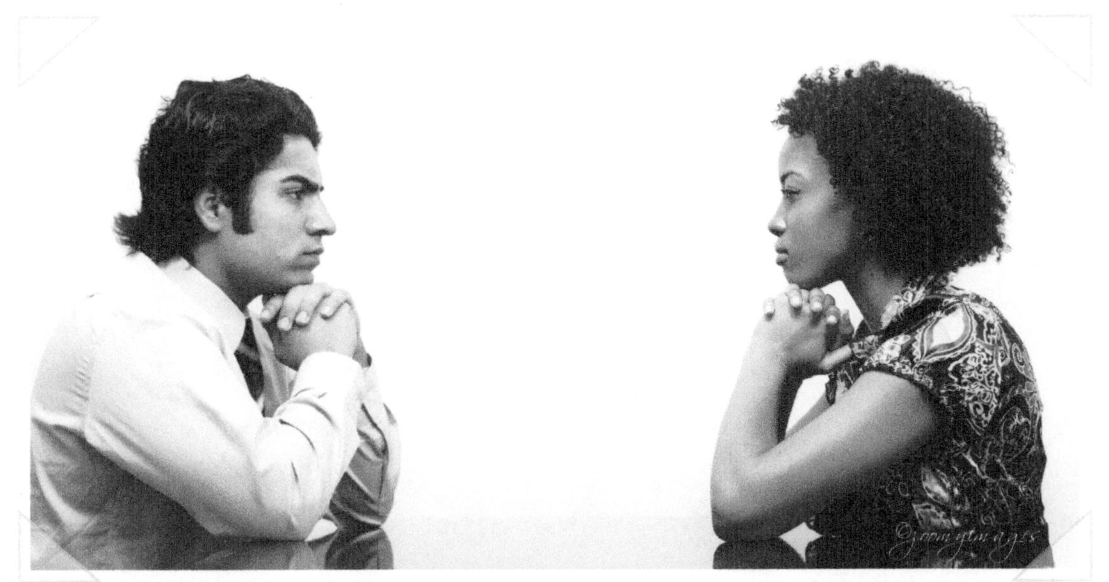

Fig 7.5: Often our greatest fears about wearing natural hair in the workplace are unfounded.

actually faced direct, personal discrimination because of their hair. The overwhelming majority hadn't faced any direct discrimination at all.

The Most Important Thing To Remember

Ultimately, your professionalism on the job lies in what you bring to the table: your ideas, creativity, skill sets and experience with the tasks and demands of the job. Remember, professionalism is about what's *in* your head, not what's *on* your head. Many professional men and women all over the world report to work each day with their natural hair styled and ready to meet the demands of the day. Today's workplace is largely results-driven and productivity-oriented. Assuming that your hair is kept neat and clean and is styled in a way that does not physically hinder the fulfillment of your job responsibilities, you should not face flack in the work environment.

Some people, of course, will never appreciate your natural hair, no matter how neat or business-ready it is—the same way that some people may not like your skin color or background. You cannot change those kinds of people. All you can do is continue to be the best possible you. You are valuable. Your skills are valuable, and your time is valuable. A workplace that discriminates against you simply because of your hair texture and style is not a place deserving of your service and career loyalty. You have the ability to dictate to others how they can and will treat you. If your work environment is not elevating or grow-

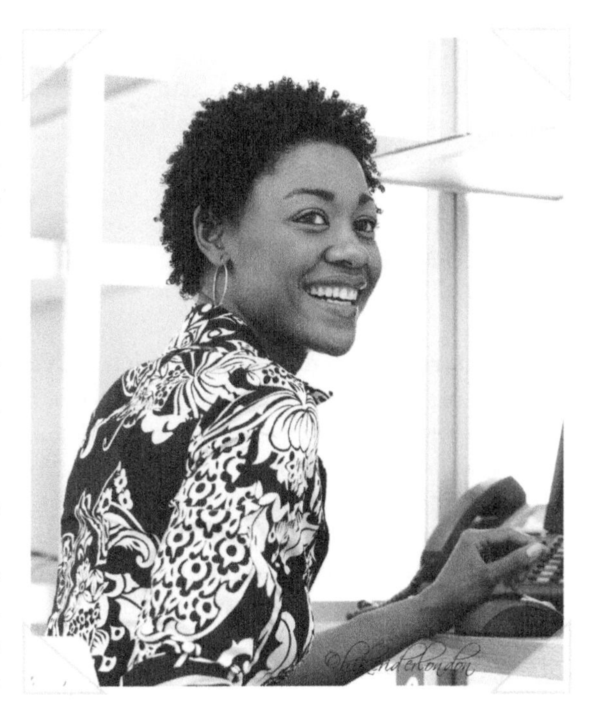

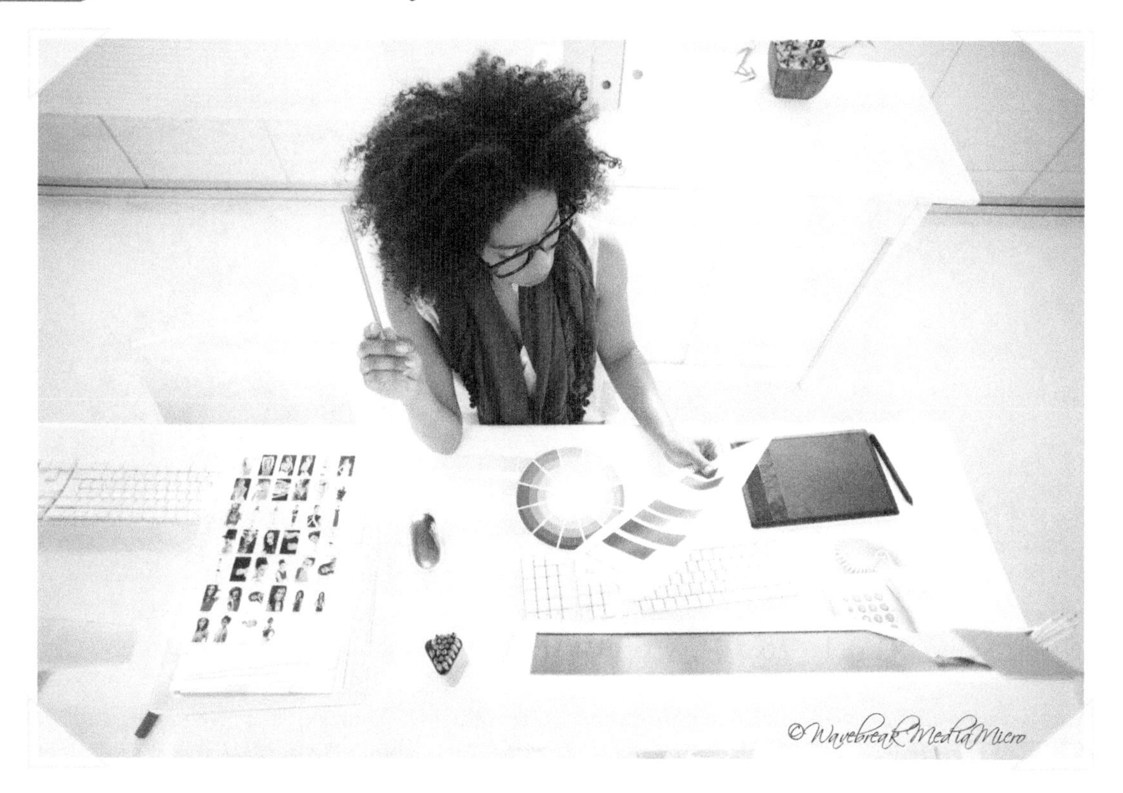
©WavebreakMediaMicro

ing you, take your skills, gifts and talents where they will be respected and esteemed.

Stay positive and focus on why YOU are choosing to go natural. You are, after all, doing this for you. More often than not, the negative comments you feared would pour in will actually come in as compliments. Natural hair is truly unique in its beauty, and naturally, people will be taken by it. That's a promise.

7.4 On Really, Really Loving Yourself—Hair and All

- **Understand that YOU deserve to have the best.** It's true. Many times we live our lives for others, and we try to live up to their views of how we should be. But you are in control! Eliminating or reducing your exposure to potentially harmful chemicals in your beauty routine could never be a bad thing, and it's a step toward improving the overall quality of your life. Realize that you have the power to create an amazing life for yourself, and that you have the power to decide whether or not to allow others to control you. Those who truly love you and have your best interests at heart will encourage you to seek ways to make your life healthier, and you should do the same for them.

- **Speak life!** You may have heard it said that "life and death are in the power of the tongue." This is true for almost everything in our lives—hair included! Speaking happiness and encouragement over your situation—even when it really looks rough—can go a long way. If you don't feel beautiful, attractive or worthy enough—speak it anyway. Eventually, you'll start to move confidently into the positive world that you have spoken to life. It really does work, *and it works both ways*. If you speak negativity and defeat, you will also encourage it to grow and grab a foothold in your life. A good friend of mine put it very simply: You will always have what you say—so speak life!

- **Get a change of scenery, or try something new.** Although for you going natural is something already pretty new in and of itself, sometimes it's good to add another positive distraction to the mix. Plan a trip to some place new and interesting, volunteer with the less fortunate, try a new restaurant or food, or redecorate a room in your home. These positive distractions will help you take your mind off any negativity you are feeling and give you something else to think about.

- **Surround yourself with positive, like-minded people and images.** This is where online blogs, video-sharing sites like YouTube and local meet-up groups come in handy. They will give you a sense of community and eliminate any isolation you may feel should you not have the support of those closest to you. The more you feed yourself images of beautiful textured hair, the more you will feel and see it.

- **Be grateful.** The journey back to natural hair can be hard. If it were easy for everyone, there'd be no books like this one, no meet-ups or groups dedicated to helping newbies navigate the process. But in the grand scheme of things, going natural is really a walk in the park. Let's always keep our perspective. Compared to the other more serious issues that we may face in life, such as losing a job or losing a loved one, going natural is something you can look forward to!

7.5 Relaxer Relapse

Although many women successfully transition to natural hair on the very first try, this is not the case for everyone. Relaxer relapse is often a part of transitioning and "new naturaldom" for many of us. While none of us like to feel like we've "failed," relaxer relapse is a valuable part of the learning process.

For transitioners, weeks six to eight after a relaxer seem to be the most trying weeks, with things escalating from there. For new naturals, the chance of a relapse in the weeks and months following the Big Chop is also high. We may be confronted with a hair texture we didn't expect or with less supportive reactions than we expected from family members. These things may lead us back to the relaxer, and back into the earlier stages of change.

Our poll of transitioners and new naturals who'd thrown in the towel showed that styling issues, breakage and shedding were the top reasons for relapse.

Styling problems were cited by almost 82 percent of our participants as a determining factor in their relapses. When it comes to styling transitioning and natural hair, remember that there will always be a learning curve. Just think back to your very first attempts at styling and handling your own hair as a child. It probably didn't go too well for a while! Hair was new territory altogether—but you kept at it over the years until you had something you could work with! Your relaxed hair also took some time, trial and error before you were comfortable enough to work with it—and this is true even if your highest styling achievement is just a ponytail! When it comes to styling transitioning and natural hair, the same truth applies: Speed and skill come only with time and practice.

Think about the styling process like learning how to walk. When we first learn how to walk, our first steps are always going to be slow and wobbly. But with practice (and some falls), we eventually gain the confidence to keep stepping forward. If you keep at it, you'll soon be able to run.

Here are some of the other reasons they gave us for throwing in the transitioning towel:

- "I just wasn't ready."

- "Too time consuming."

- "I just did not know my hair, and had no understanding. I felt lost."

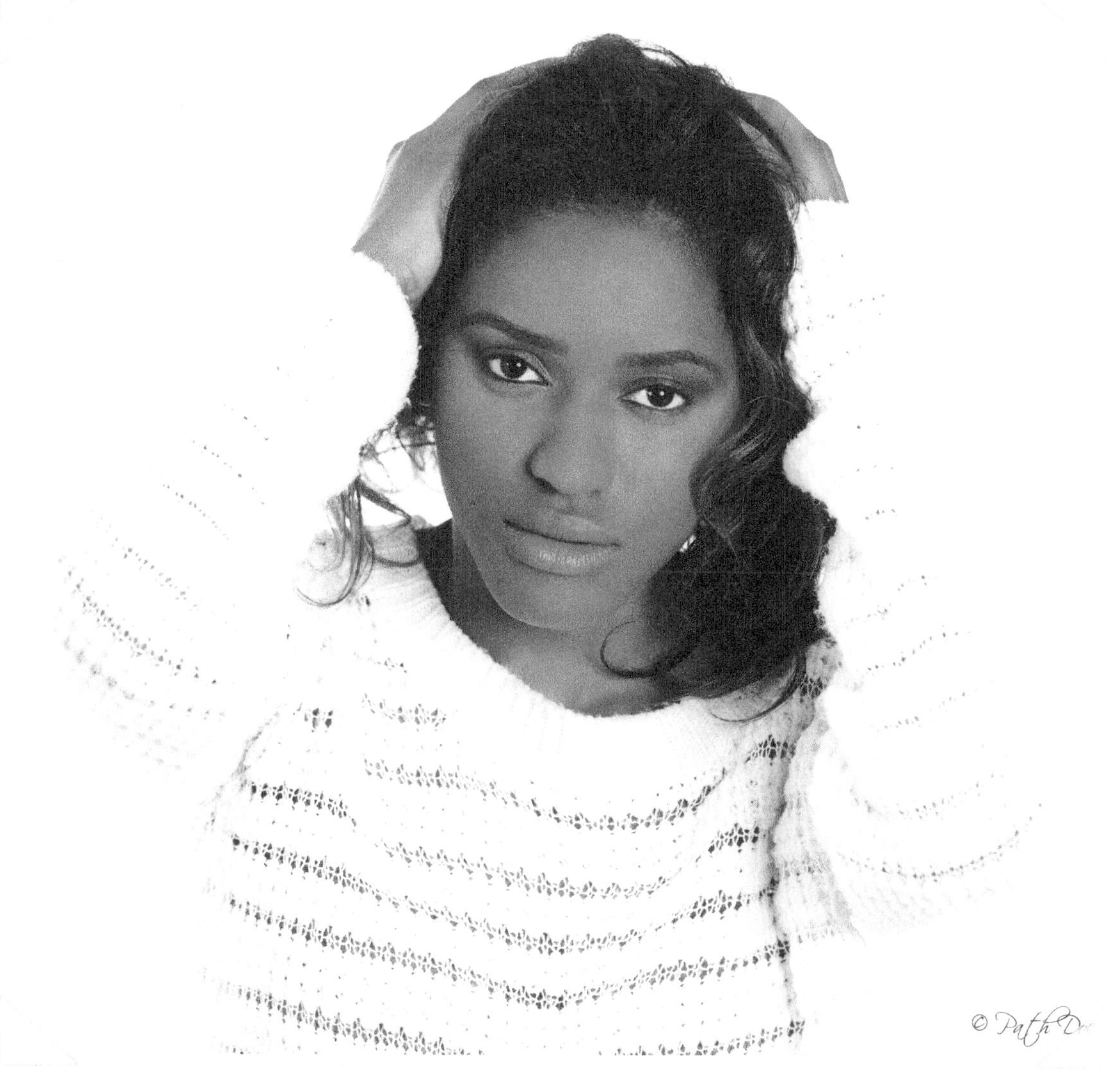

Fig 7.6: Relaxer relapse can be a valuable part of the transition learning process.

- "I was worried about what others might think."
- "My hair dresser kept talking me out of [going natural]."

If you are facing a relaxer-relapse situation, just remember these things:

You're not a failure! It happens. Don't beat yourself up. You can always pick yourself up and try again. Remember, your transition starts again immediately after your relaxer is applied because your hair is always trying to find its way back to natural!

Appreciate your accomplishment. Feel good about the time away from the relaxer. It wasn't a waste! That time counts for something and no doubt put your hair in better shape for that relaxer service.

Reflect and learn. Really think about the reasons, feelings and circumstances that led you back to relaxing again and learn from that experience. What didn't work for you? What did? What would have helped you stay the course?

Your Chapter 7 Take-Aways

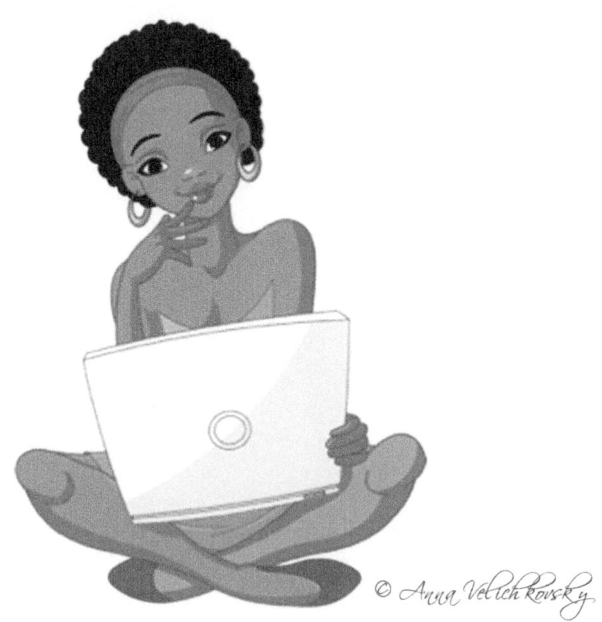

- ✓ Transitioning can bring up a wide variety of emotions and feelings (anger, joy, pity, love, sadness, pride)—all of which are normal.
- ✓ Remember your own personal reasons for making the journey, and stick to your goals.
- ✓ Sometimes the negativity we expect to experience from others is us projecting our own fears about being natural.
- ✓ If at any time during your transition or newly natural journey you don't feel beautiful, attractive or worthy enough—speak it anyway! You will eventually begin to walk in that!
- ✓ If you have a relaxer relapse, remember: Don't beat yourself up. Feel good about the time away from the relaxer, and really try to think about the reasons, feelings and circumstances that lead you back to relaxing again. Learn from it!

In the next chapter, we will discuss the ins and outs of the Big Chop experience.

unit 4

Living the Natural Life

Chapter 8: Arriving at Your Destination

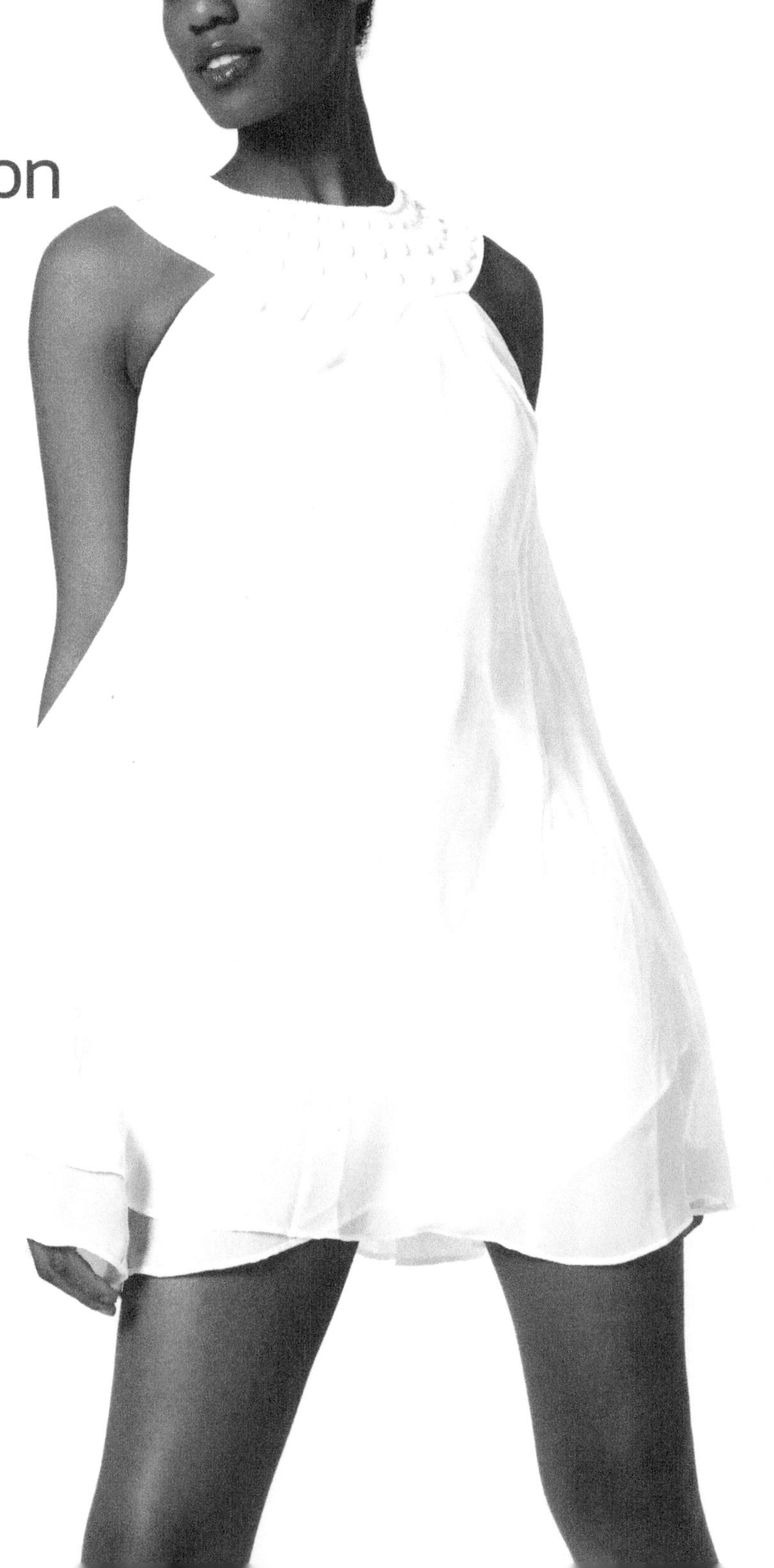

8. How To Big Chop!

Visiting the Stylist

Many transitioners visit a stylist to help them with their Big Chop, or Transitioning Chop. Your stylist will shampoo and condition your hair as needed and proceed to remove the remaining relaxed ends. He or she, more than likely, also will give you a light trim to ensure that your hair is shaped well and that you aren't carrying any damaged hair into your natural hair journey.

A stylist is a great option for Big Chopping because a professional can see and reach parts of your head that you'd have to really do some stretching to get to properly. Plus, you'll also get a nice cut and shape from a stylist that would be hard to duplicate on your own unless you have amazing cutting skills.

Doing It Yourself

If you are a do-it-yourselfer, the Big Chop is definitely something you can do on your own. Many women find it very empowering to be the one who does the actual cutting. Some women do the initial chop on their own and then have a stylist clean it up sometime later.

Just as with the transition itself, there is no one correct way to go about doing your Big Chop. Some women like to do it in the privacy of their bathrooms, while others enlist friends or significant others to do the honors. You can make as big or as small a deal out of it as you want! My own Big Chop was very unplanned and very quiet. I did it myself in the bathroom and snapped a few pictures when everything was done—nothing spectacular.

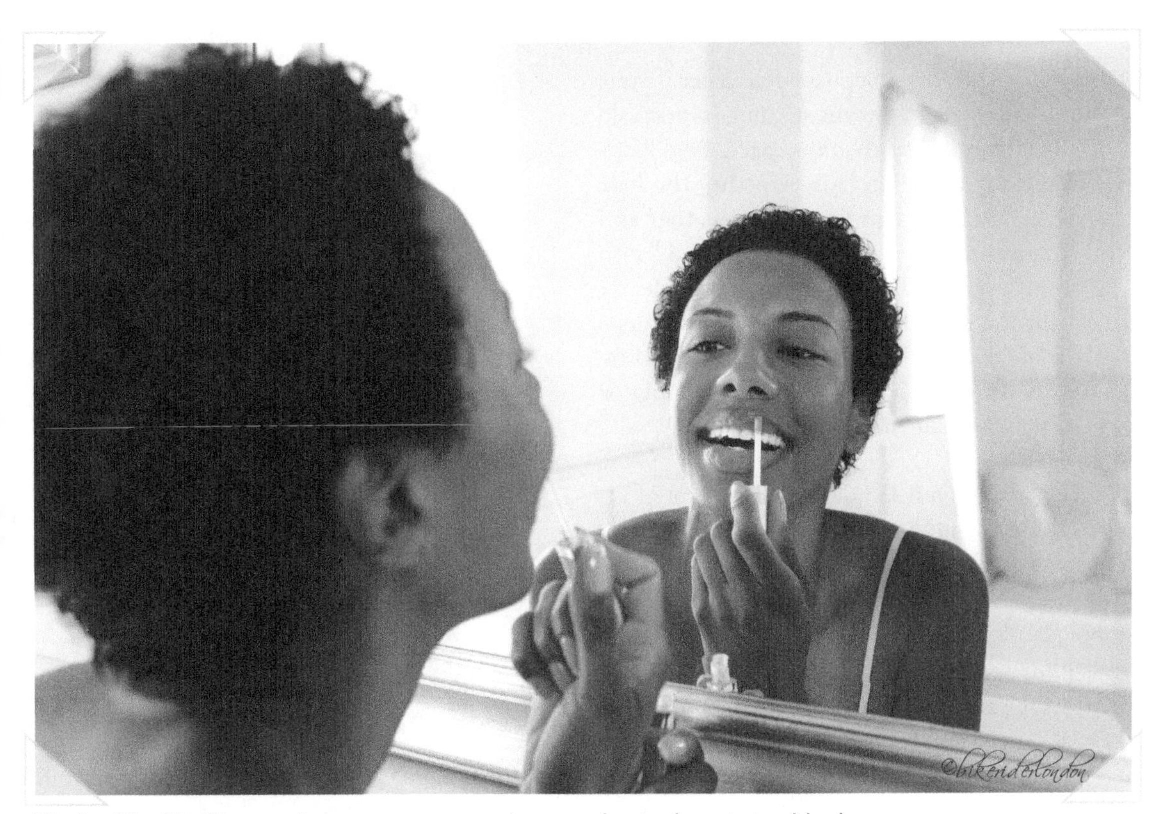

Fig 8.0: The Big Chop really encourages your inner and outer beauty to shine!

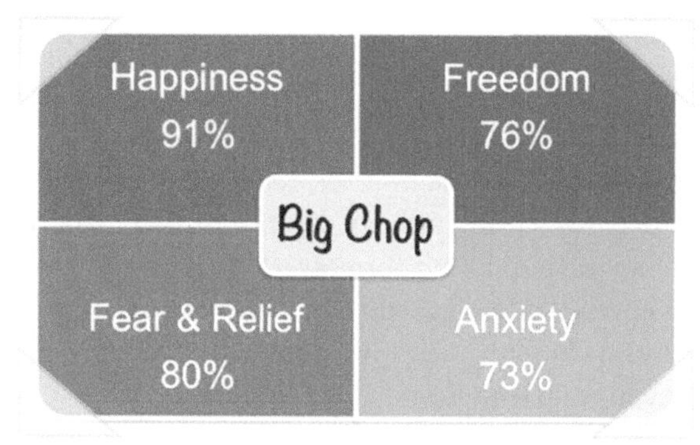

Fig 8.1: We asked our transitioning survey participants: ***When you think about your upcoming big chop, how does it make you feel?*** Participants were allowed to select as many emotions as they wished. The emotions that ranked highest were all relatively positive, but there were negative and neutral emotions expressed as well. **Indifference** was selected by 33% of the group, **discouragement** by 31% of the group, and **anger** by 9% of the group.

Here are some tips to help you jump start your chop!

Getting Started

Doing your own Big Chop is much easier if your natural hair is lengthy, but it's not impossible with shorter hair. For the most part, Big Chops are best done on damp hair. Wetting the hair causes your relaxed hair to clump together and your natural new growth to curl and fold into its natural pattern. This will help you to clearly make out the point where the relaxed hair ends and the natural hair begins. The Big Chop is one of the few times when I recommend cutting or trimming your hair in its wet state.

NOTE: Although it is not a requirement, I always recommend shampooing and conditioning the hair prior to doing a Big Chop. It is just easier to work with clean, conditioned hair (although some people prefer not to waste perfectly good conditioner on relaxed hair that will just end up on the floor). As long as your hair is damp prior to your cut, shampooed or not, you will be okay!

To do your own Big Chop you'll need:

Materials

- Moisturizing shampoo
- Deep conditioner
- Leave-in conditioner
- Spray bottle
- Hair shears

1. Start with clean, conditioned hair that has been separated into four to six sections.

2. Starting with the first section or quadrant, use your fingers to gently divide the quadrant into smaller sections.

3. Spray your small section with plain water, or a water/conditioner combo to encourage your curl pattern to form.

4. Gently stretch out the small section and locate the line of demarcation (where the relaxed hair meets your natural hair). If the section has started to dry, repeat STEP 3.

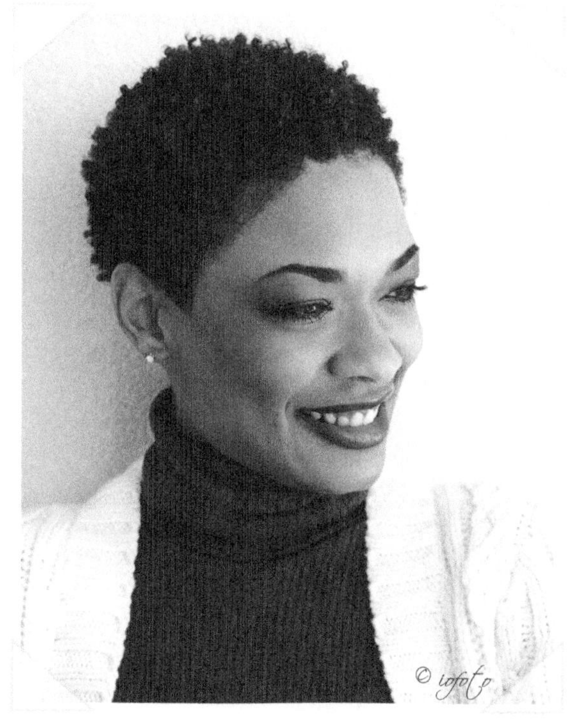

Fig 8.2: Having a professional stylist perform your Big Chop is a great option. You'll walk out with a nice edge-up, plus a cut and shape that fits your face.

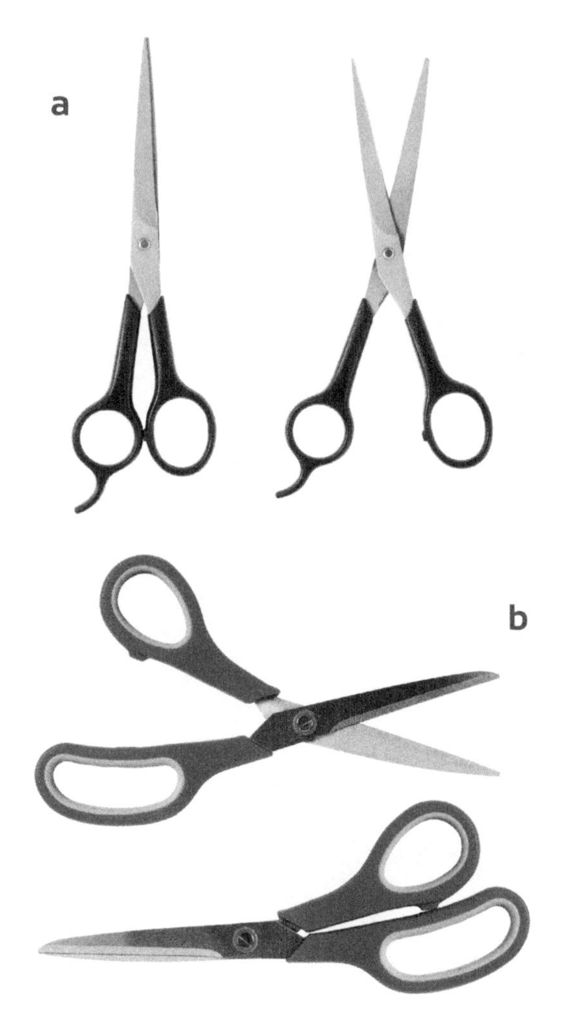

Fig 8.3: The scissors you choose for your own Big Chop are very important. Always use hair shears (Figure 8.3a) to maintain your hair. The scissors in Figure 8.3b can damage your freshly trimmed ends.

5. Trim at or just above the line of demarcation.

6. Continue steps 2–5 to trim your entire head.

Optional

After you've completed the trimming, rinse your entire head of hair with water, and reapply your conditioner or leave-in conditioner. This will allow you to see any remaining straight pieces that you may have missed the first time. Simply snip them out of the way.

You may run into random straight pieces days or even weeks after doing your Big Chop. That's normal. Continue to snip these strays as you see them.

Caring for a Short Crop or Fade: Quick Tips

If you've done a Big Chop that has resulted in a super short crop or low fade, it is still important to keep your hair and scalp moisturized and protected.

1. Co-washing (washing your hair with conditioner instead of shampoo) will keep your short crop super conditioned.

2. For additional daily moisture, mist your hair with a water-based product and follow with a light cream or oil-based product to seal it in. If your hair is very thick, you may find that butters work better as sealants than oils.

3. Apply any moisturizers and oils in the pattern your hair grows in, working with the natural direction of your hair. This will prevent frizzing and stray strands from popping up.

4. A satin pillowcase at night will protect your super low cut against nighttime dryness and friction from your pillow.

> Since relaxed hair is more porous than natural hair, your ends can dry out quickly. Keep a spray bottle nearby so that you can re-mist any sections of hair that dry out before you get to them. (For more on porosity, see page 47.)

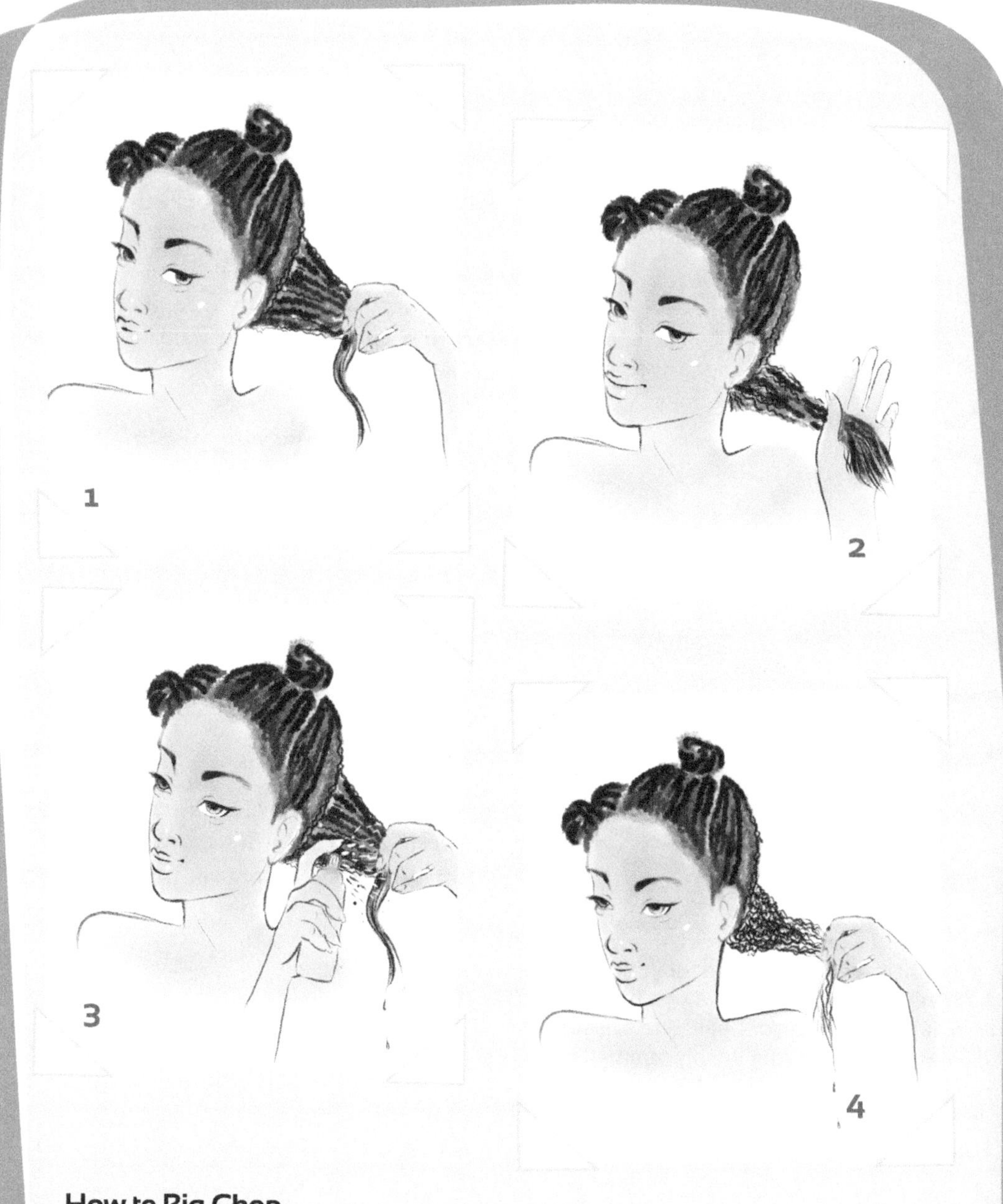

How to Big Chop

STEP 1. Start with sectioned, freshly washed and conditioned hair.

STEP 2. Isolate a small section from one of the larger sections.

STEP 3. Spray with water or leave-in conditioner to bring out your curl pattern.

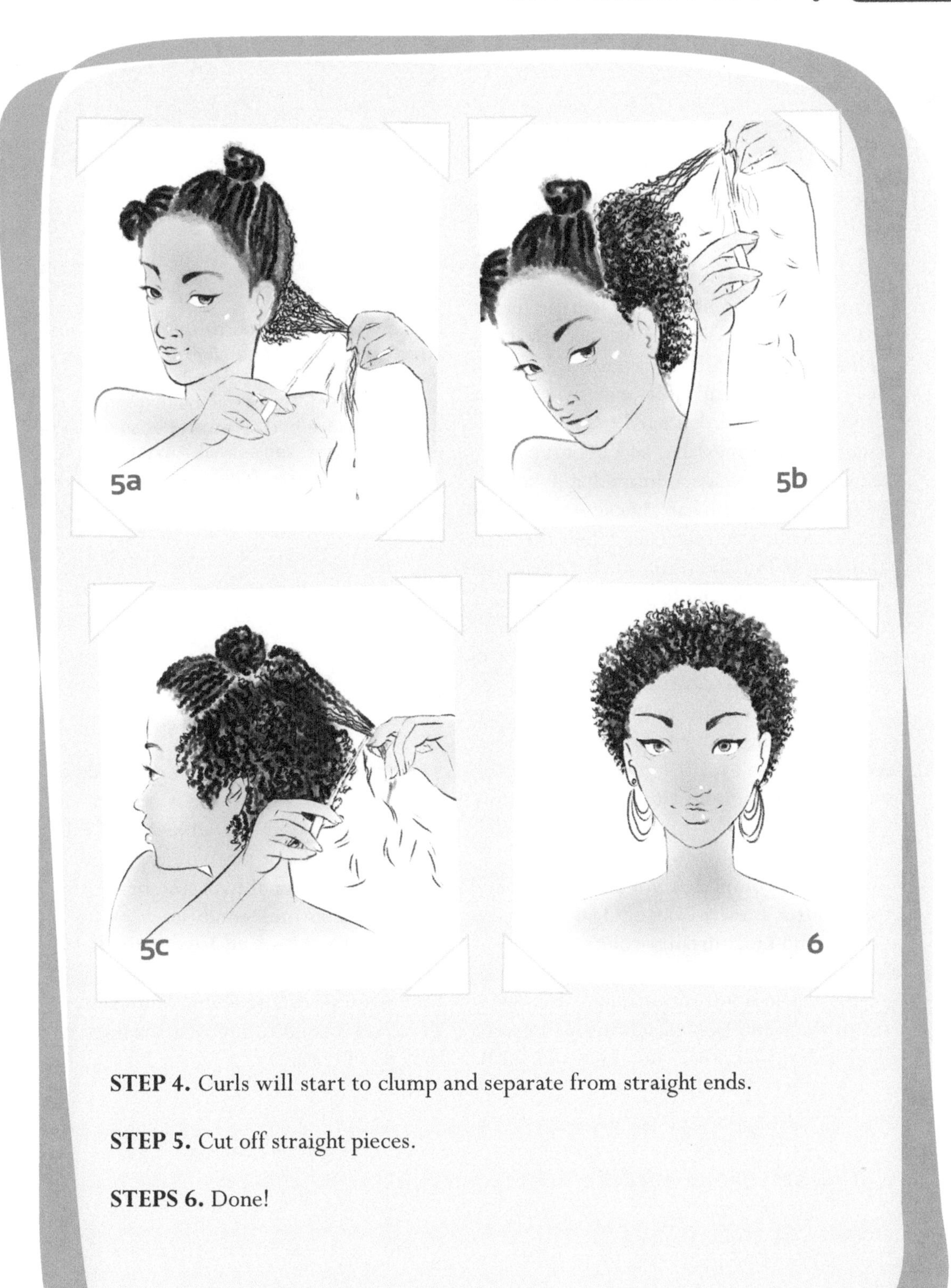

STEP 4. Curls will start to clump and separate from straight ends.

STEP 5. Cut off straight pieces.

STEPS 6. Done!

Dry Hair. No Curl Pattern. Do I have Scab Hair?

Mention "scab hair" in a crowd of naturals, and you'll get some understanding nods and some disapproving glares. Scab hair, or what we refer to in Chapter 1 as "transitional hair," refers to the first one or two inches of new hair that grows in immediately after your last relaxer. Scab hair is not a medical or scientific term–it is a term that originated on Internet hair-care forums to describe new natural hair that is super dry and has an oddly undefined texture and/or curl pattern. It's hard to tell whether the immediate dryness and lack of curl pattern some women experience immediately after a Big Chop is truly scab hair, because many new naturals have never experienced their own natural textures and don't know what their hair is supposed to look and feel like.

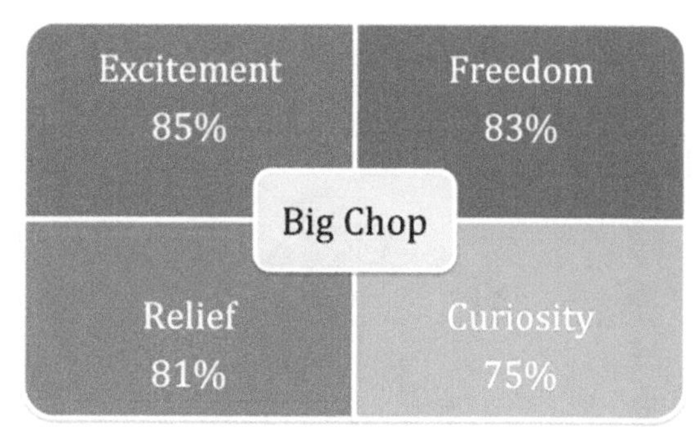

Fig 8.4: We also asked our natural survey participants: ***Which emotions did you feel after your big chop?*** Participants were allowed to select as many emotions as they wished. The emotions that ranked highest were all positive, but there were negative and neutral emotions expressed as well. **Anxiety** was selected by 58% of the group, **fear** by 44% of the group, and **indifference** by 30% of the group.

Ultimately, the scab hair phenomenon is one of those things that can only really be recognized in retrospect, after hair has been allowed to grow out for some time without chemical treatment. Basically, you can't really know if you have experienced scab hair until after your real texture begins to grow in!

If you've just completed your Big Chop and find that after a few weeks of cleansing, conditioning and moisturizing your tresses your hair is relatively unresponsive, you may be dealing with scab hair/transitional hair. However, if the dryness and lack of definition continue beyond several months, you could indeed be working with your final natural texture and simply need to adjust your regimen to match your hair's needs.

The existence of scab hair is difficult to prove or disprove because there is no published research available on the subject as of this writing. If you believe that you are experiencing scab or transitional hair, the best solution is to simply continue conditioning your hair as normal. If you indeed have scab hair, it will eventually grow out and be trimmed away. If your natural texture is simply in need of some TLC, your conditioning will bring your hair back to life again!

Your Chapter 8 Take-Aways

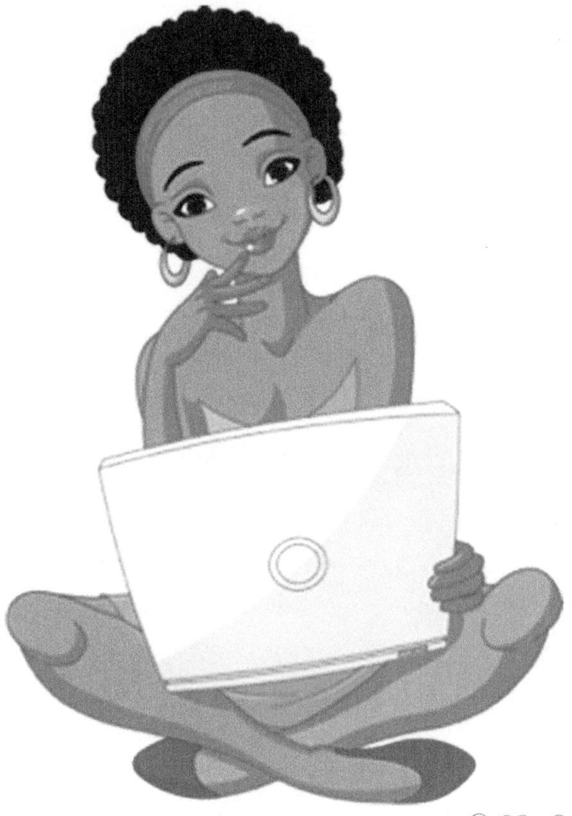

- ✓ Many transitioners visit a stylist to help them with their Big Chop, or Transitioning Chop.
- ✓ Others find it very empowering to be the one who does the actual cutting.
- ✓ Just as with the transition itself, there is no one correct way to go about doing your Big Chop.

In the next chapter, we will discuss the features and properties of natural hair. We'll also provide tips for handling and caring for your new natural tresses!

Chapter 9:
Working with Your New Hair

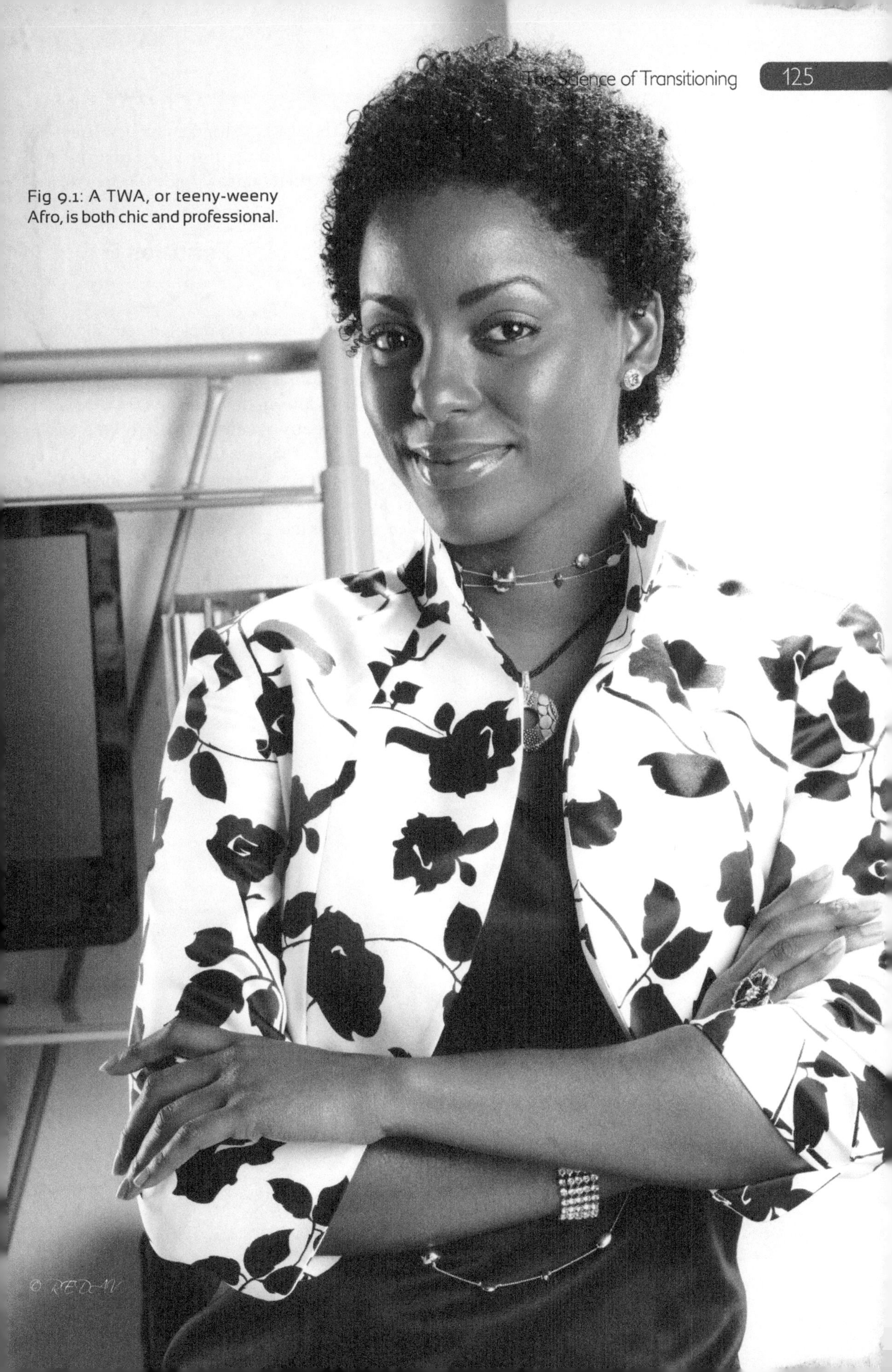

Fig 9.1: A TWA, or teeny-weeny Afro, is both chic and professional.

And now . . . you're natural!

You've survived the physical transitioning process, you've chopped and now you are living your life as a new natural. There is an entire community of women just like you who've passed on the relaxers and have opted for more chemical-free ways of living. You may still have some things to work on as far as the mental aspects of transitioning are concerned—but to the world, you are now natural.

No two naturals will look exactly the same after their chop. Some of you will Big Chop to discover flat, silky waves, or loopy curls that will gain character with length. Others may discover a low, shrunken crop of cottony-textured coils. Some of you will have a mix of textures and types going on! Your hair may also be uneven, and you'll probably continue to have a few straight pieces popping up over the next few weeks. This is normal. The regular bends and twists along our natural hair fibers make our strands extremely vulnerable to breakage, so handle your new hair with care. Our hair is indeed strongest in its natural state, but it still requires a gentle touch to thrive.

9. Natural Hair Features & Properties

If you've just recently completed your Big Chop after a short transition—or jumped immediately into your natural journey—you'll be presented with what's known in most hair-care circles as a **TWA, or teeny-weeny Afro**. A TWA is longer than a fade but shorter than a full-fledged Afro. Of course, if you've transitioned for longer than eight to ten months, you may be working with a length that is much longer than a standard TWA.

For some women, this new hair is the shortest hair they've ever had in their lives, and if you've never worked with short hair, there is definitely a learning curve.

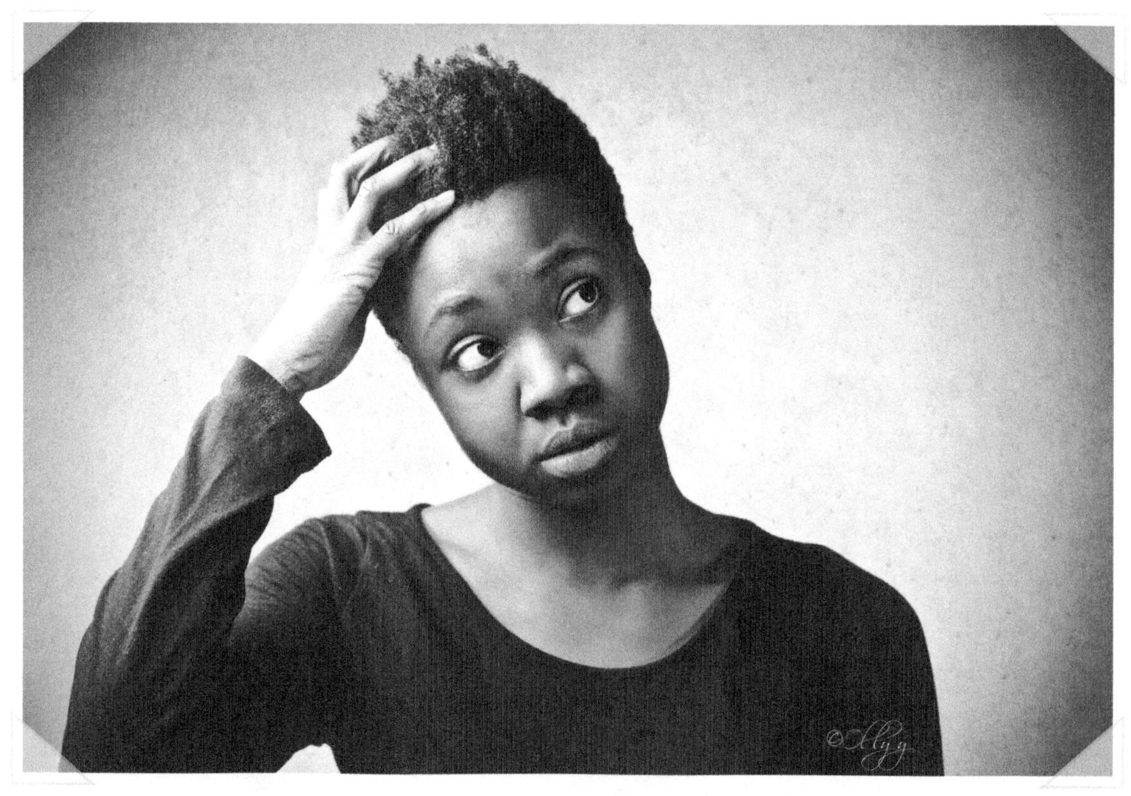

Fig 9.2: For some women, their new natural hair is the shortest hair they've ever had in their lives.

Now, let's get one misconception out of the way quickly! Many women welcome shorter hair because it gives them what they believe will be maintenance-free hair—but no hair is 100 percent maintenance free. While it is true that the shorter-length stages are generally the lowest-maintenance natural hair stages, short hair still requires care—especially if it is your goal to grow longer!

Knowing your hair's basic properties is essential if you are going to make a successful partnership with your natural hair. If your hair is highly textured, your post-chop new hair will very likely look dry. Rather than shine, it will tend to have a dull but healthy matte *sheen*—especially when held taut.

This is probably also a good time to tell you not to trust your eyes.

9.1 Healthy Natural Hair: Touch and Visual Cues

I'm sure you've heard the adage, "Looks can be deceiving." *It's true!* Our eyes tell us much about the world around us, but they aren't very good at assessing the quality or health of natural hair. Some natural hair types look very dry, even though they are completely moisturized and conditioned. This is particularly true for those with the tightest, coiliest hair types. On the flip side, your natural hair can also look "okay" and still be damaged to high heaven. This is where your hands come in. Your hands almost need to become your new eyes and your sense of touch your new sight!

Your fingers can pick up on cues that give you much more information about the state of your hair than your eyes ever could. Natural hair's volume and organic shape make *touch cues* such as "hard," "crunchy," "brittle" or "soft" more valuable and helpful for natural tresses than *visual cues* such as "dry," "dull" and "uneven" that work well for relaxed hair. To successfully read your hair, you'll need both types of cues, with an emphasis on the touch cues.

How Should It Feel?

So, how *should* your new hair feel?

Your hair should feel strong yet soft, fluffy, cottony and/or springy. Hair that feels hard, tangly or scratchy needs moisture. One way to naturally improve your hair's moisture is to eliminate common causes of hair dryness from your hair-care regimen. You may, for instance, see an improvement in your hair's moisture levels if you remove sulfates, heavy proteins, oils and silicone ingredients from your regimen. Additionally, making sure to address any hard-water issues you have at home will also ensure that your tresses maintain their optimal moisture levels.

Shrinkage

In its natural state, our hair is prone to considerable fiber shrinkage. Natural hair's tendency to draw up tightly and hug the scalp when dry makes it appear much shorter than it truly is. Many people get their first real dose of reality about shrinkage after their Big Chop. Imagine going into your chop expecting to see four inches of new growth, only to find a two-inch crop of hair! The weight of the relaxed hair on transitioning strands can give a false expectation of length.

Shrinkage is advantageous for some hairstyles with compact shapes (Afros and puffs), but if you are one who loves to show off her length—shrinkage will be your worst enemy. While shrinkage affects all curly-haired people to some extent, some textured hair types are more affected by hair shrinkage than others. Hair with a looser, wavier curl pattern may retain more of its natural length when going from wet to dry than naturally coiled or kinky hair. This shrinkage is normal, healthy and is simply a part of our hair's natural character.

Using the Banding Method To Stretch Out Natural Hair

STEP 1. Start with loose natural hair (short, shrunken Afro).

STEP 2. Separate and comb out a section.

STEP 3. Apply a small ponytail holder from roots, and weave along length to the ends. If your hair is longer, you can place several ponytail holders along your section at one-inch intervals.

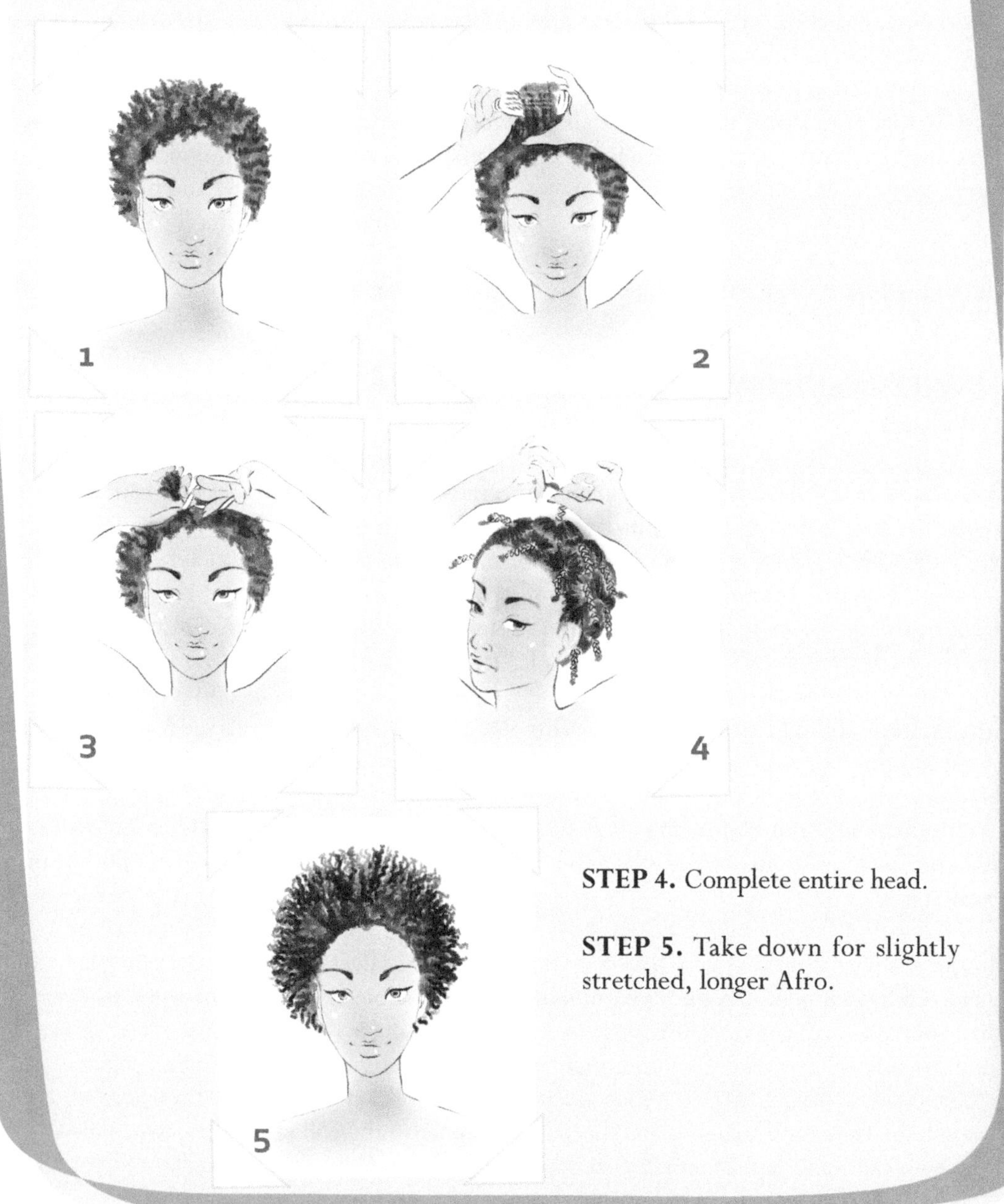

STEP 4. Complete entire head.

STEP 5. Take down for slightly stretched, longer Afro.

Knotting, Coiling & Tangling

Shrinkage does have a downside. When we wear our hair in its shrunken state for extended periods of time, we increase the chances for severe tangling and knotting that can lead to unwanted hair breakage. To reach maximum lengths, we must work around natural hair's tendency to tangle and knot on itself. The best way to avoid severe knotting and tangling is to keep the hair in stretched or protective styles such as braids or two-strand twists. Try not to rely too heavily on styles such as Afros, puffs and undefined twist-outs that allow the hair to swell, shrink and mat over a period of days.

Single Strand Knots

Occasionally, natural hair will develop tiny single-strand knots (SSKs) along single fibers. These knots occur when naturally coily or curly hair bends or folds back onto itself. Left unchecked, these little knots can tangle your relatively healthy neighboring coils and curls into a huge, matted mess. Unlike other knots that tend to involve multiple strands and can be carefully picked apart, single strand knots are so small that they cannot easily be undone. These knots should be dealt with by snipping the strand just above the place where the knot has formed.

We can't prevent all knots from occurring, but we can try to keep them contained. Try these tips for drastically reducing the number of single-strand knots and other tangles in kinky- curly hair.

Keep It Hydrated!

The single best solution for single-strand knots is simply to keep the hair hydrated. Tangles are more likely to form in dried, shrunken hair than in moisturized, elastic, and stretched-out hair. Regular deep conditioning with moisture-rich products also goes a long way toward combatting knots and tangles with natural hair. You will quickly find that the one thing that natural hair needs more than anything is water. Because of this, you should get in the habit of supplying the moisture your hair craves on a regular schedule. You cannot wait for dryness to respond with moisture.

Detangle Your Hair Thoroughly

While it is undeniably time consuming, careful detangling will save you lots of hair stress and trouble down the road—especially as your coils and curls grow longer. You should always apply a softening product (moisturizer/conditioner/oil) to the hair before detangling to reduce friction.

To avoid additional damage, start the detangling process using your fingers first. Always work on the hair in small, manageable sections, isolating individual hairs as you move along.

Start detangling the hair at the ends, and work up from the bottom toward the scalp. Once the hair is detangled with your fingers, you can work your way down to progressively smaller combs until you've detangled to your taste. If your hair can tolerate it, try a detangling brush like the Denman to polish off your detangling efforts. Continue to work slowly in sections until the entire head is thoroughly detangled.

Condition the Hair with a Vengeance

Regular attention to your hair's moisture balance will keep most single-strand knots at bay. You really want to strive for conditioner coverage (See Chapter 10, *Supernatural Maintenance Tips & Strategies, pg 152*). Here's why: Typically, we condition our hair as one large unit, paying the most attention to the top and sides and barely scrunching product through the middle of the head. Add to this the fact that conditioner products on the whole aren't as spreadable on the hair as shampoos, and it's easy to leave certain parts of the hair needing a moisture boost! Be sure that you are getting conditioner to all areas of your head.

If you have a problem with knotting, moisturize or lightly mist your hair once a day to keep your curls fresh and hydrated. Follow up by sealing your hair with an oil product to prevent friction between the strands that can lead to knotting.

Keep It Stretched!

Shrunken hair styles are Knot Central. When curly and coily hair is allowed to shrink into its tightest (default) configuration, the hair is primed for knotting! Curls and coils love to intermingle with their neighbors and even coil back onto themselves. Afros, puffs, and wash-n-go curls are the number-one single-strand-knot culprits—especially if the styles are worn for several consecutive days. Try stretching out your hair as much as possible with twists, braids, and fluffed-out variations of these styles.

At night, protect your hair by plaiting or twisting it to lengthen the curls and coils. Cover the hair with a satin scarf or bonnet to reduce friction between your hair and bedding.

Wear It Shorter

If all else fails, consider wearing your hair at a shorter length (less than 3 to 4 inches) to reduce the occurrence of single-strand knots and tangling. Shorter hair is much easier to work with and is less likely to knot on itself than lengthier tresses.

Curl Consistency

Some visual cues can be helpful for understanding your hair. If your hair is curly or coily, your curls, spirals and coils should exhibit their general curliness from root to tip. Hair that starts curly and then straightens or goes flat in sections, especially near the ends, is likely damaged. Heat use is one of the main causes of an inconsistent curl pattern. Curls and coils that start flatter from the roots and build curl toward the ends, however, may be perfectly healthy; the weight of the hair may simply distort the curl pattern near the roots. Although your hair should maintain its general curliness from root to tip, this is not to say that your curls and coils will be perfectly uniform from root to tip! Textured hair may kink, fold and perform a number of reversals along the hair fiber and still be completely healthy.

Ensuring that your strands are thoroughly moisturized will also allow you to bring out all of the natural characteristics and features of your hair's unique texture pattern. Dry, thirsty hair doesn't curl, coil or radiate the sheen that hydrated strands do. Of course, if your hair is not naturally curly or coily, even with adequate moisture you won't be able to create curls and coils where there are none. Keep in mind that with some kinkier and wirier hair types, the kinks and bends that you have are all individuals. They

A Multitude of Textures: Loving What's There

No two heads of natural hair are the same. Some of us come into this world with large, springy curls, while others are born with tight, compact coils and spirals. Curls and coils may change over the course of a lifetime or even from one section of scalp to another.

Before you start off on your quest for those perfect curls and coils, take a moment to fall in love with what's already there. Remember, your natural hair may not look or behave the same way that your favorite blogger or even your own mother's hair does. You may not have the perfect Afro that stands tall—yours may grow down and floppy. You may not have perfect spirals but a soft, unorganized nest of wiry coils. It's best to seek inspiration from all types of natural textures, but remember to really look to those ladies who are rocking a texture that seems similar to your own. Love what is naturally you!

may not clump together to form uniform ringlets and curls; instead, they may weave together and form a mesh pattern. This is normal and part of the character of some of our hair types.

Sheen

Many new naturals wonder why their natural hair does not shine, but the truth is, whether relaxed or natural, textured hair rarely ever shines outright. Rather, most healthy black hair types tend to have sheen and a matte appearance. Although shine is related to the ideal, flattened orientation of the cuticle layers, the inability to produce or maintain shine among some textured hair types is not always a reflection of poor condition.

Shine is a direct result of light bouncing from the hair's surface and being directed toward the eye. Tightly wound curls and intertwining coils, however, simply do not reflect light in the same manner that straighter hair shafts do. Because most textured hair does not shine in the usual sense unless aided by oils or serums, this hair may appear to be quite dry at first glance. Touching often reveals its true softness and health.

Color Consistency

Your natural hair also should have root-to-ends color consistency unless you are graying or you've colored your hair during your transition. If your hair starts to become lighter as you approach the ends, this usually is a sign that the ends of your hair are stressed or worn. Color is an especially important visual cue for those who have naturally frizzy, undefined curl patterns who can't rely on visual cues that indicate root-to-tip curliness.

What Happens When You Are Not a Curly Girl?

When you hear words such as *curly, defined* or *wavy* with regard to our hair, what comes to mind? For most people, the association is usually pretty positive. Now think about words such as *frizzy, puffy* and *undefined* as applied to our hair. What comes to mind? If you are like most people, these last words don't seem positive, and many associate them with hair problems. Unfortunately, the problem with this association is that, for many naturals, these words accurately describe their hair's texture in its healthy natural state.

In a natural-hair renaissance that prides itself on embracing all natural textures, these types of negative associations (good=curly and defined and bad=kinky and undefined) are a huge problem. Instead of straight hair being the ultimate goal, curly hair is now often pegged as the goal—at least in the natural community. Now, of course, this isn't a problem for you if your hair is indeed

Mane Messaging

We've turned the tables on companies who've pushed the mantra that natural hair is unmanageable and undesirable, but we're still allowing subtle messaging to creep into our hair community that says: Wavy and curly natural hair are the ideal natural hair types. Those kinkier natural textures are still on the "unmanageable" and "undesirable" side of the natural-hair spectrum. But no worries, you can fix them. Bring your hair in line [with our product]! Of course, product manufacturers don't say this outright, but they do say it—with images, subtle suggestion and even silence. If we allow our discourse to be controlled in this way, we will be right back at square one without ever really learning to appreciate what we were born with.

curly! But what about the millions of you who are reading this book right now who are wondering what happened to the curls you spent months in transition waiting to see? What happens when you find out that you are really *not* a Curly Girl?

Most new naturals enter the natural-hair arena not really knowing the capabilities or innate tendencies of their unique hair type. Many transitioners spend months reading blogs, watching YouTube videos and scrolling through Instagram, Pinterest and Facebook feeds in which they see nothing but curly natural hair (or other natural hair types styled in curly twist-out and braid-out styles). After all of the moisturizing, conditioning, gelling, shingling and defining recommended to help new naturals style their tresses, it's not surprising that many women feel some kind of way when they finally realize that their frizzy, undefined texture is really . . . just their texture. Add in the slew of products geared toward new naturals and the relaxer-free pushing the idea that curls and waves are the real goal, and it's hard to look at undefined kinks and feel like your hair is still all that it should be.

While it seems that product companies have slowly lost ground in their ability to convince us that our hair needs to be permanently stick straight for us to have any chance at this thing called beauty, these companies are regrouping and subtly repackaging their old messages. This time, they seem to be promoting a hierarchy of hair textures within the natural community. Instead of broadcasting a wide range of natural textures in the spirit of inclusiveness and texture diversity, they are doing what businesses do best— zeroing in on the most profitable texture: curls. Curly Girls buy into curls, and non-curlies buy into curls as well. Marketing simply doesn't flow the other way.

The Power of Language

We always need to be mindful of the power of words and language. In the war for people's minds, hearts, souls and purse strings, words are the most powerful tools and weapons. Companies come armed with biases that they express through the monologue of advertising and marketing language—and they are very clever. Product companies know that they make money when they convince us that we have a problem that they can fix. There just isn't that much money to be made with pride and acceptance. As women, we are especially vulnerable to this type of marketing.

Even innocent-sounding language can be a slippery slope. The marketing pitch TAME AND DEFINE YOUR CURLS simply means BRING YOUR HAIR IN LINE with "acceptable" natural hair types and practices. To those who are genuinely curly, the pitch says that your curls need to be this specific way. To those who are fabulously non-curly, it says that you should be curly and that those curls (which you don't have) should be this specific way. And since you don't have curls and they don't look like this, then, well—too bad for you

If you fall into the non-curling group, this language can perpetuate the myth that some natural textures are better or preferable to others, and that if your hair is natural at all, your goal should be curls. Remember, we are all natural in different ways. There is no one natural texture. There is no one prized or ideal natural texture. Being natural is about embracing and loving what your hair was born to do. If it's curls, it's curls. If it's kinks, it's kinks! And honestly, if you are like many people, you will probably have a little of all of the above.

Be wary of people and companies who suggest to you that your natural is not good enough. This type of advertising does nothing to promote the message that your hair—be it fine, thick, frizzy, undefined, kinky, wavy, curly or a combination of these natural types—is just fine. Natural hair isn't defined by having the perfect curls or by having the perfect Afro, by having sleek, silky waves or by having big, springy tresses. What

SURVEY SAYS!

When we asked women in our super hair survey how often they washed and conditioned their hair, the answers were pretty clear! Seventy-two percent had wash days at least once per week, with 18 percent of that group having days scheduled at least twice per week.

makes natural hair beautiful is that it's an original, and the original doesn't concern itself with rules, limitations, boundaries or other people's hangups. It simply is.

9.2 Regimen Pointers for New Naturals

Much of the basic hair care advice given for transitioning hair will apply to newly natural tresses as well—with some adjustments of course.

On Wash Day

How often you cleanse and condition your natural hair is a personal choice—but there is a balance to strike. Since our hair is weakest and most easily damaged when wet, cleansing too frequently (more than two times per week) can keep your hair in a vulnerable state. Frequent wetting requires extra detangling manipulation, and those with longer or thicker natural hair may even find that their natural hair never quite dries fully from wash to wash. On the other hand, cleansing and conditioning too infrequently (less than once every two weeks) can lead to dryness and hair breakage issues too. If your natural hair doesn't get the moisture it needs, the fiber will begin to split, peel and crack. Frequent cleansing and conditioning regimens are best for those with shorter natural hair (fade to TWA stage—or less than four inches of natural hair). Frequent wash-day manipulation may prove to be too much for those with longer natural hair—and it simply isn't practical.

In general, if you are new to healthy hair care and just getting started with a regimen, it is best to cleanse and condition your hair every three to five days in the very beginning. This frequency helps improve and restore your hair's natural moisture balance—a process that can take two to three weeks. After this point, you can cleanse and condition your hair every seven to ten days to keep your hair's moisture balance maintained. Others, depending upon their particular hairstyle, may need to adopt a more infrequent cleansing and conditioning schedule. If you are having problems with your hair, your cleansing and conditioning frequency or infrequency may be something to consider.

Conditioner Washing: For a midweek moisture boost, conditioner washing is very helpful. It's a great way to cleanse your hair and maximize the moisture your hair receives. Simply rinse your hair with warm water and apply a conditioner to the hair. Work conditioner into the hair, and rinse after five to seven minutes. Style as desired.

Fade to TWA

Cleansing and conditioning a fade or TWA is very simple—and the ease of this process is often what makes the busiest of us fall in love with hair at this stage! Frequent, even daily, cleansing and conditioning during this stage is possible—and possibly beneficial. During the fade/TWA stage, the risk of your hair tangling and knotting is minimal, so working in sections is not as important now as it will become when your hair begins to accumulate length. In fact, at this point, sectioning your hair in any meaningful way is pretty much impossible!

To boost your hair's moisture throughout the week, simply rinse your hair with warm water and apply a squeeze of lightweight conditioner the size of a quarter to your hair. Use more conditioner if your hair is longer or very thick. Since the hair is still quite short at this stage, there is no real need to work in a shampooing step unless the hair is seriously dirty or product-laden.

After five to seven minutes, rinse the conditioner out in cool water. If your hair is prone to drying out quickly, feel free to leave just a touch of conditioner behind on the hair when rinsing.

Beyond TWAs

Cleansing and conditioning hair that is longer than a TWA takes a bit more time and organization. Simply follow the steps outlined in the cleansing and conditioning section for transitioning hair (page 89-90). As a natural, you must still pay attention to your hair's protein/moisture balance and the cues your hair gives. Please refer to page 52 for more information on managing your hair's balance.

TIP: Instead of using a towel to dry your natural hair, opt for an oversized tee-shirt. Tee-shirts are super absorbent and will dry your hair without creating frizz.

Detangling Your Natural Hair

Natural hair loves being finger combed and finger detangled. Detangling and styling natural hair is all about feeling your way through the hair and navigating around bends, tangles and knots. Your fingers are the absolute best tool for doing this. They were made for this!

Very few people enjoy detangling their hair, relaxed or natural, but you can make it a much more enjoyable experience by preparing your hair for the challenge. The two key things to remember when detangling natural hair are 1) to work with your hair in four to six sections to maintain organization, and 2) to work only with hair that is thoroughly moisturized and conditioned beforehand. Never attempt to work with your natural hair as one large unit, and never attempt to dry detangle your hair.

1. Start with your hair separated into four sections. (You can always break these sections

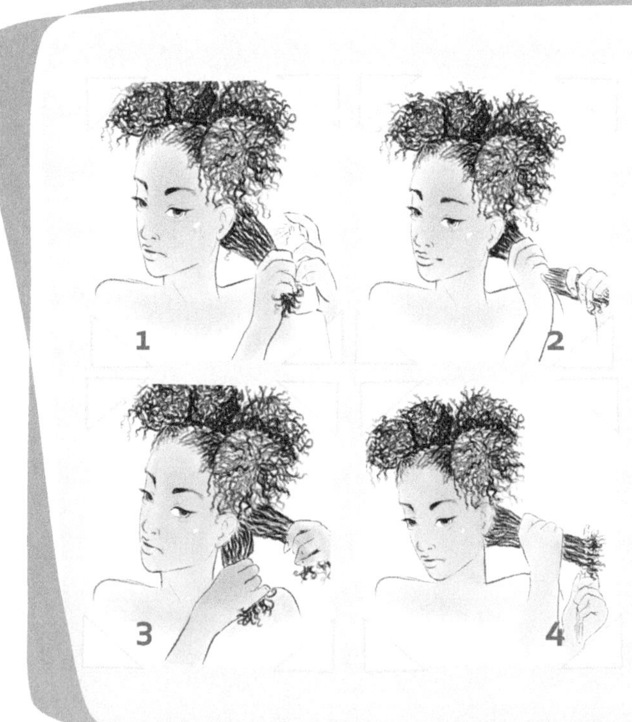

Detangling Your Natural Hair

STEP 1. Section hair, mist with water

STEP 2. Smooth and lengthen out hair.

STEP 3. Gently free and remove tangles from section with your fingers.

STEP 4. Use large-tooth comb to detangle, starting from bottom of section.

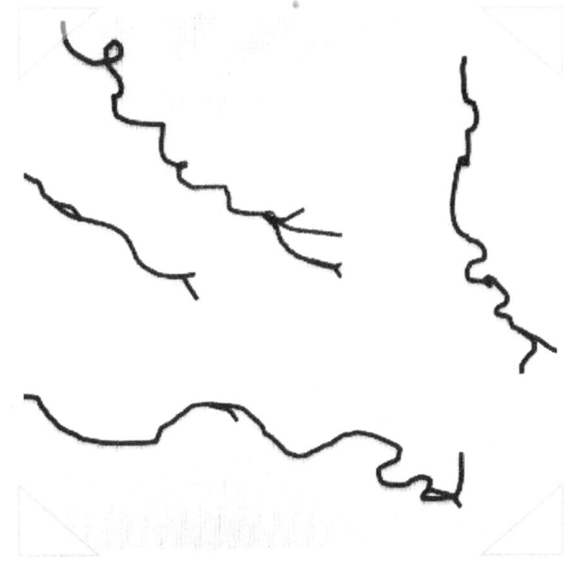

Fig 9.3: Natural hair's split ends can take on a number of shapes and configurations.

down into smaller ones if it helps keep things better organized for you!)

2. Apply a moisturizer or other conditioning product to the hair to soften it and prepare it for detangling.

3. Use your fingers to carefully lengthen out the hair (which is likely hugging the scalp due to shrinkage!) and remove any large tangles from each section.

4. Detangle with a large-tooth seamless comb or a Denman detangling brush if desired. Start from the bottom of your natural hair and work your way back up toward the scalp until your comb or brush passes easily through the hair.

5. Twist the detangled section out of the way, and move on to the next section.

Trimming Your Natural Hair

Staying on top of your trimming schedule is also important, and of course, your schedule will vary depending upon your goals. Some naturals prefer to perform maintenance trims on a set schedule (i.e. every six to eight weeks), while others prefer to trim a handful of times a year, or whenever they see actual damage.

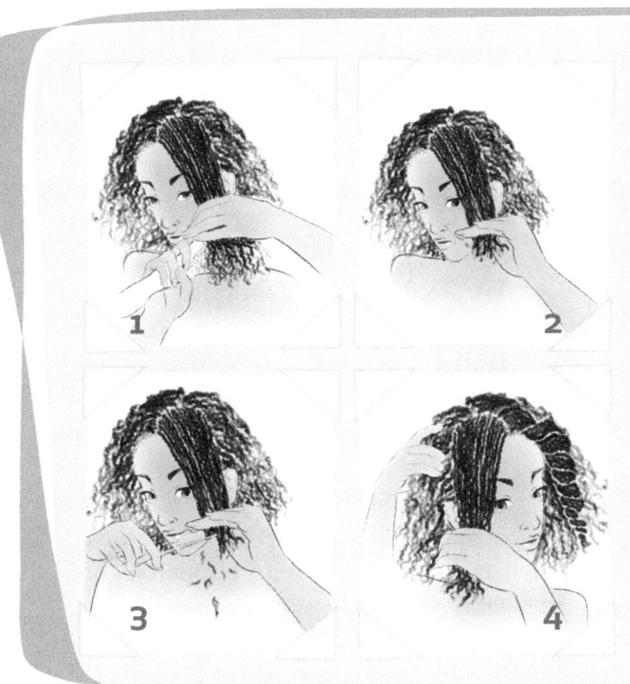

Trimming Your Natural Hair

STEP 1. Detangle and lengthen hair.

STEP 2. and STEP 3. Smooth hair down to about an inch above where you will trim.

STEP 4. Trim hair just above the old damaged hair.

STEP 5. Twist hair, and move to next section.

While natural hair may not need to be trimmed as often as relaxed hair, it still needs occasional maintenance in order to look its best. Pay attention to strands that seem to be on their last leg, with many splits and knots. These strands tend to be scratchy feeling, very dull, lighter colored and dry. You'll know them when you see them. If you allow those types of hairs to linger simply because they have not broken off on their own, they will eventually create tangling problems for you.

One thing you may find out about your natural hair is that it is very resilient. You may even see split-end combinations that you didn't think were possible. In fact, split ends that would have easily broken a strand of your relaxed hair will often linger in your natural hair without ever breaking. Resist the urge to keep such hairs. They will only encourage trouble for you later!

Staying True to the Balance

It is important to maintain a proper balance between protein and moisture by alternating your products accordingly. If we fail to maintain our balance, we will experience hair breakage: Too many protein products, and our hair will produce a dry, snappy breakage; too many moisture products, and our hair will produce a weak, stretchy kind of breakage. In general, hair-care regimens for natural hair should lean more heavily toward the moisture side of the balance.

And we're back to the protein/moisture balance again! Getting a really good understanding of this concept will save you a lot of time, stress and money with your hair. Although protein comprises 70 percent of the hair fiber, the most important part of the protein/moisture balance is the 30 percent water component. Why? Because water is fickle! Water enters and leaves our hair strands twenty-four hours per day, seven days a week. This moisture must be replenished constantly.

Protein, on the other hand, has more staying power. Protein is only lost or depleted when we damage our hair. And, of course, anything that depletes protein will deplete moisture because the two are so interdependent. If our hair's protein structure remains shoddy, moisture will simply pass in and out at a faster rate than normal, leading to extreme dryness and breakage.

If your hair is natural, you will not need to reach for your protein conditioner as often as someone who is chemically-relaxed or color-treated, because much of your hair's natural protein stores are undisturbed and intact. However, since those bonds are also always under attack from the sun, heat use, styling and regular wear and tear, it's still a good idea to have a protein-based conditioner in your arsenal. Most naturals can get away with using protein about once every 1 to 3 months—but, of course, your individual situation may differ. Some naturals go months and months, even years without a protein conditioning. Keep in mind that your other products (shampoos, leave-ins, butters) may also be giving you the small touches of protein you need to stay balanced without the need for a dedicated protein conditioning session.

Throughout the Week

Daily Moisturizing: With natural hair, moisturizing and conditioning are absolutely key. Very often, however, the moisturizing process is rushed, skipped or done haphazardly, almost as an afterthought to the style. This is definitely a recipe for disaster! Your unique hair type, your hairstyle and your outside environment will determine how often you will need to moisturize your hair—but a good rule of thumb is to apply moisturizer at least once or twice daily. Listen to your hair—it will definitely tell you when more moisture is required!

When you are moisturizing natural hair, consider employing a couple of simple techniques to ensure that you are giving your hair the moisture it truly needs.

1. **Section it!** The most important thing to do is to work with your hair in sections whenever possible. Sectioning the hair ensures that each strand, especially those that are in the crown area, receives the moisture coverage it needs. Moisturizing in this manner adds time to the moisturizing process, but it also prevents problem areas from forming later in your hair-care journey.

2. **Stretch it out!** To ensure maximum coverage, it's also a good practice to gently stretch and lengthen out your natural hair as you are moisturizing. Lengthening out the strands ensures that moisture reaches the strand inside of your hair's natural bends, twists and curves, not just on the ends or the exposed part of each curve or bend. Simply scrunching and patting moisturizer through your hair will ensure that you are missing quite a lot of the hair fiber in your moisturizing process. It's tempting, but don't do it!

Feel free to use your favorite water-based spray mixture or water-based cream moisturizer for hydration, followed by an oil or butter of your choice to seal the moisture in. Water-based spray mixes work best on styles that can handle direct moisture: short Afros, puffs, braids or two-strand twists. These styles aren't affected too much by direct application of water. Simply use a spray bottle to mist your hair once or twice daily to keep the hair moist and supple. A good misting mixture will contain water and a bit of conditioner and oil—but feel free to be creative. You can always take an off-the-shelf product spray and add your own bit of goodness to it. My personal favorite mix is ½ cup Water + ¼ cup Kenra Daily Provision Spray (off-the-shelf) + 1 tablespoon or so of Suave coconut conditioner (off-the-shelf) + 1 tablespoon of sweet almond oil or castor oil. Feel free to adjust these amounts or ingredients to your liking.

NOTE: If your mixture includes water and natural ingredients but no off-the-shelf products, you will need to refrigerate your mix to prevent it from going rancid. Off-the-shelf products contain preservatives that help fight off nasty microbes!

Cream moisturizers work better on styles that will frizz or "shrink" with direct water contact. Most loose styles (twist-outs, braid-outs, pressed/flatironed styles) fit into this category and fare better with creams. Creams will moisturize your hair without disrupting your style in most cases.

After moisturizing your hair, gently pat the hair with a light coating of oil to help the moisture stay with the hair longer. Oil acts as a natural barrier to moisture loss. Your hair's texture will determine which types of products (heavy oils vs. lighter oils) you should use on your hair—and whether that extra barrier to moisture loss is even needed. For example, if your hair is fine, you may have to use lighter ingredients or skip the oil barrier so that an excess of product doesn't weigh down your hair. If your hair is thicker, you might consider using a butter product rather than an oil to seal in your moisture.

Styling as a New Natural

Super Short!

If your natural hair is six months old (two or three inches) or less, styling will come pretty easily. Hair at this length is pretty much wash and GO! Styling your hair at this point is simply a matter of keeping it conditioned, moisturized and sealed. Accessories tend to figure in pretty big during this stage. Popular hair accessories include decorative clips, bands and flowers.

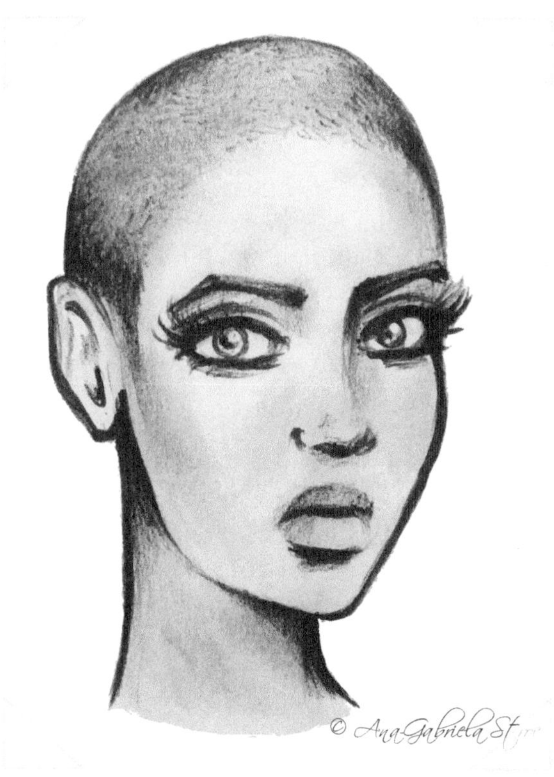

Fig 9.4: Hair at this length is fuss free and truly wash and go!

Accessorized TWA: There quite a few ways to style a TWA, and it is truly one of the lowest-maintenance styles available. Even a carefully placed front parting can add the right bit of spice and interest to a basic TWA or fade. [Fig. 9.5]

Comb Coils: When your TWA starts to gain a bit of length, comb coils (finger coils) [Fig. 9.6a] are one of the first natural hairstyles that become achievable. While comb coils can be done on longer natural hair, they look their absolute best on very short natural hair. Comb coils can be worn for up to four weeks without issue; if left to their own devices for longer, however, the coils will begin to form dreadlocks. (For this reason, comb coils are also often used as a starter loc style.) To cleanse your hair while in comb coils, you can simply place a stocking cap over the hair to preserve the hairstyle. The water will seep through the cap but won't disturb your coil pattern. Unravel coils to create a coil-out style. [Fig.9.6b]

The Wash-and-Go a.k.a. Wash-and-Wear a.k.a. Shake-and-Go. The wash-and-go is just as it sounds. You wash, condition, shake and, ideally, you go! This style was the go-to style of choice for about 12 percent of our hair survey respondents, second only to twists and twistouts.

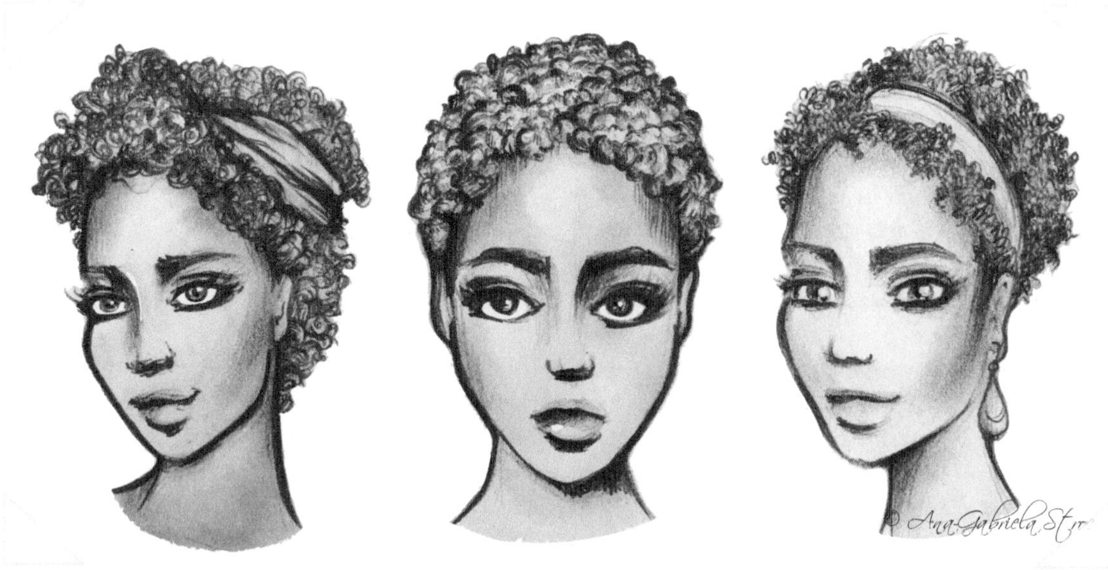

Fig 9.5: At this length, many of your style options will include accessorizing your TWA with headbands or flowers and accentuating your kink, coil or wave pattern.

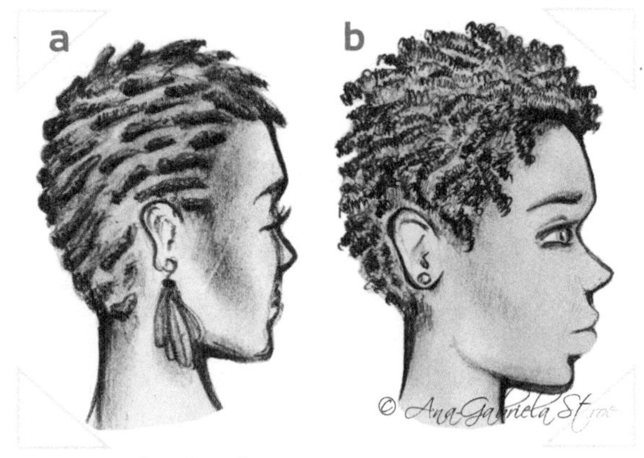

Fig 9.6a: Comb coils.

Fig 9.6b: Coil-out.

Shaking the hair encourages the hair's natural pattern to emerge. After shaking, very few products are used on a wash-and-go. Typically only a shine serum or anti-frizz product is used to add polish to the style. With shorter hair, it's much easier to have a true wash-and-go routine, but as your hair grows and its various textures and patterns emerge, things may get trickier. Although true wash-and-gos are great low-manipulation protective styles, the style has its downsides. Knotting and tangling are two common problems associated with wash-and-go styling, especially when the hair begins to pick up length.

The wash-and-go can also serve as a preparatory step to achieve other "curls-on-the-go" types of styles. For many new naturals with considerable transitioning time under their belts (i.e., more hair!), their wash-and-go process is more like: wash, condition, detangle, rake through gel

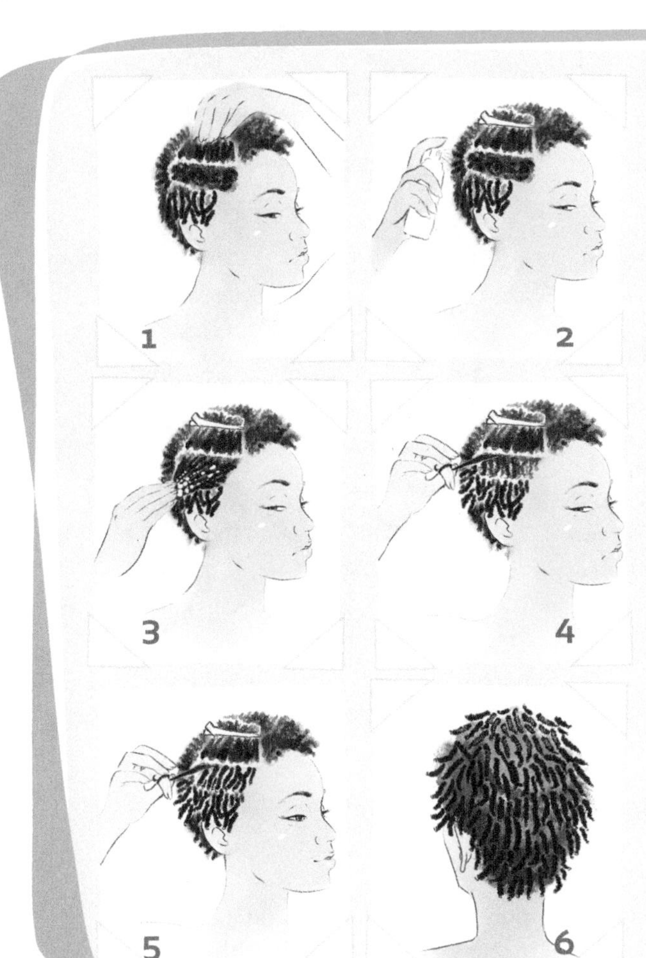

How To Create Comb Coils

STEP 1. Section hair with comb.

STEP 2. Spray hair with water.

STEP 3. Apply gel or other styling product to hair from roots to ends.

STEP 4. Take a small section of hair and coil around fingers. Release.

STEP 5. Continue twisting hair.

STEP 6. Done!

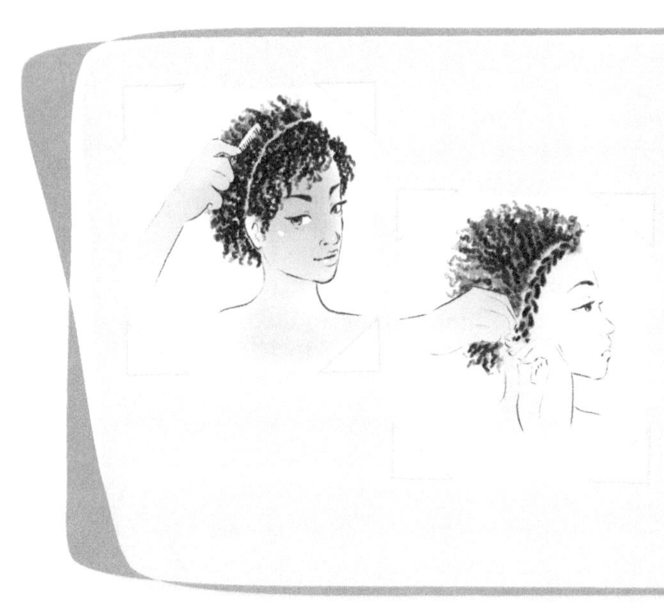

The braided headband is a style that can be created on short to medium-length natural hair.

Simply part the hair about one inch back from the hairline. Create a side part to separate the front section into two sections. Braid or flat twist your hair along the front section to create a headband. Pin braid behind ear, and repeat on other side.

or other curl-defining products, shake, dry and then go. If you are having to add tons of product and go through several additional steps and techniques to bring out your curl pattern, then your wash-and-go is technically not a wash-and-go but a wash-and-go plus style.

The wash-and-go plus style is difficult for some to master because it usually involves finding the right combination of curl-defining products, putting them on in the correct order and praying that the weather cooperates with your hair plans! If your hair's natural pattern is not curly, coily or particularly defined, it will be difficult, if not impossible, to replicate your favorite curly blogger's wash-and-go—even with top-quality gels and defining products.

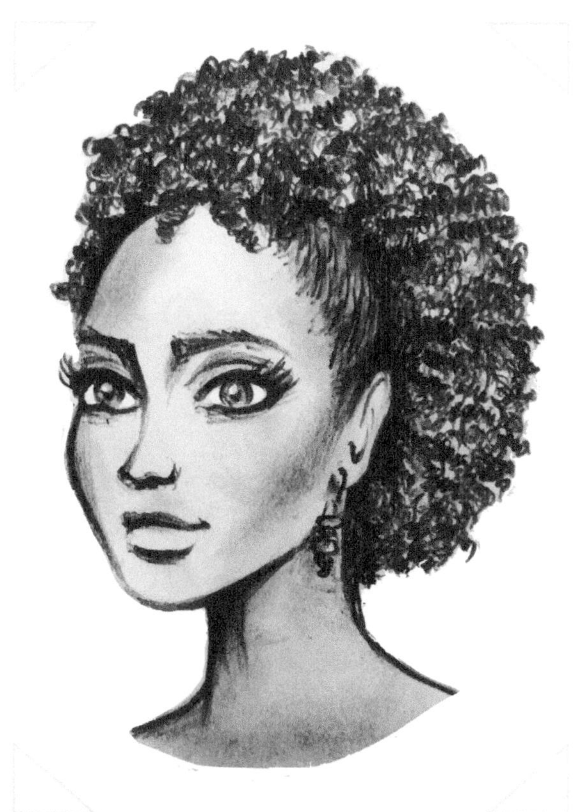

Fig 9.7: The side pinup can be worn on one side or both.

Mid-Length Strands

After about three inches of growth, many new naturals enter an in-between phase of length. In this phase, the hair is too long to be a TWA but not long enough to be styled as much else. Having your hair professionally shaped during the in-between phases is a good pick-me-up and will eliminate some of the styling challenges that come up during this time. If you have at least six months of new growth (more than two or three inches of hair), there are still quite a few styles that you can achieve at this length.

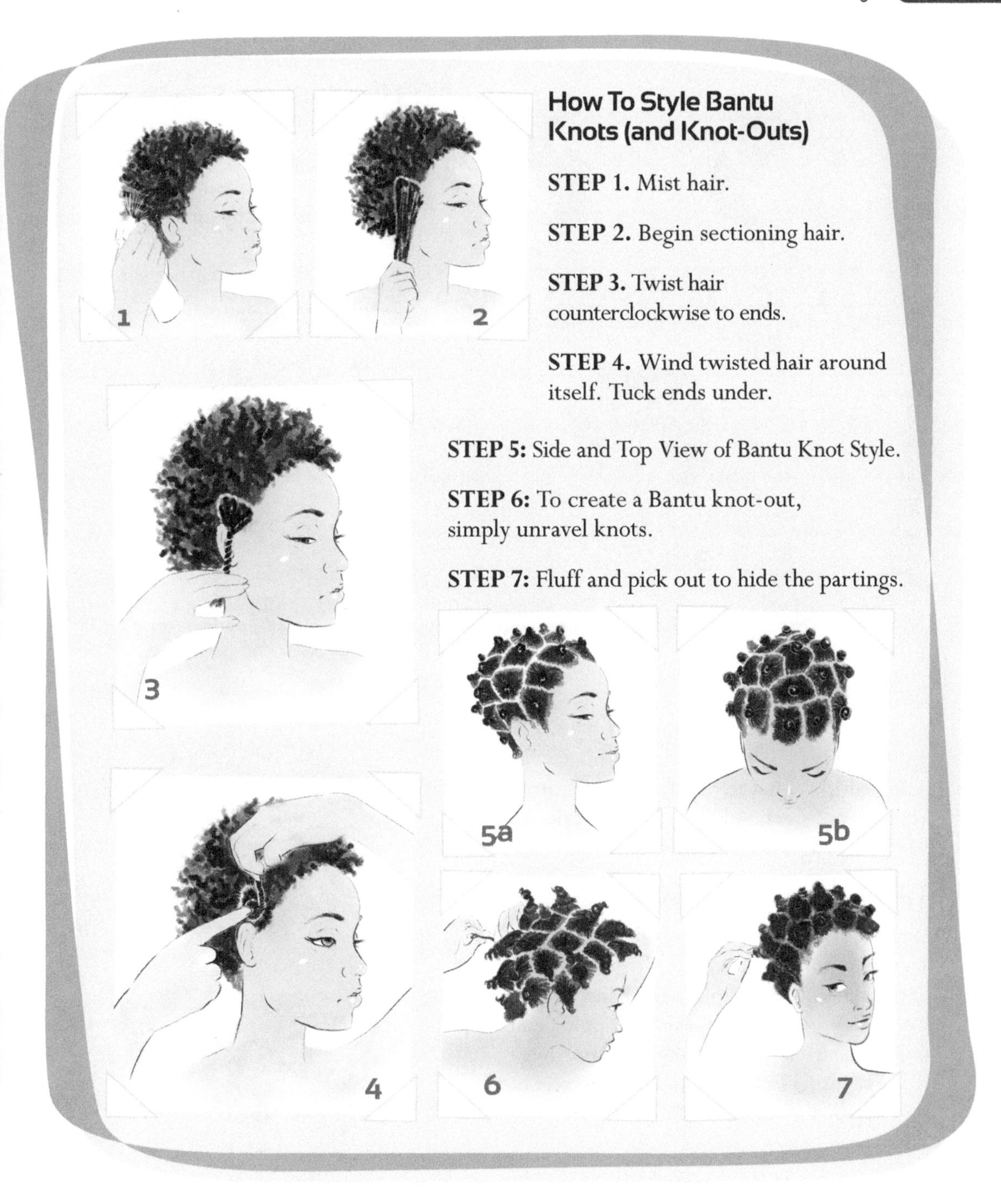

Afro Puffs: If your natural hair is kinky-curly, you'll be able to pull off an Afro or Afro puff style. When many women think of natural hair, these are the styles that often come to mind. They are both natural-hair classics! The puff is a great go-to style for when your twist-out or another style is ready to be redone and you are not quite ready for wash day.

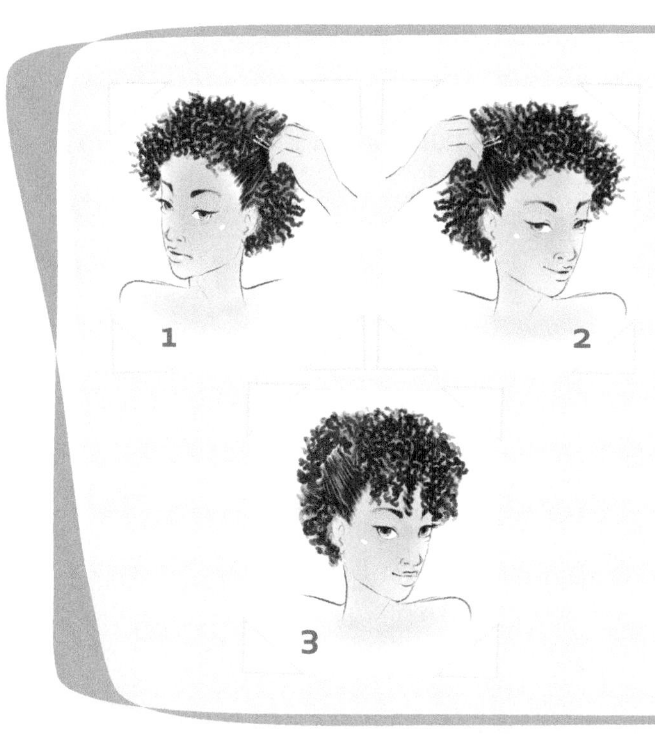

How To Style a Side Pinup

STEP 1. Gently pull a section of hair just above the ear straight up. Secure with bobby pin.

STEP 2. Repeat on other side if desired.

STEP 3. Done.

Creating Your Puff

There are a few simple ways to create a puff. In nearly all variations, you'll need to mist your sides and edges with water and apply a moisturizer before you start. Adding gel or a styler to lay down the edges is optional.

OPTION 1: The "headband puff" method works by using an oversized Ouchless® headband (important to minimize breakage!). To get the band around your hair, simply place the band around your neck first (double it for a snugger puff), and then slide the front of the band up to your forehead. Next, using both hands, work the rest of the band up and around the hair.

OPTION 2: Alternatively, you can use a cut leg of hosiery, or a silky knee-high stocking to secure your puff. This option works well for those who want to fully control the tension created by their puffs. After moisturizing and brushing your sides:

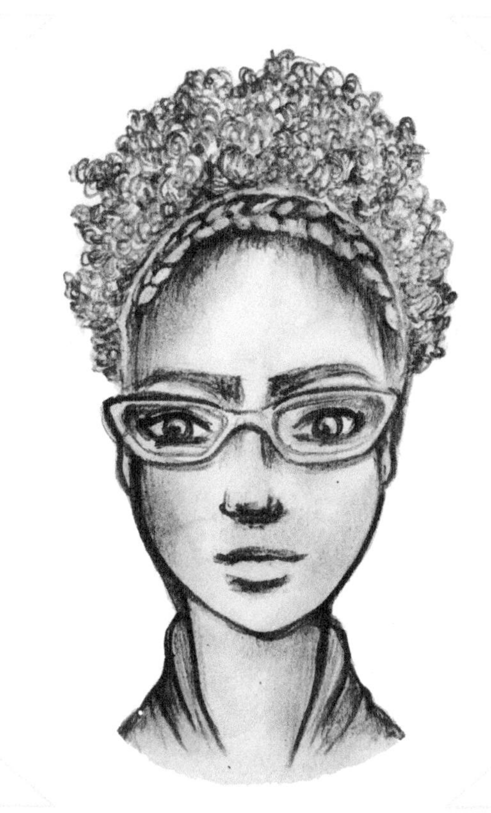

Fig 9.8: Add some jazz to your puff by incorporating a braided headband.

To ensure that you get maximum length or height from your puff, avoid using the headband as a reg-

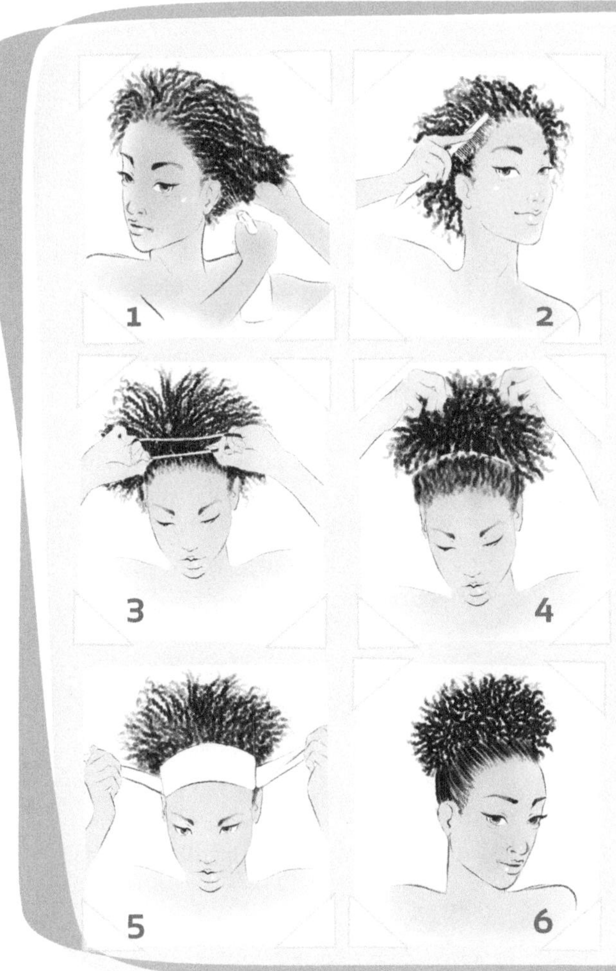

Puff Style

STEP 1. Spray edges and sides of hair. Apply moisturizer to soften the hair.

STEP 2. Using a soft-bristle brush, gently brush the sides of your hair back and up toward the top of your head.

STEP 3. Place a large, stretchy headband (Ouchless®) around the hair. Loop twice for a tighter fit.

STEP 4. Fluff with fingers.

STEP 5. Tie a satin scarf around your edges to smooth them.

STEP 6. Done!

My Go-To Style

Twists are by far my absolute favorite style. I often wear my hair in minitwists (half a pencil width) that I style in various ways for about seven days. I cleanse my hair on the seventh day and braid my twists into four to five plaits. Once my hair is dry, I unravel the plaits and wear my new curly minitwists for another several days. Next, I unravel the minitwists entirely to wear a twist-out for another few days. My final day is spent in an Afro puff, and then the process repeats itself!

ular ponytail holder. Instead, take advantage of your headband's large size and allow the volume of your hair to fill in the space. To add even more length, you can plait or band your hair on wash day, or lightly blow dry your freshly washed and conditioned hair. Be careful not to pull too hard on the delicate hairline when drawing your puff. Many new naturals make their puffs very tight in an effort to achieve maximum sleekness along the front part of the puff, and also to smooth short hair into the style. To create a sleek finish at the hairline, simply mist the hair with water and apply a defining cream, butter or lightweight gel (not the brown, protein-packed extra-hold styling gel!) to the front and sides. Tie down your hair with a satin scarf and allow it to stay on the hair for about ten minutes. Gel is optional, but

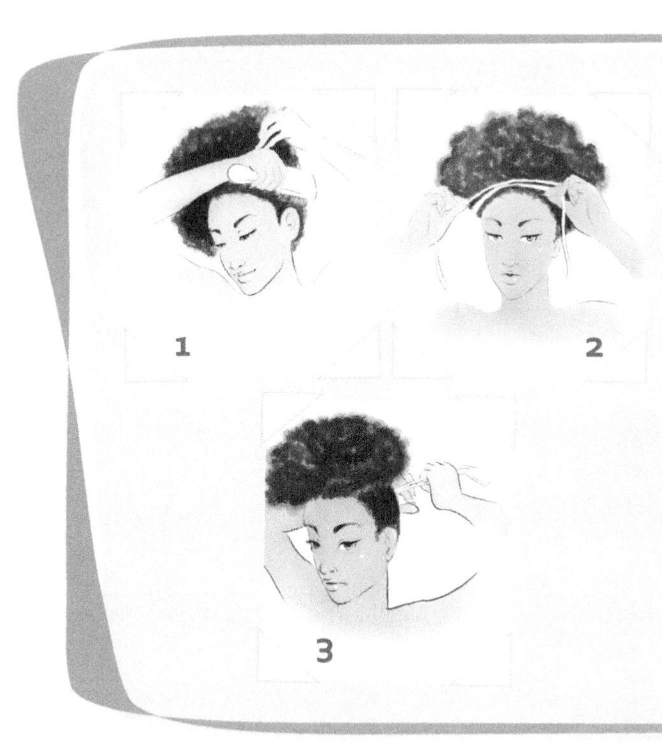

Puff Style Alternate

STEP 1. Simply place the length of the stocking tie along the back hairline.

STEP 2. Grasp the ends of the tie and wrap them around to the front of your head, creating a circle around your hair.

STEP 3. Pull on both ends of the tie to tighten the puff. Wrap the ends of the stocking tie around the puff and tuck them underneath the circle band you've created.

it will give you a faster, firmer hold. Ecostyler gel and Fantasia IC gel are popular, crunch-free gels that work well for this style.

Twists: Twists are an extremely versatile protective style. They can be worn for their own merits or used to set the stage for future styles throughout the week. Twists can be unraveled to form twist-outs or kept intact and manipulated to create updos and virtually any hairstyle you can create on straight hair. Twists can even be braided together and roller set to create wavy and curly styles. Because twisting is much easier than braiding for most people, they are a quick, DIY-friendly way to style natural hair. In fact, 44 percent of our survey respondents listed twists and twistouts as their go-to style.

Although you can successfully twist your hair either wet or dry, you will always get the best curl definition (and greatest shrinkage) when twisting on wet or damp hair. If you twist on dry hair, you'll have longer twists that won't shrink as much—but any twist-out that you create with these twists will not have as much definition unless they've been misted and allowed to dry first.

How To Twist Your Hair

1. Start with freshly cleaned, conditioned and detangled hair (or clean, dry hair, if you prefer).

2. Use your fingers to carefully isolate a section of hair. (Use larger sections for bigger twists with less definition or smaller sections for smaller twists with lots of body and definition.) Be sure to keep your twists at roughly the same size for best results.

3. Finger-detangle each section one more time to ensure that the hair will be smooth in the twist.

4. Divide the section into two equal parts and twist two sections of hair together, crossing left over right until you reach the ends. If you make your twists with a left-

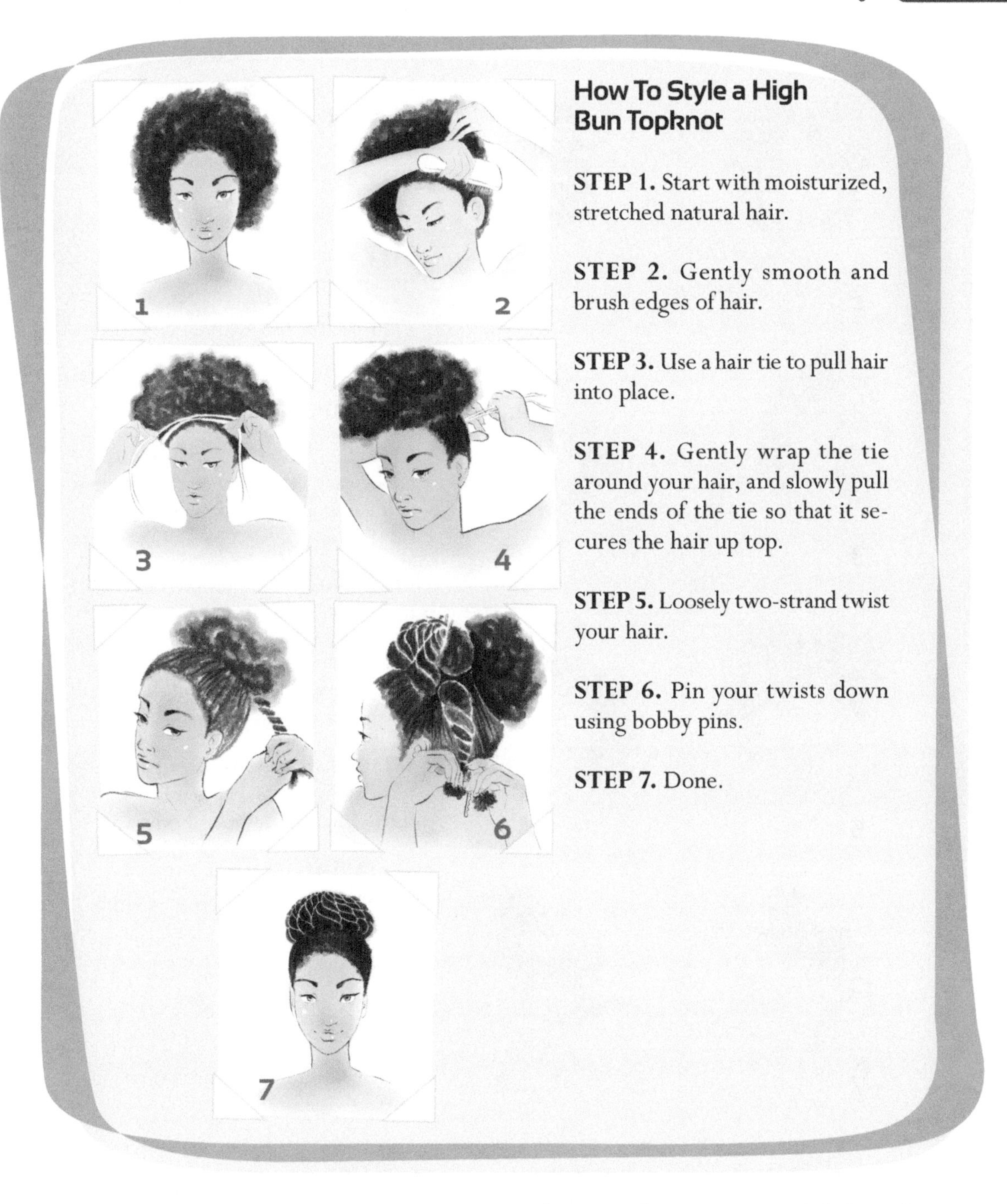

over-right twisting motion as you move downward, your twists will hold together better than if you twist only with a downward motion.

5. Twirl the ends of the twist around your finger to encourage your ends to curl. Ends that do not curl with gentle encouragement may be a sign that a trim is needed if your hair is naturally a curly or coily type.

Twists begin to gain character as they age, usually swelling a bit in size and shrinking in length. If you intend to wear your twists as a style, you may occasionally need to retwist some sections to keep your set looking fresh.

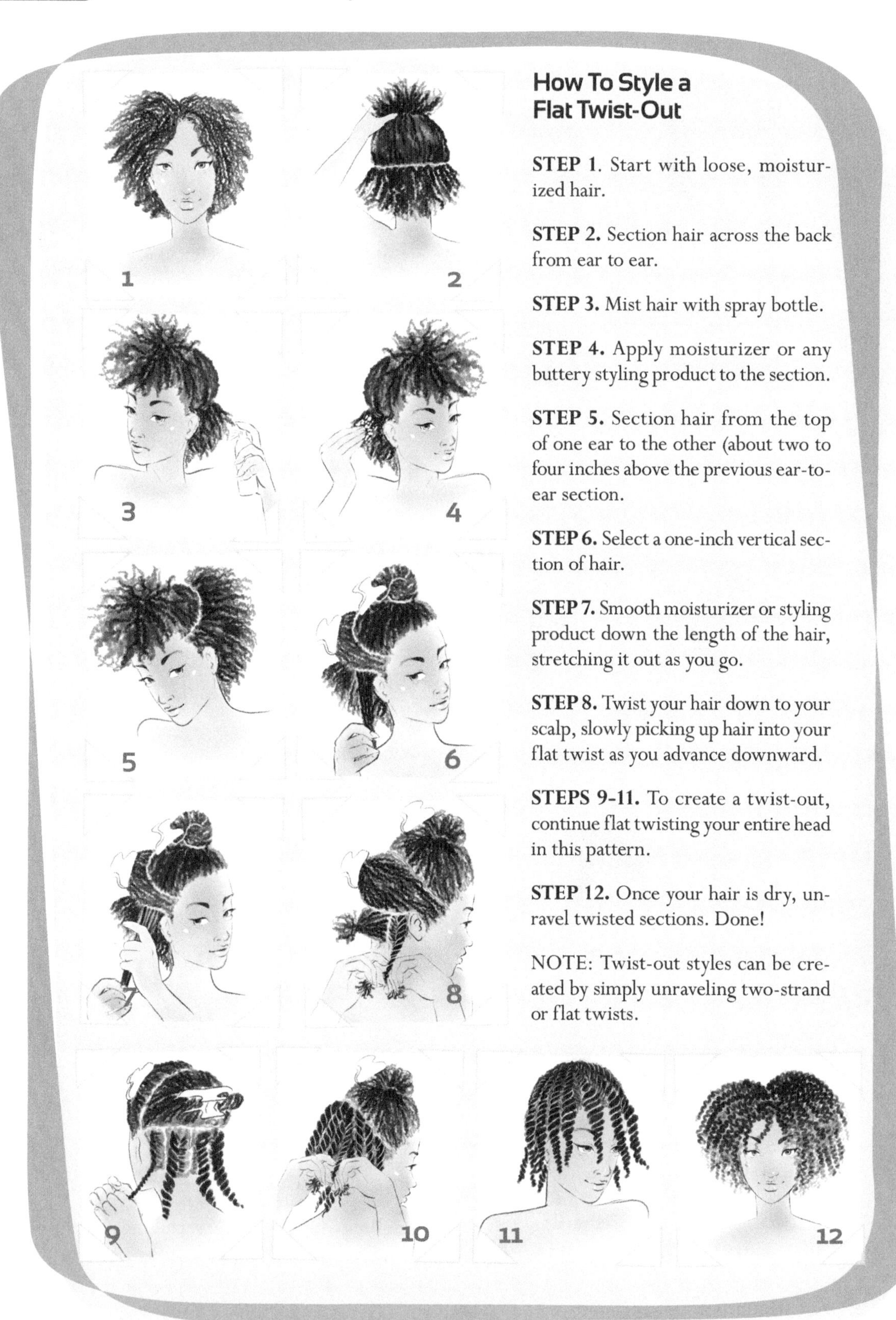

How To Style a Flat Twist-Out

STEP 1. Start with loose, moisturized hair.

STEP 2. Section hair across the back from ear to ear.

STEP 3. Mist hair with spray bottle.

STEP 4. Apply moisturizer or any buttery styling product to the section.

STEP 5. Section hair from the top of one ear to the other (about two to four inches above the previous ear-to-ear section.

STEP 6. Select a one-inch vertical section of hair.

STEP 7. Smooth moisturizer or styling product down the length of the hair, stretching it out as you go.

STEP 8. Twist your hair down to your scalp, slowly picking up hair into your flat twist as you advance downward.

STEPS 9-11. To create a twist-out, continue flat twisting your entire head in this pattern.

STEP 12. Once your hair is dry, unravel twisted sections. Done!

NOTE: Twist-out styles can be created by simply unraveling two-strand or flat twists.

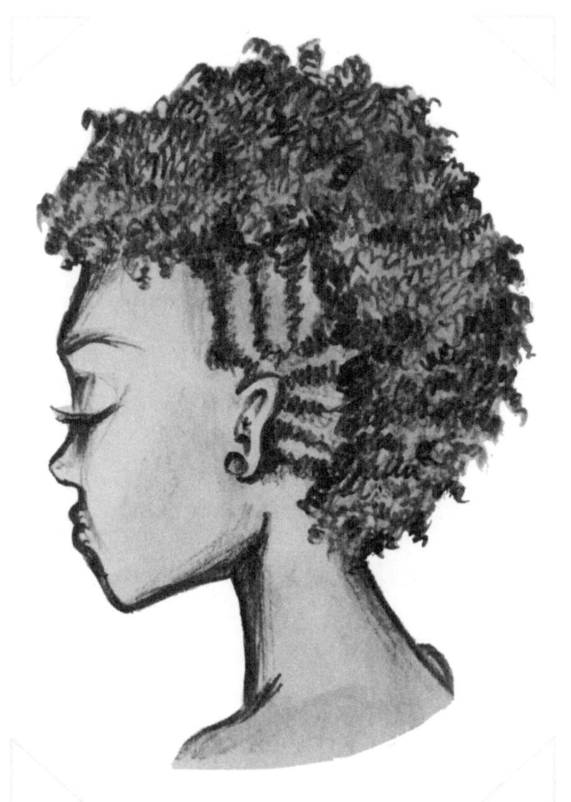

Fig 9.9: Flat twists can be added to the side of Afros or twist-outs to add character to the style.

For those with more than six to nine months of natural new growth, even more styles are possible. YouTube is a great video resource for step-by-step styling instructions for nearly any style that you can think of!

Night Care

Although it is often overlooked, the nighttime routine is very important for those of us with natural hair. Protecting your hair before you go to bed will ensure that you wake up to soft, supple hair that is ready for styling the next morning. A disorganized or nonexistent nighttime regimen often leads to tangling and matting that ultimately cause breakage and frustration with your natural hair in the long run. Take just a few moments each night to pamper your tresses, and you'll be glad you did!

Here are your three nighttime prep steps:

1. **Moisturize and seal it**. Simply apply a water-based moisturizing product to your hair before bed as needed. Follow the moisturizer with an oil to help seal in your moisture and preserve your hair's conditioned state. Do not go to bed with thirsty hair!

2. **Set it and forget it.** To reduce tangling, matting and shrinkage at night, you will need to "set" your hair at night. The setting method you choose will vary, depending upon how you plan to wear your hair the following day. If your morning style will need a bit of hold, apply a styling cream with light to medium hold after your moisturizer or oil to keep things together. Depending on how neatly you create your set, some of these nighttime protective styles can even be worn out and about for a few days. Bonus!

    a. *Chunky twists:* Separate your hair into four large sections. Loosely twist (or braid) each section into four or five smaller sections. The smaller the twists, the more texture, definition and volume your hair will have. The thicker your twists are, the more stretched and undefined your hair will be. Stretch the twists out and pin them down for maximum length in the morning, pincurl them for a curly look or simply tie them down as is. Cover your hair with a bonnet or scarf. In the morning, remoisturize if needed and fluff. This sleep preparation method works best for twist-outs, pinned updos that require stretched hair and Afro puffs.

    b. *Cornrows and flat twists:* Braid your hair into two to four large cornrow braids or flat twists rather than braids. This preparation method stretches the hair and creates a looser, wavier look than chunky twists. As with the pre-

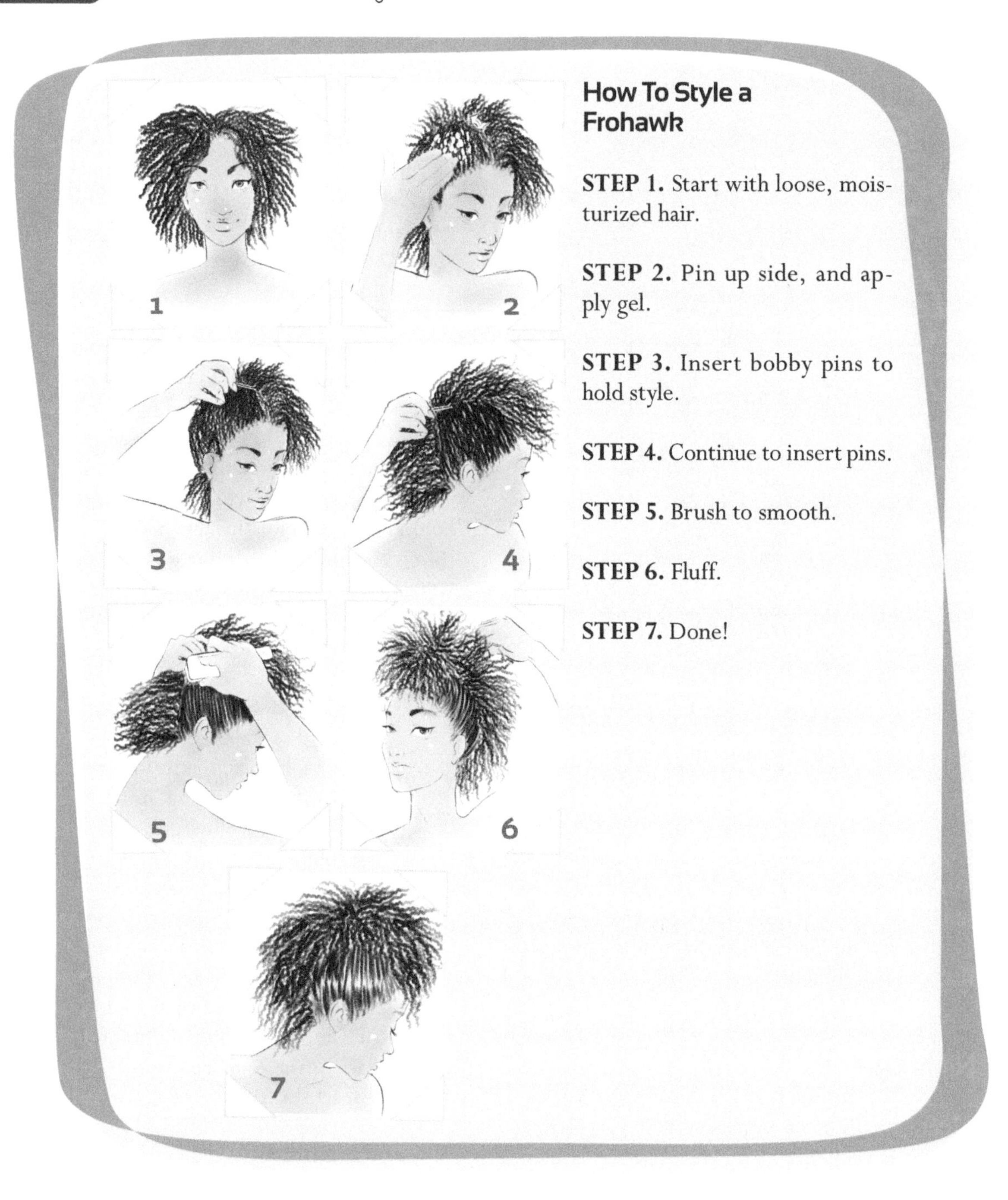

How To Style a Frohawk

STEP 1. Start with loose, moisturized hair.

STEP 2. Pin up side, and apply gel.

STEP 3. Insert bobby pins to hold style.

STEP 4. Continue to insert pins.

STEP 5. Brush to smooth.

STEP 6. Fluff.

STEP 7. Done!

vious prep method, the smaller the cornrows or flat twists, the tighter and more defined your hair's waves will be. Of all the night preparation methods, this is one of the easiest to sleep on at night! This prep method is best for creating stretched updo styles, Afro puffs and wavy styles on hair that is already styled in twists or minitwists.

c. *Bantu knots:* Bantu knots are not actually knots but minibuns. To create Bantu knots, simply twist or twirl a section of hair around in your fingers two to three times. Next, wind the

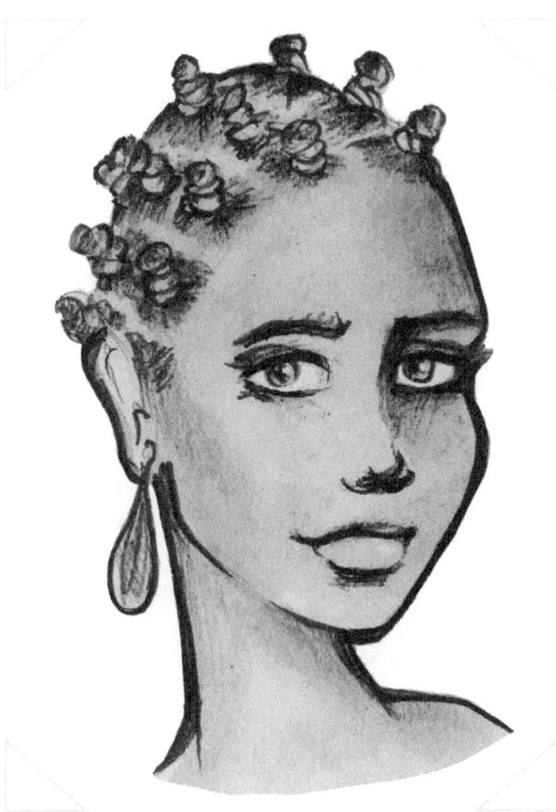

Fig 9.10:Bantu knots are also known as "China bumps" and "Zulu knots."

hair around itself into a minibun. You can tuck the ends under the bun or pin the little bun into place. Bantu knots will give you a playful, curly look the following morning. For large curls, eight Bantu knots will do the job. For a tighter, springier and more defined look, ten to twelve knots will work. If you are simply using Bantu knots to stretch out your hair, up to four knots will accomplish this goal. Longer hair tends to need fewer knots than shorter hair to achieve a full, voluminous look. The downside: Bantu knots can be a challenge to sleep on at night!

d. *Pineapple method:* If your hair is longer, you can set your hair with what is referred to as the "pineapple method." To do this, simply bend forward at the waist and gather your hair into a high ponytail. Fold your headscarf into a triangle, and secure the scarf around your head, tying the knot in the front

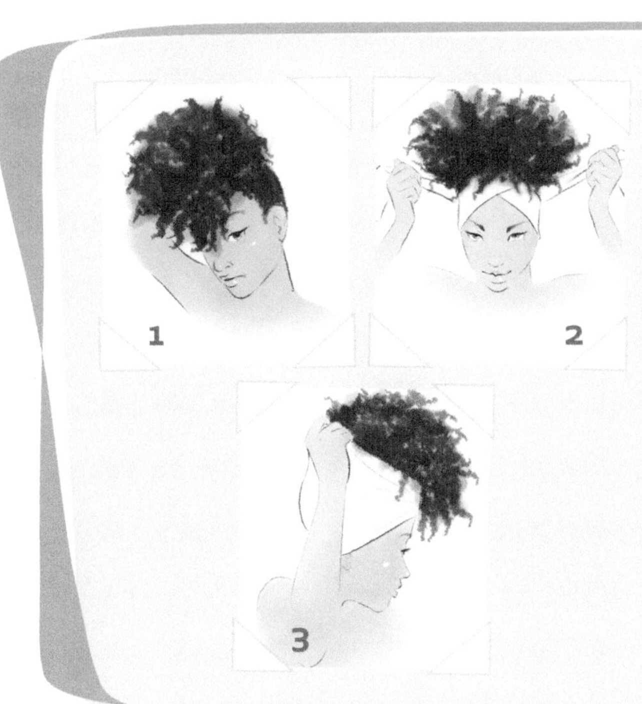

How to Create a Pineapple

STEP 1. Gather hair to the top of the head, or secure in a high ponytail.

STEP 2. Fold scarf into triangle and secure across the back of the head. Tie in front.

STEP 3. Slide back part of scarf upward to cover more of the back of the head.

of your head. The large part of the scarf should be covering the back portion of your head. The pineapple allows you to sleep on your hair, and provides incredible volume for wash-and-gos, twist-outs and braid-outs the following day. In the morning, simply remoisturize as needed and scrunch the hair.

e. Bun: If your hair is already straight or stretched, a simple bun is a good way to preserve your hairstyle at night. High buns work very well for keeping your hair together and stretched without affecting your style.

3. **Cover it.** No matter how you choose to set your hair, always be sure to protect your hair at night by covering it in a protective satin bonnet or scarf. Cotton pillows and sheets are extremely absorbent and will sap the natural moisture from your hair. The difference after employing a satin head covering is one that can be felt. Hair that has been protected under a scarf or bonnet almost always feels more moisturized and healthier than hair that has been allowed to rub around on pillows and sheets all night. If this happens night after night, over the long term you'll have drier hair that is always more prone to breakage the following morning. You could even slowly rub out your delicate edges due to the combination of friction and dryness. Always, always protect your hair at night. It's okay if your scarf doesn't stay with you during the entire night. The goal is to have more nights than not with protection for your hair!

Your Chapter 9 Take-Aways

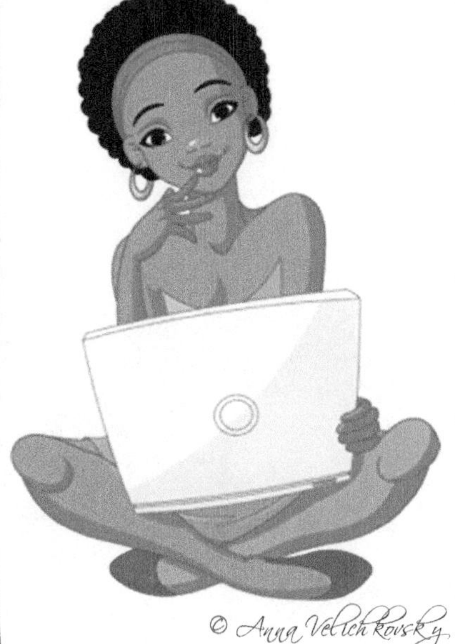

- ✓ No hair texture, length or style is 100-percent maintenance free.
- ✓ Our eyes tell us much about the world around us, but they aren't very good at assessing the quality or health of natural hair.
- ✓ Our hair is strongest in its natural state, but is still requires a gentle touch to thrive.
- ✓ Natural hair's tendency to draw up tightly and hug the scalp when dry makes it appear much shorter than it truly is.
- ✓ The best way to avoid severe knotting and tangling is to keep the hair in stretched or protective styles.
- ✓ Whenever our hair's protein structure is damaged by relaxing, coloring, heat use or photochemical damage (sun damage), our hair increases in porosity, and we have to include protein conditioning products in our hair-care regimen to restore the protein balance.
- ✓ How often you cleanse and condition your natural hair is a personal choice—but there is a balance to strike.
- ✓ To ensure maximum hair-product coverage, it's also a good practice to gently stretch and lengthen out your natural hair as you are moisturizing or applying product.
- ✓ Protecting your hair before you go to bed will ensure that you wake up to soft, supple hair that is ready for styling the next morning.

Chapter 10: Supernatural Maintenance Ti & Strategies

Fig 10.0: You've made it! You are now supernatural!

In the maintenance phase, you've been natural for at least a year. Your change has become habit now, and the chances for relaxer relapse are significantly lower. This is especially true if your mental transition has gone smoothly, and you've grown more comfortable with your new hair. Here are some tips and things to keep in mind as you work through the maintenance phase.

Keep It Simple

As you get comfortable with your natural hair, you'll soon find that extra-complicated regimens just don't work. Why? It's the same reason that really complicated diets don't work. They are just too hard to follow for the long term! It's best to identify a few key principles that work well for you and execute them flawlessly, rather than try to do a little of everything that works for everyone else. When it comes to hair care, doing a few things right all of the time is better than doing a lot of things right some of the time. Believe it or not, boring, repetitive regimens tend to be some of the most effective regimens out there! Now, I'm not saying to put a bag over your head and lose all hope! But keep in mind that the less manipulation your hair encounters, the easier it will be to minimize breakage and tangling situations and maximize your hair growth. Cut out the fluff, and you'll be well on your way.

Anticipate Adjustments

As your hair gains length and thickness, you'll have to change some aspects of your regimen. You will need to make adjustments based on issues that come up with your hair and living routine, as well as the specific demands of your hairstyle. For example, if you were cleansing and conditioning once a week at one time, your parched strands may mean you'll have to step up the conditioning frequency. Or, if your hair is holding up well in a certain style, you may choose to back off on some planned cleansing and conditioning for a while longer. These are judgment calls that you'll have to make.

10.1 On Dividing & Conquering

One tenet will become more and more important as your hair begins to thrive and grow: Divide and conquer. This means working on your hair in manageable sections. This is extremely important when it comes to detangling and applying conditioners to your growing natural hair. Many women don't increase the amount of conditioner they are using as their hair grows bigger/longer. They also neglect the hair deepest in the center of the head and crown area—with longer hair, these sections can be pretty hard to reach. Coincidentally (or perhaps not), these sections also tend to be some of the driest sections of hair. They desperately need regular, dedicated moisture, or they will succumb to breakage. The best way to ensure proper conditioner coverage is to use the CCC (or comprehensive conditioner coverage) method when you are conditioning your hair. In this method, you simply part your hair at one-inch intervals using your fingers. Then, take each section of hair and apply conditioner to both sides of the section. Lengthen and stretch out the section of hair as you apply the conditioner product. These steps will ensure that the entire strand and the ends are treated. Sure, it's tedious, and it uses a lot of conditioner product, but it is so worth it for your hair.

10.2 On Moisturizing

When you're moisturizing your natural hair, it's always important to stretch the hair out to ensure that the full length of the strand is being treated with product. As natural hair shrinks and folds back onto itself, it leaves many areas of the strand inaccessible to the quickie method of dabbing moisturizer over the surface of your hair. An easy way to ensure that you cover the total length of the strands is to apply the moisturizer or oil to your hands and rub your palms together. Gently clasp your hair between your hands and smooth your hands together downward along the strands. This method of product application is often referred to as the "prayer method" because of the hand positioning.

When you are selecting moisturizer products, always look for products that contain water as a first ingredient and are free of heavy, hair-shaft-coating oils such as petrolatum and mineral oil. See pages 53-55 for more information on choosing a great moisturizer.

10.3 On Maintenance Trimming

Don't let your ends go without your attention. Every three months or so, do a quick scan of your ends to see how you are doing. Keeping your ends manicured can go a long way toward ensuring that you are seeing the best length retention possible.

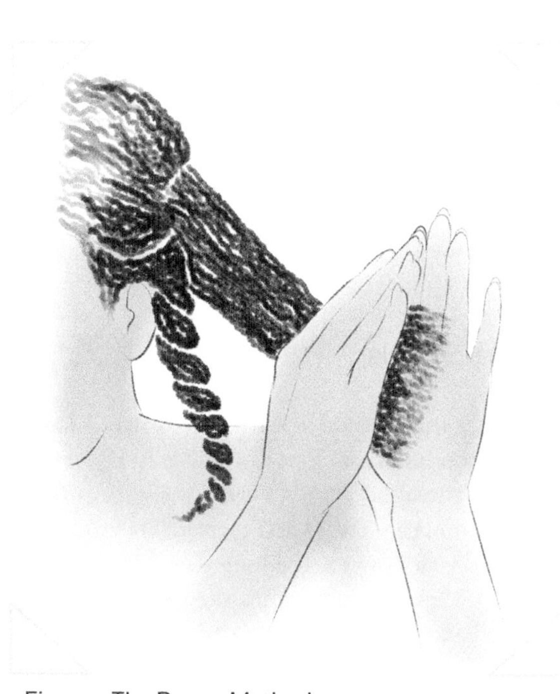

Fig 10.1: The Prayer Method.

If you've been styling protectively, you should not see as much stress showing up at the ends of your hair. This is not to say that there won't be some pretty awful-looking strands here and there, but if you are keeping your hair well-hydrated, the amount of damage to be cleaned up should be minimal. If you are finding that you have a lot of split ends, knots and shredded looking ends, that's either an indication that your ends aren't getting moisture with the needed frequency or that some ends are just worn out and it's time to let them go.

Some people say that trimming grows the hair or promotes hair growth. This is only partially true. Trimming does promote hair growth in that it helps prevent the unnecessary loss of hair at the ends. This means that you can see your hair growing longer over time much sooner. Trimming, however, does not have any effect on the speed at which your hair emerges from the scalp, on the quality of the hair that comes from the scalp or on the ability of your hair to grow from the scalp. Your body controls all of these processes internally. Trimming simply makes your ends look nice and reduces tangling and splitting that can lead to breakage.

For best results, natural hair trims should only be done on dry hair. It's easy to see why this makes sense if you've ever attempted to cut a piece of paper while it's wet. Try it! Even the best shears cannot cut wet paper cleanly. The same thing goes for your hair. Always trim your hair while it is dry.

There are other good reasons for only trimming and cutting the hair while it is dry. Consider the fact that when we wet our hair, it stretches out with the weight of the water and appears much longer. Depending on your hair's porosity, which will vary from section to section, your hair will absorb more or less water in some parts than in others. When our hair dries, this excess water is removed and our hair shrinks back to its normal length.

For this reason, dry length is a much more stable indicator of where your hair measures up. When you cut wet or damp hair, you never get the length you saw when it was wet. We always get our truest indication of length when our hair is fully dry.

Finally, with kinky, curly and wavy hair types, the wet hair shape is often drastically different from the dry hair shape. Those of you who have curls when the hair is wet, and nothing when the hair is dry know exactly what I'm taking about! Cutting the hair based on its wet state is just asking for trouble—lopsided, shapeless and probably much-shorter-than-you-imagined kinds of trouble!

For best results, trim your hair in the style or state in which you wear it. If you are a natural who'll be wearing your hair straight all of the time, you'll need to trim when your hair is straightened. Find a stylist who is experienced in working with a range of different kinky, curly and wavy-textured hair types.

10.4 On Protective Styling

Wearing protective styles is one of those things that some either love or hate. But one thing is for sure: Protective styling is a quick path to lengthier strands that don't need to be trimmed as often. Exposure to the air and regular brushing, combing and styling all quickly deteriorate the ends of the hair, leading to splitting, peeling and breakage. Keeping your hair in styles like twists, buns and pinups helps to keep manipulation down to a minimum. When low manipulation is combined with a moisture-rich and protein-balanced hair-care regimen, your natural hair will thrive!

If you are in growth mode, then protective styles can really fast-track you to your goals. The problem with protective styling is that it can get to be a bit boring for even the most dedicated women out there. There are only so many buns a woman can do—right? Wrong! Protective styling doesn't have to be boring! You'd be surprised at the level of creativity some of your fellow naturals have! There is no lack of inspiration for protective styling out there. A simple search of "natural hair styles" or "natural protective styles" on YouTube brings up more than 100,000 video search results!

If you're still not that into protective styling, why not give your hair a boost by incorporating low-manipulation styles into your routine during the week and save your out-and-about styles for the weekend, holidays and other special occasions?

10.5 On Using Heat

No matter how you choose to wear your hair, protecting your hair against heat damage is extremely important. Your kinks, curls and coils depend on it! Overzealous heat use can permanently destroy your natural curl pattern, leaving you with weak, limp straight pieces of hair. With so much at risk, it is no wonder that 27 percent of naturals who responded to our hair survey said that they never use heat on their hair! Another 44 percent told us that they only rarely use heat, and many months pass between uses. Hooded dryers are a good exception to the heat rule. These appliances deliver an even, controlled form of indirect heat that is much easier on the hair.

Remember, we are all different. Just because your sister can fire up her irons daily with very little damage, doesn't mean that you're cleared, too. Responsible heat use now will prevent you from having to complete another Big Chop later! Here are some quick tips for using heat responsibly.

> **The Science of Black Hair Super Survey**
>
> **Survey Says! 27%** of our super survey respondents NEVER use heat on their natural hair.

Check Your Strand Size

The size of your hair strands can tell you quite a bit about their natural heat tolerance. Some hair types (usually coarser, thicker, naturally straight or wavy heads) can handle heat styling better than finer, curly and kinky-coily strands. Asian hair is perhaps the most heat tolerant/resistant. These strands are usually packed with extra cuticle layering that is tightly oriented from root to tip. The individual strands tend to be the same size or larger than a standard sewing thread, and so they are able to take quite a bit more heat before damage becomes apparent. Asian hair makes the perfect hair for weaves and extensions—it's so forgiving!

Fine, kinky-coily strands do not have cuticle layers that are oriented as tightly. Our cuticles gently lift around our fiber's natural bends, twists and coils—and our individual strands are the same size or smaller than a standard sewing thread. Because our hair's curling and coiling ability is so dependent on its moisture levels and internal protein structure, damage to either of these from heat use will affect our curl pattern. Chemical processing of any kind also affects the cuticle, and reduces our hair's heat tolerance.

Hydrate Like Your Life Depends On It

Start with hair that has been deep conditioned within the last day or so for best results. Hair that has been recently conditioned is extra hydrated and will be able to properly buffer itself against the heat you are applying. Water takes on a very special role deep inside the hair fiber. Its naturally high heat capacity slows the temperature increase of the strand in the presence of heat. Water can absorb a large amount of heat without increasing its own temperature. Damaged, dehydrated hair does not have the internal mois-

Did You Know?

We can see the effects of water's amazing heat capacity by looking at Earth's oceans. Our oceans' ability to absorb massive amounts of heat without increasing drastically in temperature is what keeps our planet's climate temperate and livable.

ture available to slow the temperature increase of the hair strand. These dehydrated strands heat up rapidly, and it is this rapid heating that ultimately damages the strand.

Put on the Full Armor

You wouldn't walk into a battle without your protective gear, would you? Always apply a thermal/heat-protectant spray, cream or serum to the hair prior to heat styling. Silicone-based products offer the very best heat protection. Remember how important it is to have fully hydrated tresses prior to heat use? Well, silicones help to keep the strand's natural moisture levels steady. The protective film that silicones create on the hair strand makes it tough for water to easily evaporate. Slowing moisture evaporation from the hair allows us to better regulate the hair's heating process.

Make it Measurable

Healthy hair burns at just over 450F. This means that if your hair is compromised in any way (dehydrated, color-treated, etc.), you can be sure that your heat tolerance is much lower than 450 degrees.

If your hair is fine or fragile, use temperatures no higher than the upper 200s or low 300s. If your hair is a medium texture and fairly healthy, 300 to 375 should work. If your hair is coarse (thick strands), you can venture above 350F to the low 400s fairly easily, but don't push it. Hair is a fiber, and fibers will wear down with time and mistreatment! Start your appliances on the low end of the range and work upward until you find a comfortable temperature zone.

Always work with appliances, especially flat irons, that have dedicated temperature dials with actual, measurable readings—not just High and Low, or On and Off! This way, you'll know immediately how much heat you're working with.

Keep Your Distance and Keep it Moving

The more direct the heat contact, the more potential for hair damage in the long run. Hold blow dryers about 6 to 10 inches away from your head, and direct the air down the hair shaft—not at the head. Use a diffuser attachment when possible for a more even heat distribution. When straightening the hair with an iron, slowly decrease your ironing tension as you move along the hair shaft. The hair nearest the very ends is the most vulnerable to heat damage and has a much a lower heat tolerance, so ease up!

Allowing heat to concentrate or linger in sections will dry your hair faster and straighten it better, but it will also lead to high, mid, and low-shaft split ends. Keep your heat source moving! Do not leave heat appliances on the hair for more than a few seconds.

Make a Clean Sweep

Never use heat on hair that is dirty or laden with product buildup. Starting with clean, conditioned hair will give you a fresher, longer lasting style. Also, make sure that your flat iron or curling iron plates are clean before running them through your hair. Product crud can easily snag and abrade your hair.

10.6 On Coloring Natural Hair

In the maintenance stage, many naturals begin to experiment with color. Color can provide a welcome change as well as be a nice way to add some spice and flavor to your natural 'do. But before you take the plunge, there are some things that you will need to keep in mind. First, know that your color-treated hair will be very sensitive to things that you may have taken for granted before— (i.e., water, the sun, heat etc.) Color-treating your hair is not the time to get lackadaisical with your hair. If you are lazy, put down the box! If you plan to take the color plunge, keep in mind that you may experience:

Curl pattern changes

Did you know that coloring your natural hair can sometimes result in unpredictable changes in your hair's curl pattern? Sometimes, these changes are permanent. This unintended straightening tends to happen with permanent coloring products that lift or lighten the hair several shades, but it can also occur with safer, plant-based colors including henna. Whenever you alter or manipulate the hair's protein bonding arrangement a slight relaxing effect can occur. In the case of henna, the weight of the henna deposited along the hair shaft application after application can result in a flattening of the hair's natural texture.

While some people find that after applying henna their texture does begin to return over time, this is often not the case for those who are using permanent coloring products. It is best to have these types of hair colors applied by a professional whenever possible to ensure the proper degree of processing for your hair. Another transition or Big Chop may then be needed to get back to where you were.

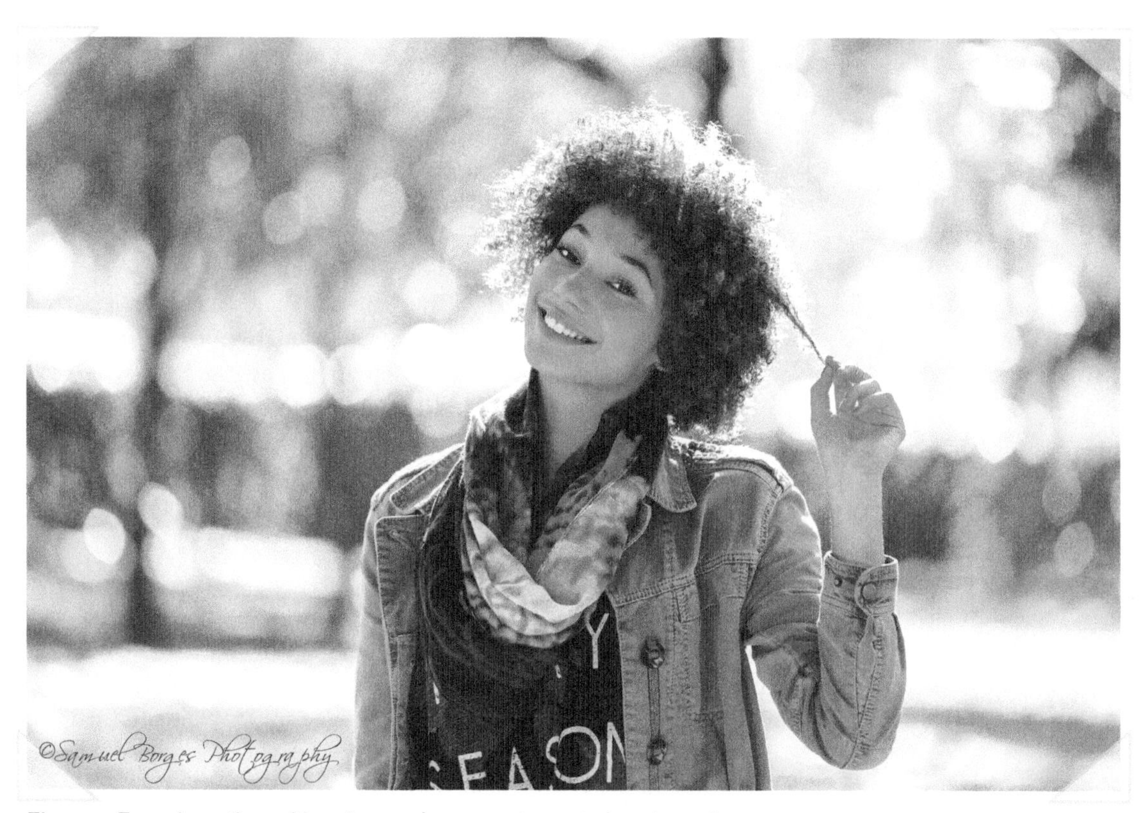

Fig 10.2: Experimenting with color can be a great way to break up the monotony.

Curl pattern changes are less likely to occur in those with coarser hair textures (thick individual strands), and are more likely to occur in those with fine to medium hair textures. Prior damage may also influence whether or not you experience changes in your curl pattern. Using a protein reconstructor after coloring may help some lost curls find their way again, but it is not a guarantee.

Increases in hair porosity

Products that lighten the hair always require direct access to the hair's cortical layers. When the hair's cuticle is breached in this manner the hair's natural porosity increases, leading to a dryness that hardly ever lets up. When porosity increases, dryness becomes a major complaint because moisture is next to impossible to hold securely within the fiber. Your hair becomes like a bucket with holes poked in the sides. Color-treated hair can be unforgiving, too. Miss a regularly scheduled deep conditioning and you may find yourself parting with your colored strands prematurely. A strict, moisture and protein-focused regimen is absolutely essential if the hair is to thrive in this condition. If you never cared before, now is definitely the time to learn how to balance protein and moisture sources in your regimen!

Loss of Elasticity

Because color-treated hair has lost much of its natural moisture (and its overall ability to retain supplemental moisture given), the hair may lose some of its elasticity. Elasticity refers to the ability of our hair fibers to stretch gently and return back to their normal shape and character without damage. The elastic quality of our hair is what makes putting our hair in a ponytail or drawing a puff effortless. When hair lacks elasticity, it does not move or bend and recover when pressured like healthy hair does— it simply gives up under pressure and snaps in its fragile condition. Again, moisture and protein balancing become critical for establishing elasticity because it is that careful mix of moisture and strength that gives our hair the ability to resist breakage from being stretched and handled day to day.

Horrific Color Result

Color is very, very unpredictable and all the swatches, box comparisons and focus groups in the world can't prepare you for the result you should expect. Why? Because color uptake is dependent on a number of factors— namely your hair's current color, porosity and texture (strand size). At best, the hair color on the box is just the product manufacturer's best corporate guess at what your hair will look like (with a bit of photoshopping thrown in for good measure.) Sometimes, multiple steps will be needed to get your color right. It is always best to have an experienced professional stylist take color more than three shades out of your natural color range. Chances are, they've seen numerous heads of hair with textures like yours and varying degrees of porosity—plus they have the added bonus of experiences with various colors and looks to bring to the table. The numbers game is in their favor. You standing there in the store aisle with a box and maybe 0-5 colorings under your belt really can't compete. (Okay, okay— maybe some of you can!) Don't let your color job be the first time you are sitting in this stylist's chair— especially if the color change is drastic. You want someone who knows you and your hair and who'll be available if you have questions.

Extra-Temporary Colors

If you are simply looking for a quick color change that will wash out in a few days, then temporary colors may be for you. These colors are deposit only and less damaging than permanent hair colors that have to break through the hair fiber to gain their staying power. To increase their staying power, lightly blow dry the colors in or set them with a light hold hair spray. These temporary colors can be purchased from beauty supply stores like ULTA, Sally's, Target, Sephora and Amazon.

Hair Chalk Pens: Simply apply your desired pen color to dry hair and wash out with shampoo. These creamy colors last about five to seven days. (Brands to try: Lashes and Cosmetics Neon Shimmer Hair Chalk, EDGE Metallic Glitter Hair Chalks, and Navayah Blendable Hair Color Pens)

Spray On: Spray-on colors like Beyond the Zone Color Bombz are great temporary color options. Apply spray color to dry, styled hair in a well-ventilated area. Also, be sure to protect your clothing, furniture and other surfaces from the spray! Stay away from the spray-on colors that tend to show up on shelves around Halloween time. These sprays tend to make hair quite crispy!

"Hair Shadows" and Eye Shadow Color (Cream and Powder): Yes, there is a such thing as "hair shadow"! Shadows make a great temporary color option for natural hair. Simply smooth the color onto your desired sections of hair for a little pop of color!

Cream shadows last longer than powder ones, and tend to not fade as much when you go to moisturize your hair later on. Creams also tend to not be as drying as powders. With cream colors, oils will definitely fade the color fast! (Brands to try: COLORSMASH Hair Shadow by Condition Culture, Kiko Milano and any basic eye shadow make up brand.)

Temporary colors are best for one or two days of dramatic color. Applying moisturizers or styling products on top of the colors, especially powder-based colors, will almost always cause them to fade. Because temporary colors are only superficially attached to your hair, they do tend to flake, rub off or get on your hands when you mess with your hair. To get around the fading and flaking, it's recommended that you use cream-based colors instead of powders, and use the colors as a final touch after you've already applied your other hair products and have completely finished styling your hair. Some temporary color brands can make the hair feel crunchy and hard, mostly because they are just sitting on the outside of your hair strand.

For curly color inspiration, check out hair shadow pioneer *Naturallytash* on Instagram and Youtube! www.irockmynatural.com

Natural Alternatives

As a supernatural, you are probably looking for a more natural way to color your hair. Here are a few natural options:

Coffee (darker)
Lemon (Lighter)
Henna (Red)
Honey (Lighter)
Tea Rinses (Darker)

The downsides? If you are looking for color variety and flexibility, the limitations are many. It is difficult (nearly impossible!) to achieve lighter tones on darker hair reliably using only natural products. And of course, spunkier colors are simply out of the question! Many of these natural colorants require multiple applications before they really show up on the hair, and their results are not always consistent from head to head.

A temporary solution for jazzier colors (blues, greens, purples, etc.) is to apply a liquid or cream-based eye shadow to your hair. There is no commitment with these funky colors because they rinse out quickly in just one shampoo.

Chapter 11: Final Thoughts

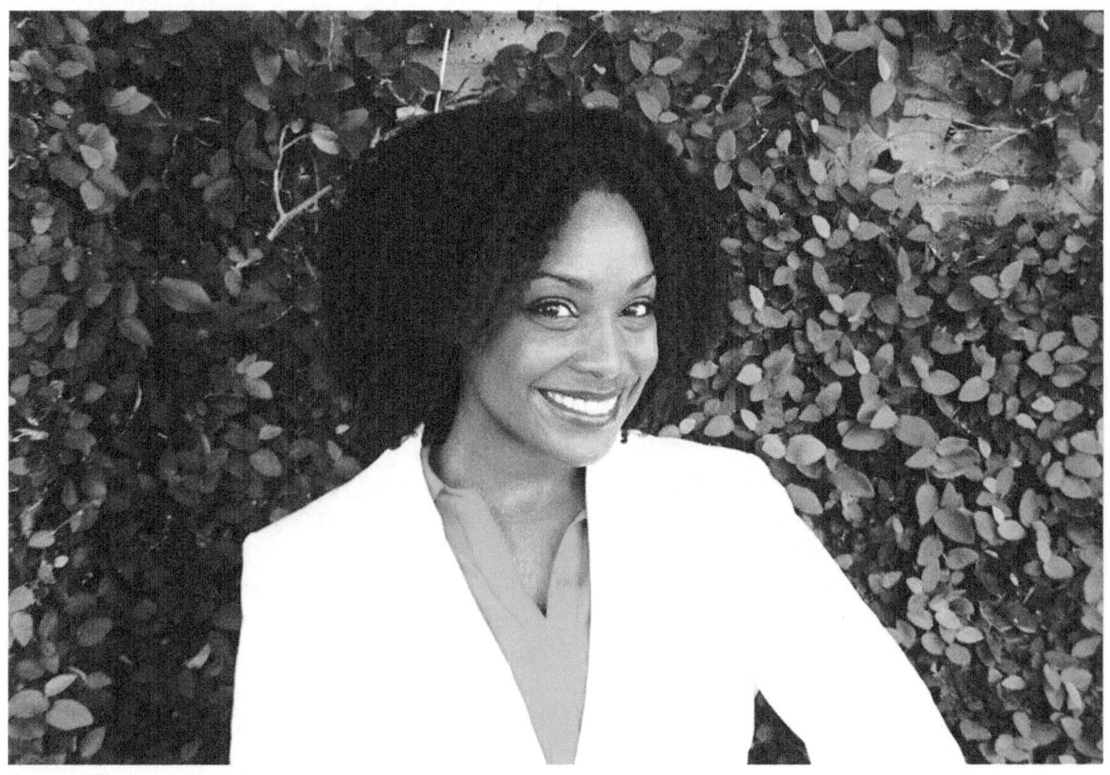

Audrey Sivasothy

I was the relaxed girl whom everyone thought would never go natural. Why? Because I'm sure I yelled it from the rooftops on a number of occasions. I was very vocal and adamant about never, ever wanting to be seen with natural hair. My plan was to grow long, healthy hair that could cascade, feather out in layers, hang or flip on command. All of this hair would be relaxed, of course, because in my mind natural hair was just too "limited" to perform any of those tasks. Natural hair wasn't the plan. But, what they say about God laughing at our plans is definitely true! And boy, did he ever get a good laugh!

The very first time that I felt the coolness of relaxer near my scalp, I was five years old. To me, relaxers were as normal and necessary as toothpaste. In fact, they were a necessity of the highest order, and anyone who cared about her appearance would and should have one. In my mind, relaxers were a required part of a woman's personal hygiene. Everyone in my family had one, and nearly everyone in my realm of influence did as well.

During my teen years, I continued to relax my hair on schedule, year after year, despite the dryness and breakage I dealt with. I never missed an application. Those puffy, coily roots just would not do under any circumstances, and I knew what always needed to be done. They were like weeds, unwanted and unstoppable, and I was more than willing to do my part to keep them in check. "Going natural," as it was called, was never really an option for me. In fact, even when my relaxed hair was in its absolute worst condition, I wore it with pride. In my mind, that fragile, breaking hair was still better than the puffiness that kept trying to grow underneath it.

When I went off to college, I started doing my own relaxers and never missed a beat. I knew that I wasn't exactly helping my hair with the relaxers (and burns couldn't be good, right?)—but I continued to use them. I told myself that since my hair was still somewhat lengthy and in acceptable condition, giving relaxers up to explore natural hair was crazy. Going natural became even less of an option for me when I finally learned how to take care of my relaxed hair, and it started to pick up incredible length. In my mind, this whole hair thing was solved. Why throw away all of that progress to have short hair again? Ironically, one of the ways that I worked around relaxer damage was by not using them as much. I learned that having the healthiest relaxed hair meant not relaxing my hair as often. By spacing out my relaxer applications from every eight weeks to every ten, and then to every twelve and so on, my hair drastically improved. The farther out I stretched the relaxers, the better my hair looked and felt. But still, wearing natural hair never occurred to me.

Some of you may be thinking, *Now, Audrey, that sounds pretty backward.* And it *was*! In fact, I'm almost too embarrassed to put this in print, but I'm doing so with the hope that it reaches someone who is now where I was. Looking back, I was broken. I was not one of those enlightened individuals who could separate my hair from myself or view my hair as "just a style." Hair, to me, has always been deeper. Natural hair for me was about embracing the beauty of blackness—and I just wasn't there yet. Although this isn't the case for everyone, I will freely admit that I was a relaxed child and eventually a relaxed woman who was not comfortable in her own hair or skin. For me, my hair and skin communicated my blackness to the world. It is so difficult to say this now in such a public place, but I simply did not want to be reminded of my blackness. My hair and skin were both "faults," and I was oh so thankful for relaxers for allowing me to "minimize" those faults—if even for only a short time. I was in such a difficult place. I so wish that I had had a mind like some of you who felt pride and confidence from Day One. It took me almost the entirety of my twenties to really, truly love me. We all explore natural hair for different reasons. My journey was about self-awareness, self-discovery and self-love.

A Journey Like No Other

While it may seem insignificant and even obvious now, in the wake of our current natural hair renaissance, the idea that there is a choice outside of chemical straightening is a new one to many women with textured hair. Despite the fact that natural hair has gained popularity and a larger foothold in society, natural hair is *still* considered to be outside the box or trendsetting in many circles. Perhaps the most encouraging thing about the scores of women choosing to reclaim their natural hair is that this movement challenges the longstanding position that chemical relaxers have held in our hair-care discussions. Once viewed by many as a hair-care *requirement* and the only real choice for presentable hair, relaxers have increasingly been assigned a different role in our hair-care discussions. Relaxers are no longer a necessity, but an option. That's powerful.

Time for a Change

Two major changes in my life brought natural hair to the table: working on my first book, *The Science of Black Hair*, and the birth of my curly-haired daughter. Together, they triggered a curiosity that led me back to my natural hair. Once I fully understood what I was putting my hair through by subjecting it to the relaxing process, I realized that even though my hair was in acceptable condition, I still was not seeing or maximizing my hair's full potential; I was just amazingly successful at patching up damage. If you think about it, working with relaxed hair is very much like trying to pour water into a leaky bucket. If you work hard enough, you can get the water level high, but of course, the work required to keep it there is pretty exhausting. Why not start over with a leak-free bucket? A bucket that's in better condition in the first place? Natural hair is as close to a leak-free bucket as you can get.

Working with my daughter's curls for the first time also turned on a light in me. I loved the versatility of her hair and wanted her to grow to love her curls, too. But the idea that I was not setting a good example for her haunted me. How could I reassure her that her curls were beautiful the way they were when I wasn't embracing my own? I did not want her to grow up thinking that some curls were okay and other curls were not—like I did. We teach our children to celebrate diversity and not discriminate against other people on the basis of their skin colors, heights, religions and other unique features. Why not start with ourselves and celebrate our own diversity?

So, a journey that for me started as a fourteen-week relaxer stretch became a full-scale transition to natural hair. I transitioned for *nearly eleven months* before officially cutting off the relaxed ends.

The Learning Curve

I wish I could say that every part of my personal transition was wonderful and just full of breathtaking, awe-inspiring moments. But it wasn't. Those ten months—which started out so promisingly, I must say—did not go smoothly. They were hard. Toward the final months of my transition, my hair just did not cooperate. My edges wouldn't lie down, flat-ironing ended in failure and my hair was neither here nor there. Truth be told, I felt ugly, and I seriously wanted to hide. I think I even I even stopped writing *The Science of Black Hair* for a while because I felt like a complete fraud. *How could I encourage other people to love their hair when I was barely comfortable looking in the mirror at my transitioning self?*

And, that's when it dawned on me that I'd been approaching transitioning in the wrong way. The transition from relaxed to natural hair is much more mental than physical. You have to change along with your hair. If your hair changes without you, every day will be an uphill battle.

Well, despite those down days, I pressed on, worked on myself and completed my transition. Sure, I still have those days when I have to convince myself that I am beautiful and wonderfully made. Don't we all? I am not perfect, and I freely admit that I am still a work in progress. And you know what? That is completely okay.

I certainly hope you've found this book helpful to your hair journey in some way. For some of you, reclaiming your natural hair will be a journey that tries your very soul—but for others, it'll still simply be just another date with a pair of scissors. No matter what brings you to the natural path you choose to tread, your hair will be happier and healthier for it.

If you've found even one helpful thing here, I would like to ask a huge favor! Please be sure to tell us what you think—what you liked and what you didn't—by leaving a review for us on the website or via the venue where you picked up the book! We read and consider each and every single review, both positive and negative. They are all helpful, and we do appreciate them so much! In fact, this book would not be here if it weren't for those *Science of Black Hair* book reviews calling for more information on transitioning. Again, we appreciate you all so very much and hope that we've succeeded in producing another high quality book that you can count on and be proud of! Thank you!

Audrey Sivasothy

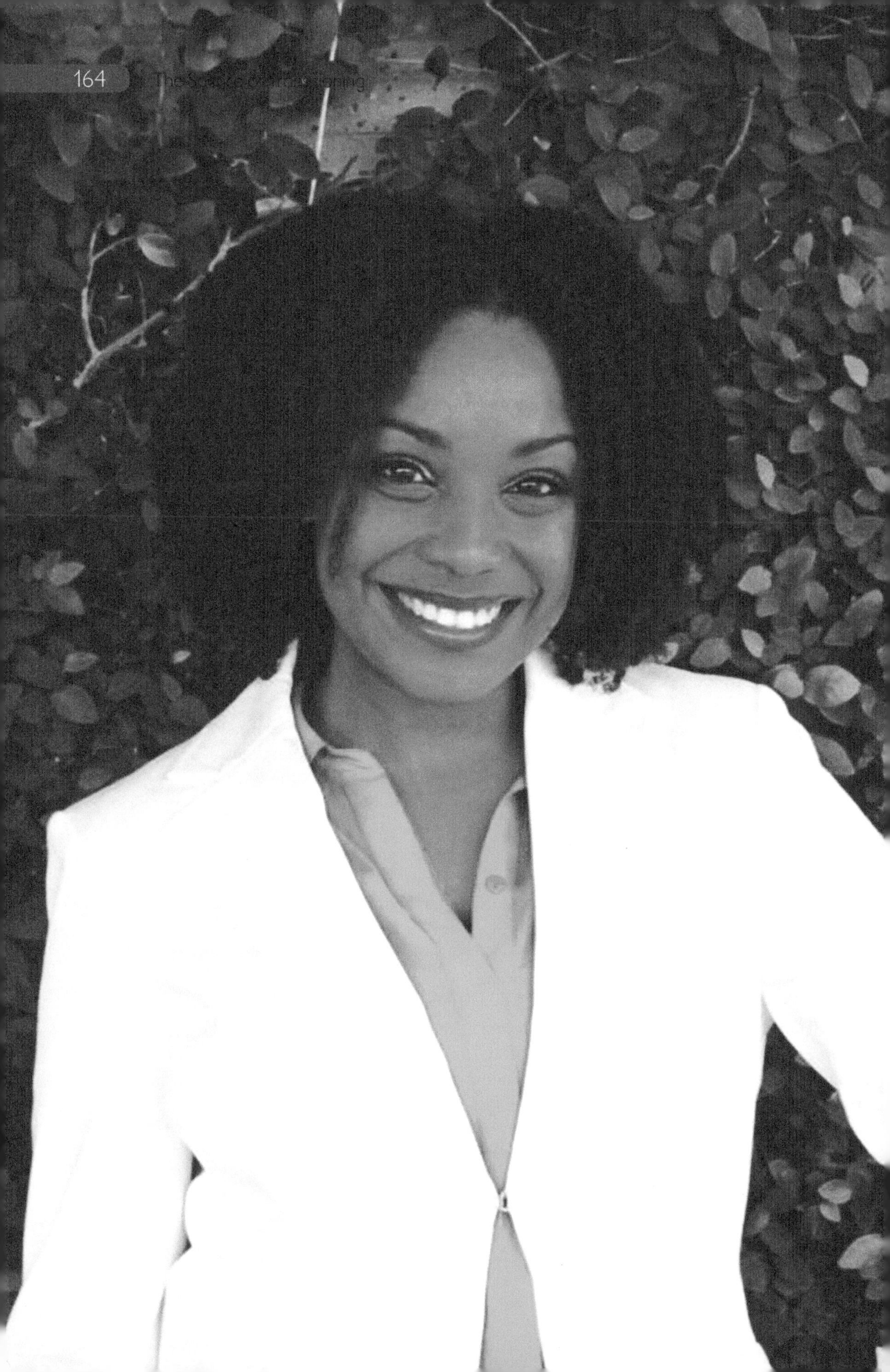

About Audrey!

Audrey Davis-Sivasothy is a Houston-based freelance writer, speaker and consultant to the cosmetology industry. As a trained health scientist, Sivasothy has written extensively on the intricacies of caring for hair at home. Her work has been featured in *Good Housekeeping, Woman's World, The Huffington Post, Essence, Sophisticate's Black Hair* and *Hype Hair* magazines. *The Science of Black Hair* has also been adopted for training courses in cosmetology and continues to maintain international bestseller status in the U.S., Canadian, U.K. and French fashion and beauty book markets.

Keep Up with Audrey!

If you enjoyed this book, please let us know by taking a moment to write a review http://amzn.to/19zkjWJ. Your review makes a difference. We read each and every one. Thank you for reading and supporting this work.

If you'd like to be notified when Audrey releases new books, sign up for her newsletter here: http://bit.ly/17YyiHw. The mailing list ensures that you never miss an update and gives you exclusive access to subscriber-only perks!

ANTISPAM PROMISE: We hate spam as much as you do, so news is infrequent and always relevant. Your information will never be used for any other purpose. Promise!

On the Web

You can visit www.blackhairscience.com for more healthy hair tips and advice.

On Facebook: www.facebook.com/blackhair101
On Twitter: @blackhair101
On Instagram: @blackhair101
On YouTube: The Science of Black Hair

More Books by This Author

The Science of Black Hair: A Comprehensive Guide to Textured Hair Care by Audrey Davis-Sivasothy (April 11, 2011)

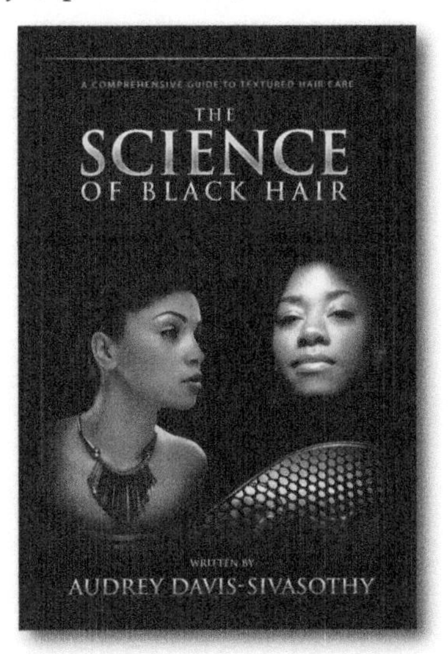

Kindle Edition (http://amzn.to/19zkjWJ)
Paperback (http://amzn.to/14BQ0QA)
Audio (http://amzn.to/19ziUzx)

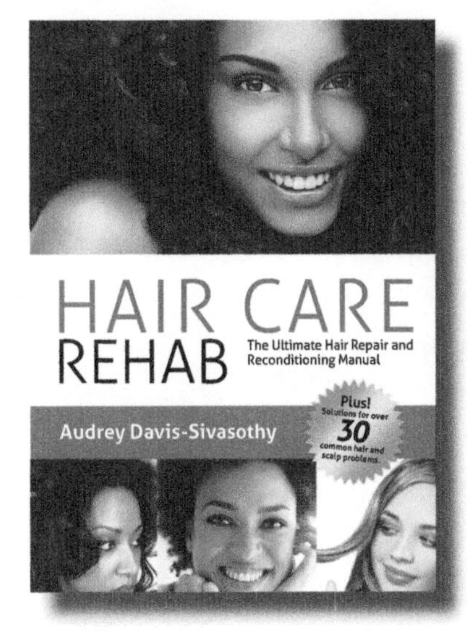

Hair Care Rehab: The Ultimate Hair Repair & Reconditioning Manual by Audrey Davis-Sivasothy (April 11, 2012)

Paperback (http://amzn.to/17CELse)
Kindle (http://amzn.to/1aaSU)

unit 5

Hair Product Index & Additional Resources

Hair Product Index

Disclaimer

The information provided here is true to the very best of our knowledge at the time of this writing. The list of products and brands represented here is not exhaustive and is only included for informational purposes. Before you commit to buying a product, always double-check the ingredients first. If you have any doubts, contact the company directly for the most correct and up-to-date information.

Sulfate-free Shampoos

If you have decided to include shampoo in your hair-care regimen, it is recommended that you select the gentlest formula for your textured tresses. Natural and sulfate-free formulas are typically easier on textured hair, but in hair care there are few absolutes. The best way to determine if a product will be gentle enough for your needs is to try it on your own hair.

Also keep in mind that just because a shampoo is sulfate-free, this does not mean that the other ingredients in the formula are outstanding. If you are avoiding specific ingredients—including parabens, silicones or others—you'll still need to check labels to verify that the other ingredients meet your standards.

Abba Gentle Shampoo
Abba Moisture Shampoo
Abba Color Protection Shampoo
AfroVeda Foundation Pumpkin & Pomegranate Herbal Shampoo
AfroVeda Monoi De Tiare Cleansing Cream
AG Hair Cosmetics Colour Savour Sulfate-Free Shampoo
AG Hair Cosmetics Fast Food Sulfate-Free Shampoo
AG Hair Cosmetics Recoil Curl Activating Shampoo
AG Hair Cosmetics Smoooth Sulfate-free Argan Shampoo
Alba Botanica Cocoa Butter Dry Repair Hair Wash
Alba Botanica Coconut Milk Extra Enrich Hair Wash
Alba Botanica Gardenia Hydrating Hair Wash
Alba Botanica Honeydew Nourishing Hair Wash
Alba Botanica Mango Moisturizing Hair Wash
Alba Botanica Plumeria Replenishing Hair Wash
Alba Botanica Daily Shampoo
Alikay Naturals Bentonite Me Baby
Alikay Naturals Black Soap Shampoo
Alikay Naturals Caribbean Coconut Milk Shampoo
Alterna Color Hold Repair Shampoo
Alterna Color Hold Shine Shampoo
Alterna Color Hold Straight Shampoo
Alterna Scalp Therapy Shampoo
Alterna Clarifying Shampoo
Alterna Color Hold Repair Shampoo
Alterna Volume Restore Shampoo
Anita Grant Babassu Amla Shampoo Bar
Anita Grant Babassu Lavender Rose Shampoo and Shower Bar
Anita Grant Peppermint Babassu Shampoo Bar
Anita Grant Organic Kelp + Ylang Babassu Shampoo Bar
Aubrey Organics BGA Protein + Strengthening Shampoo
Aubrey Organics Egyptian Henna Shine-Enhancing Shampoo
Aubrey Organics GPB Glycogen Protein Balancing Shampoo
Aubrey Organics Green Tea Clarifying Shampoo
Aubrey Organics Honeysuckle Rose Moisturizing Shampoo
Aubrey Organics Island Naturals Replenishing Shampoo
Aubrey Organics J.A.Y. Desert Herb Revitalizing Shampoo
Aubrey Organics Rosa Mosqueta Nourishing Shampoo
Aubrey Organics White Camellia Ultra-Smoothing Shampoo
Au Naturale Sulfate Free Shampoo by Dark N Lovely
Auromere Ayurvedic Sulfate-Free Aloe Vera-Neem Shampoo

As I Am Cleansing Pudding
As I Am Coconut CoWash Cleansing Conditioner
Avalon Organics Awapuhi Mango Therapy Deep Moisturizing Shampoo
Avalon Organics Biotin B-Complex Therapy Thickening Shampoo
Avalon Organics Clarifying Lemon Shampoo
Avalon Organics Grapefruit & Geranium Smoothing Shampoo
Avalon Organics Nourishing Lavender Shampoo
Avalon Organics Olive and Grapeseed Extra Moisturizing Shampoo
Avalon Organics Shine Ylang Ylang Shampoo
Avalon Organics Strengthening Peppermint Shampoo
Avalon Organics Tea Tree Mint Therapy Scalp Normalizing Shampoo
Avalon Organics Tea Tree Scalp Treatment Shampoo
Avalon Organics Tear-Free Baby Shampoo & Body Wash
Avalon Organics Volumizing Rosemary Shampoo
Aveda Scalp Benefits Balancing Shampoo
Aveda Damage Remedy Restructuring Shampoo
Aveda Dry Remedy Moisturizing Shampoo
Aveda Invati Exfoliating Shampoo
Aveda Men's Pure-Formance Shampoo
Bed Head Foxy Curls Frizz-Fighting Sulfate-Free Shampoo
Bed Head Superstar Sulfate-Free Shampoo for Thick Massive Hair
Bee Mine Botanical Moisturizing Shampoo
Blended Beauty Silky Swirls Shampoo
Blended Beauty Soy Cream Shampoo
Body Shop Rainforest Moisture Shampoo
Bumble and Bumble Color-Minded Shampoo
Bumble and Bumble Straight Shampoo
Burt's Bees Baby Bee Shampoo
Burt's Bees More Moisture Baobab Shampoo
Burt's Bees Super Shiny Mango Shampoo
Burt's Bees Very Volumizing Pomegranate Shampoo
Camille Rose Caramel Cowash
Camille Rose Clean Rinse
Camille Rose Crème Restore Conditioning Cleanser
Carol's Daughter Black Vanilla Shampoo
Carol's Daughter Hair Milk Co-Wash Cleansing Conditioner
Carol's Daughter Monoi Repairing Shampoo
Carol's Daughter Tui Moisturizing Shampoo
CHI Color Therapy Shampoo
CHI Hydrating Therapy Shampoo
CHI Infra Shampoo
CHI Ionic Color Protection System Sulfate Free Shampoo
Curl Junkie Curl Assurance Gentle Cleansing Shampoo
CURLS Creamy Curl Cleanser
CURLS Peek-A-Boo Tearless Baby Shampoo
CURLS Curlicious Curls Cleansing Cream Sulfate Free Cleanser
CURLS Curlie Cutie Cleansing Cream Sulfate Free Cleanser
Curls Unleashed Lavish in Lather Sulfate Free Shampoo
CUSH Creme de Palm Smoothing Shampoo
CUSH Hydration Supreme Conditioning Shampoo
Darcy's Botanicals Daily Cleansing Conditioner Cream
Davines OI Shampoo
DermOrganic Daily Conditioning Shampoo
Desert Essence Gentle Nourishing Organic Cleanser
Design Essentials Gentle Balance Sulfate-Free Nourishing Shampoo
Design Essentials Natural Curl Cleanser Shampoo
Design Essentials Strengthening Therapy Cleansing Sulfate-Free Shampoo
DevaCurl No Poo
DevaCurl Low Poo
DevaCurl No-Poo Quick Cleanser*
DevaCare No Poo
DevaCare Low Poo
Dr. Bronner's Almond Liquid Soap
Dr. Bronner's Citrus Orange Liquid Soap
Dr. Bronner's Eucalyptus Liquid Soap
Dr. Bronner's Lavender Liquid Soap
Dr. Bronner's Peppermint Liquid Soap
Dr. Bronner's Rose Liquid Soap
Dr. Bronner's Tea Tree Oil Liquid Soap
Eden Body Works Coconut Shea Cleansing Cowash
Eden Body Works Jojoba Monoi Moisturizing Shampoo

Eden Body Works Peppermint Tea Tree Shampoo
Elasta QP Creme Conditioning Shampoo
Elucence Moisture Benefits Shampoo
Entwine Lathering Hair Bathe (Act 1)
Entwine Cleansing Crème Hair Rinse (Act 2)
Giovanni Smooth as Silk Deep Moisture Shampoo
Giovanni Tea Tree Triple Treat Invigorating Shampoo
Giovanni 50:50 Balanced Hydrating-Clarifying Shampoo
Giovanni Golden Wheat Deep Cleanse Shampoo
Giovanni Root 66 Max Volume Shampoo
Giovanni Wellness Shampoo with Chinese Botanicals
Hair Rules Aloe Grapefruit Purifying Shampoo
Hair Rules Daily Cleansing Cream Moisturizing No Suds Shampoo
Herbal Choice Mari Natural Tea Tree Shampoo
Herbal Choice Mari Natural & Pure Scent-Free Shampoo
Herbal Choice Mari Natural Shampoo Eucalyptus & Fennel
Hydratherma Naturals SLS Free Moisture Plus Hair Cleanser
Intelligent Nutrients Total Body Cleanser
Jane Carter Solution Creamy Conditioning Cleanser
Jane Carter Solution Hydrating Invigorating Shampoo
JASON Natural Tea Tree Treatment Shampoo
JASON Natural Restorative Biotin Shampoo
JASON Moisturizing 84% Aloe Vera Shampoo
JASON Long and Strong Jojoba Shampoo
JASON Natural Smoothing Sea Kelp Shampoo
JASON Natural Volumizing Lavender Shampoo
JASON Natural Revitalizing Vitamin E Shampoo
JASON Natural Super Shine Apricot Shampoo
JASON Color Protect Henna Shampoo
Jessicurl Gentle Lather Shampoo
Jessicurl Hair Cleansing Cream
Joico Color Endure Sulfate-Free Shampoo
Joico Smooth Cure Sulfate-free Shampoo
JONATHAN Product Cleansing Hair Conditioner
JONATHAN Product Green Routine Nourishing Shampoo
JONATHAN Product Hydrating Shampoo
JONATHAN Product Infinite Volume Shampoo
JONATHAN Product Weightless Smooth No-frizz Shampoo
Karen's Body Beautiful Delicate 'Do No Poo Lather Free Hair Wash
Karen's Body Beautiful Bodacious Beauty Bar
Karen's Body Beautiful Cool Clarifying Shampoo
Karen's Body Beautiful Ultimate Conditioning Shampoo
Kenra Platinum Bodifying Shampoo
Kenra Platinum Hydrating Shampoo
Kenra Platinum Reparative Shampoo
KeraCare 1st Lather Shampoo
KeraCare Hydrating Detangling Shampoo
KeraCare Naturals Cleansing Cream
KINKY-CURLY Come Clean Shampoo
Kiss My Face Big Body Shampoo
Kiss My Face Miss Treated Shampoo
Kiss My Face Whenever Shampoo
Koils by Nature Refreshing Anti-Dandruff Tea Tree Mint Cleanser
Koils by Nature Replenishing Lavender & Eucalyptus Cleanser
Komaza Care Moja Shampoo
L'Oreal EverCrème Shampoo
L'Oreal EverPure Smooth Shampoo
L'Oreal EverSleek Shampoo
L'Oreal EverStrong Hydrating Shampoo
Miessence Desert Flower Shampoo
MOP C-Curl Enhancing Shampoo
MOP C-System Clean Shampoo
MOP C-System Hydrating Shampoo
Moroccanoil Hydrating Shampoo
My Honey Child Banana Crème Scalp Cleanser
Neutrogena Triple Moisture Cream Lather Shampoo
OGX (formally Organix) Shampoos (all)
OYIN Grand Poo Bar
OYIN Honey Wash
Pureology Essential Repair Shampoo
Pureology Hydrate Shampoo
Pureology Nanoworks Shampoo
Pureology Pure Volume Shampoo
Pureology Super Smooth Shampoo
Qhemet Biologics Egyptian Wheatgrass Cleansing Tea Shampoo
Queen Helene Mint Julep Shampoo
Scruples White Tea Sulfate Free Restorative Shampoo

SheaMoisture Coconut & Hibiscus Curl & Shine Shampoo
SheaMoisture Raw Shea Butter Moisture Retention Shampoo
SheaMoisture African Black Soap Deep Cleansing Shampoo
SheaMoisture Yucca & Baobab Thickening Shampoo
Silk Elements ColorCare Sulfate-free Shampoo
Silk Elements Moisturizing Cream Shampoo
Softsheen Breakthru Fortifying Moisturizing Shampoo
Terressentials Pure Earth Hair Washes
TIGI S-Factor Health Factor Sulfate-Free Daily Dose Shampoo
Trader Joe's Nourish Spa Shampoo
Trader Joe's Tea Tree Tingle Shampoo
Uncle Funky's Daughter Rich and Funky Shampoo
WEN Cleansing Conditioner

*Dry shampoo. Contains a denatured alcohol as first ingredient (which may be drying).

Deep Conditioners & Masks

Moisturizing Deep-Conditioning Products

Alikay Naturals Caribbean Coconut Milk Conditioner
As I Am Hydration Elation Intensive Conditioner
AtOne Botanical Reconstructor Conditioner
Aubrey Organics Honeysuckle Rose Moisturizing Conditioner
Aubrey Organics Island Naturals Replenishing Conditioner
Aubrey Organics Rosa Mosqueta Conditioner
Aubrey Organics White Camellia Ultra-Smoothing Conditioner
Aussie Aussome Volume Conditioner
Aussie Moist Conditioner
Avalon Organics Awapuhi Mango Moisturizing Conditioner
Avalon Organics Lavender Nourishing Conditioner
Avalon Organics Ylangylang Glistening Conditioner
Aveda Color Conserve Conditioner
Aveda Dry Remedy Moisturizing Conditioner
Back to Basics Bamboo Straightening Conditioner
Back to Basics Green Tea Revitalizing Conditioner
Back to Basics Moisturizing Pomegranate Conditioner
Back to Basics Rich Moisture Coconut Mango
Back to Basics Vanilla Plum Conditioner
Bee Mine Bee-U-Ti-Ful Deep Conditioner
Biolage Hydratherapie Conditioning Balm
Blended Beauty Quenching Conditioner
Bumble and Bumble Crème de Coco Conditioner
Bumble and Bumble Curl Conscious Smoothing Conditioner
Bumble and Bumble Quenching Conditioner
Bumble and Bumble Seaweed Conditioner
Bumble and Bumble Super Rich Conditioner
Burt's Bees Shea & Grapefruit Deep Conditioner
Camille Rose Algae Renew Deep Conditioning Mask
Carol's Daughter Tui Hair Smoothie
Crème of Nature Professional Nourishing & Strengthening Treatment
Curl Junkie Curl Assurance Smoothing Conditioner
Curl Junkie Curl Rehab Moisturizing Treatment
Curl Junkie Hibiscus & Banana Deep Fix Moisturizing Conditioner
Curls Unleashed No Restrictions Moisturizing Conditioner
CURLS Coconut Dream Conditioner
CURLS Curl Ecstasy Hair Tea Deep Conditioner
Darcy's Botanicals Deep Conditioning Mask
Davines Momo Conditioner
DevaCare One Condition Conditioner
DevaCurl Heaven In Hair Moisture Treatment
DevaCurl One Condition Conditioner
Dove Daily Moisture Conditioner
Dove Oxygen Moisture Conditioner
Elasta QP DPR-11 Deep Penetrating Remoisturizer
Elucence Moisture Balancing Conditioner
Frederic Fekkai Essential Shea Conditioner
Frederic Fekkai Brilliant Glossing Conditioner
Giovanni 50:50 Balanced Conditioner
Giovanni Avocado & Olive Oil Ultra-Moist Conditioner

Giovanni Smooth As Silk Deeper Moisture Conditioner
Giovanni Tea Tree Triple Treat Invigorating Conditioner
Herbal Essences BodyEnvy Volumizing Conditioner
Herbal Essences Color Me Happy Conditioner
Herbal Essences Hello Hydration Moisturizing Conditioner
Herbal Essences None of Your Frizzness Smoothing Conditioner
Herbal Essences Totally Twisted Curls and Waves Conditioner
Hydratherma Naturals Moisture Boosting Deep Conditioning Treatment
Jane Carter Nutrient Replenishing Conditioner
JASON Moisturizing 84% Aloe Vera Conditioner
JASON Smoothing Sea Kelp Moisturizing Conditioner
Jessicurl Aloeba Daily Conditioner
Jessicurl Too Shea! Extra Moisturizing Conditioner
Jessicurl Weekly Deep Conditioning Treatment
Joico Moisture Recovery Conditioner
Kenra Moisturizing Conditioner
Kenra Nourishing Masque Deep Conditioning Treatment
Keracare Humecto Crème Conditioner
Keracare Moisturizing Conditioner for Color-Treated Hair
Kerastase Nutritive Masquintense Nourishing Treatment
Komaza Care Moja Conditioner
Komaza Care Olive Moisture Mask
L'Anza Healing ColorCare Color-Preserving Conditioner
L'Anza Healing Moisture Kuikui Nut Conditioner
L'Anza Healing Nourish Stimulating Conditioner
Mixed Roots Deep Moisture Conditioner
Mizani Moisturefuse Moisturizing Conditioner
MOP Glisten Conditioner
MOP Mixed Greens Conditioner
Mop Top Daily Conditioner
Mop Top Deep Conditioner
My Honey Child Coconut Papaya Hair Paste
My Honey Child Molasses Deep Conditioner
My Honey Child Olive You Deep Conditioner
My Honey Child So Deep Conditioner
Neutrogena Triple Moisture Daily Conditioner
Neutrogena Triple Moisture Deep Recovery Mask
Nexxus Humectress Hydrating Treatment Deep Conditioner
Nexxus Humectress Ultimate Moisturizing Conditioner
Nexxus Phyto Organics Humectin Extreme Moisture Conditioner
OGX (formerly Organix) Nourishing Coconut Milk Conditioner
OGX (formerly Organix) Hydrating Tea Tree Mint Conditioner
OUIDAD Curl Quencher Moisturizing Conditioner
Oyin Honey-Hemp Conditioner
Pantene Pro-V Curl Perfection Conditioner
Pureology Hydrate Conditioner
Redken Clear Moisture Conditioner
Redken Real Control Nourishing Conditioner
Sheabutter Cottage Argan & Cocoa Butter Liquid Shampoo
SheaMoisture Raw Shea Butter Deep Treatment Masque
SheaMoisture Yucca & Baobab Anti-Breakage Masque
Silk Elements Deep Nourishing Conditioner
Tigi Bed Head Moisture Maniac Conditioner
Trader Joe's Nourish Spa Shampoo
Trader Joe's Tea Tree Tingle Shampoo
Uncle Funky's Daughter Richee Rich Conditioner
Yes to Carrots Pampering Conditioner

Light Protein Products

Aubrey Organics Glycogen Protein Balancing (GPB) Conditioner
Aveda Damage Remedy Conditioner
Carol's Daughter Monoi Repairing Conditioner
Curl Junkie Beauticurls Strengthening Hair Conditioner
Garnier Fructis Length & Strength Fortifying Cream Conditioner
Göt2B Emergency Repair Creme (so smooth, one minute)
Herbal Essences Long Term Relationship Conditioner

Joico Moisture Recovery Treatment Balm
Joico K-Pak Reconstruct Conditioner
Mane 'n Tail Original Conditioner
Motions Deep Penetrating Treatment
My Honey Child Banana Crème Conditioner
Neutrogena Triple Moisture Deep Recovery Mask
Ovation Cell Therapy Crème Rinse Moisturizer
Paul Mitchell Super Strong Daily Conditioner
Phytospecific Intense Nutrition Mask
Redken Extreme Hair Strengthening Conditioner
Rusk Sensories Calm 60 Second Hair Revive
SheaMoisture Raw Shea Butter Restorative Conditioner
SheaMoisture Yucca & Baobab Volumizing Conditioner
SheaMoisture Yucca & Baobab Anti-Breakage Masque
SheaMoisture African Black Soap Purification Masque
Silk Elements Mega Cholesterol Conditioning Treatment
Trader Joe's Nourish Spa Balance Moisturizing Conditioner
Vitale Pro Super Conditioner

Moderate Protein Products

Aphogee Keratin 2 Minute Reconstructor
Elasta QP Breakage Control Serum
Elucence Extended Moisture Repair Treatment
Frederic Fekkai Protein Rx Reparative Conditioner
Giovanni Smooth As Silk Extreme Protein Treatment
LeKair Cholesterol Plus Strengthening Conditioning Cream
Motions Critical Protection and Repair (CPR) Treatment Conditioner
Nexxus Keraphix Restorative Strengthening Conditioner
Ovation Cell Therapy Conditioner Hair Treatment
Queen Helene Cholesterol Hair Conditioning Cream

Heavy/Intense Protein Products

Affirm 5 in 1 Reconstructor
Aphogee Two–Step Protein Treatment
Dudley's DRC 28 Hair Treatment and Fortifier
Elasta QP Breakage Control Serum
Elucence Extended Moisture Repair Treatment
Joico K-Pac Deep Penetrating Reconstructor
Mizani Kerafuse Intensive Strengthening Treatment
Motions Critical Protection and Repair (CPR) Treatment Conditioner
Nexxus Emergencee Strengthening Polymeric Reconstructor
Nexxus Keraphix Restorative Strengthening Conditioner
Organic Root Stimulator Hair Mayonnaise Treatment for Damaged Hair

Silicone-Free Conditioners

Alterna Bamboo Luminous Shine Conditioner
As I Am Coconut CoWash Cleansing Conditioner
As I am Hydration Elation Intensive Conditioner
Aubrey Organics Conditioners (all)
Bee Mine Avocado Cream Balanced Conditioner
Bee Mine Bee-U-Ti-Ful Deep Conditioner
Blended Beauty Quenching Conditioner
Devacurl Conditioners
L'Oreal Eversleek Intense Smoothing Conditioner
Ojon Damage Reverse Restorative Conditioner
Ojon Dry Recovery Hydrating Conditioner
Ojon Color Sustain Color Revealing Conditioner
Ouidad Climate Control Defrizzing Conditioner

Water-based Moisturizers & Leave-In Conditioners

Moisturizing Leave-In and Water-Based Moisture Products

Alikay Naturals Shea-Yogurt Hair Moisturizer
As I Am CocoShea Spray
As I Am DOUBLEBUTTER CREAM
As I Am MOISTURE MILK Daily Hair Revitalizer

As I Am Leave-In Conditioner
Bumble and Bumble Leave-In Conditioner
Camille Rose Curlaid Moisture Butter
Camille Rose Fresh Curl
Curl Junkie Hibiscus & Banana Honey Butta Leave-In Conditioner
CURLS Curl Creme Brule
CURLS Curl Souffle Curl Cream
CURLS Lavish Curls Moisturizer
Darcy's Botanicals Sweet Cocoa Bean Moisturizing Hair Whip
DevaCurl Mist-er Right Spray
Entwine Butter Crème Hydrator
Hollywood Beauty Carrot Oil Moisturizer
Hollywood Beauty Olive Oil Moisturizer
Jane Carter Solution Hair Nourishing Cream
Kenra Platinum Color Care Botanical Detangler
Kenra Daily Provision Leave-In Conditioner
Kinky Curly Knot Today Leave-In Conditioner
Komaza Care Coconut Curl Lotion
Komaza Care Coconut Curl Milk
Komaza Care Shea Butter Hair Lotion
LUSH R&B Hair Moisturizer
Luster's S-Curl No Drip Activator Moisturizer
Neutrogena Triple Moisture Silk Touch Leave-In Conditioner
Organic Root Stimulator (Olive Oil) Moisturizer
Organic Root Stimulator (Carrot Oil) Moisturizer
Oyin's Frank Juice Nourishing Herbal Leave-In Conditioner
Oyin's Greg Juice Nourishing Herbal Leave-In Conditioner
Oyin's Hair Dew
Paul Mitchell The Detangler
Profectiv Damage Free Anti-Tangle Leave-In
Proline Lite Comb Thru Creme Moisturizer
Sheabutter Cottage Argan & Rooibos Leave-in Conditioner
Silk Elements MegaSilk Leave-In Hair Moisturizing Crème
Silk Elements Megasilk Olive Moisturizing Treatment
Soft Sheen Carson StaSoFro Hair and Scalp Spray
Soft Sheen Carson Wave Nouveau Daily Humectant Moisturizing Lotion
Uncle Funky's Daughter Midnite Train
Uncle Funky's Daughter Thirsty Curls

Protein-rich Leave-Ins and Water-Based Moisture Products

Cantu Shea Butter Grow Strong Treatment
Cantu Shea Butter Leave-In
Chi Keratin Mist
CURLS Moist Curls Curl Moisturizer/Detangler
CURLS Quenched Curls Curl Moisturizer
DevaCurl B'Leave-In
Elasta QP Mango Butter
Infusium 23 Leave-ins
Mane 'n Tail Conditioner
Profectiv Break Free Daily Leave-In Conditioner
Salerm 21
SheaMoisture Coconut & Hibiscus Hold & Shine Moisture Mist
SheaMoisture Coconut & Hibiscus Curl Enhancing Smoothie
SheaMoisture Raw Shea Butter Extra-Moisture Transitioning Milk
SheaMoisture Yucca & Aloe Thickening Growth Milk

Styling Products, Definers, Finishing Products

Hair-Friendly Gels, Jellies, Whipped Creams and Puddings

100% Aloe Vera Gel
AfroVeda PUR Whipped Hair Gelly
As I Am Curling Jelly
As I Am Twist Defining Cream
Aubrey Organics Mandarin Magic Ginkgo Leaf and Ginseng Root Hair Jelly
Aveda Light Elements Defining Whip
Beautiful Textures Moisture Butter Whipped Curl Creme
Blended Beauty Curly Frizz Pudding
Blended Beauty Happy Nappy
Curl Junkie Aloe Fix Lite Hair Styling Gel
CURLS Cashmere Curl Jelly
CURLS Curl Crème Brule
CURLS Curl Souffle Curl Cream
CURLS Curly Q Custard Curl Cream
CURLS Curly Q Gel-les'c Curl Jelly

CURLS Curls Milkshake Curl Lotion
CURLS Curls Goddess Glaze Curl Gel
CURLS Whipped Cream Curl Cream
DevaCare Arc AnGEL
DevaCurl Light Defining Gel
DevaCurl Ultra Defining Gel
DevaCurl Set it Free
DevaCurl Spray Gel
DevaCurl Styling Cream
Ecostyler Gel
Entwine Crème De La Mold
Entwine Crème Jelle Styler
Fantasia IC Polisher with Sparklelites
Garnier Fructis Cream Gel
Hair Rules Curly Whip
Jane Carter Solution Curl Defining Cream
Kinky Curly Curling Custard
Sheabutter Cottage Marula Hair Balm
Uncle Funky's Daughter Good Hair Conditioning Styling Creme

Heat Protectants

Beyond The Zone Smooth Criminal Thermo Protect Spray
Beyond The Zone Turn Up The Heat Protection Spray
BioSilk Silk Therapy
CHI Silk Infusion
Creme of Nature Argan Oil Perfect 7
FHI Heat Hot Sauce
Göt2b Guardian Angel Heat Protect 'N Blow Out Lotion and Gloss Finish
John Frieda Frizz Ease Heat Defeat Protecting Spray
Kenra Straightening Serum
L'Oreal Paris Advanced Hairstyle Boost It Blow Out Heat Spray
Mizani Iron Curl Heat Styling Cream
Mizani Thermastrength Heat Protecting Serum
Nexxus Promend Styling Spray
Redken Smooth Down Heat Glide Smoother
Sedu Anti-Frizz Polishing Treatment with Argan Oil
Silk Elements Mega Silk Heat Protection Crème
Tigi S-Factor Heat Defender Flat Iron Shine Spray
Toni & Guy Prep Heat Protection Mist

Setting Lotions/Design Foams

Design Essentials Compositions Foaming Wrap Lotion
Dudley's Fantastic Body Texturizing Setting Lotion
Giovanni Sculpting/Setting Lotion
Lottabody Texturizing Hair Setting Lotion
Jane Carter Solution Wrap and Roll
KeraCare Foam Wrap
Mizani Setting Lotion

Additional Resources

Black-Owned Companies/Companies Founded by Black Men & Women

Alikay Naturals
Bee Mine
Blended Beauty
Carol's Daughter
CHATTO
CURLS
Curl Junkie
CUSH Cosmetics
Darcy's Botanicals
Hydratherma Naturals
Jane Carter Solution
Kinky-Curly
Koils By Nature
Komaza Care
Luv Naturals
Mixed Chicks
My Honey Child
Natural Splendor
Eden Body Works
Entwine Couture
Karen's Body Beautiful
OYIN Handmade
SheaButter Cottage
SheaMoisture
Soultanicals
Thank God It's Natural

Woman-Owned

Alikay Naturals
Bee Mine
Blended Beauty
Carol's Daugher
CHATTO
CURLS
Darcy's Botanicals
DevaCurl
Eden Body Works
Entwyne Couture
Hyrdatherma Naturals
Jane Carter Solution
Jessicurl
Karen's Body Beautiful
Kinky-Curly
Koils By Nature
Komaza Care
My Honey Child
OYIN Handmade
SheaButter Cottage
Thank God It's Natural

Certified Organic (95% - 100%) Brands

These are brands that carry products that are certified organic by the USDA and carry the official seal. To be labeled certified organic, 95% of the product ingredients must be certified organic. A listing here **does not mean** that all of the products in the brand's range are certified organic, just that you can find some choice items among their selection. Also, since the seal is optional—some lines may not carry it, although they are technically certified organic. These are the top brands for passionate and engaged-level product shoppers.

Alba Botanica
Aubrey Organics
Avalon Organics
Desert Essence
Dr. Bronner's
Intelligent Nutrients
Kiss My Face
Miessence
RAW hair Organics
Terressentials

Gluten-Free

These are companies who have gluten-free offerings. Since many of these lines also make products that do include gluten, always be sure to check the ingredients lists for any form of wheat, barley or rye.

AG Cosmetics
Desert Essence Organics
Dove
Finesse
Hugo Naturals
Jason Natural
JONATHAN Product
Kiss My Face
KMS California
Morocco Method
Naturally Dah'ling
Organique
Original Sprout
Paul Mitchell
Sebastian (entire line)
Some Suave products

Vegetarian/Vegan-Friendly Brands

These are companies who have vegetarian or vegan offerings. Please be sure to double-check offerings and ingredients as everything from the line may not be vegan.

AG Cosmetics
Aubrey Organics
Avalon Organics
Dr. Bronner
DermOrganic
DevaCurl/DevaCare
Giovanni
Herbal Choice Mari
JONATHAN Product
Kiss My Face
Morocco Method
Original Sprout
Pureology

Cruelty-Free/No Animal Testing

These are companies who have pledged to not test their products (or ingredients) on animals.

AG Cosmetics
Avalon Organics
Aveda
Carol's Daughter
DermOrganic
DevaCurl/DevaCare
Darcy's Botanicals
Dr. Bronner
Giovanni
Herbal Choice Mari
Kenra
Kiss My Face
Knotty Boy Natural Dreadlock Care
Luv Naturals
Mop Top
OGX
Uncle Funky's Daughter

Bibliography

Bouillon, Claude, and John Wilkinson. *The Science of Hair Care*. Boca Raton, Fla.: Taylor & Francis, 2005.

Draelos, Zoe Draelos. *Hair Care: An Illustrated Dermatologic Handbook*. Boca Raton, Fla.: Taylor & Francis, 2005.

Engineering Toolbox."Thermal Conductivity." Accessed 2010. http://www.engineeringtoolbox.com/thermal-conductivity-d 429.html

Gwaltney-Brant, Sharon. "The Toxicology of Common Household Hazards." Veterinary Information Network. Accessed November 2, 2014. http://www.vspn.org/Library/misc/VSPN_M01290.htm

Halal, John. *Hair Structure and Chemistry Simplified*, 4th ed. Clifton Park, N.Y.: Milady, 2002.

Hatton, Lesley, and Phillip Hatton. *Perming and Straightening: A Salon Handbook*, 2nd ed. Oxford: Blackwell Scientific Publications, 1993.

Johnson, Dale H. *Hair and Hair Care*. New York: Marcel Dekker,1997.

Kamath, Y. K., Sidney B. Hornby, and H. D. Weigmann. "Mechanical and Fractographic Behavior of Negroid Hair." *Journal of the Society of Cosmetic Chemistry* 35 (1984): 24.

Kershaw, J.M. "Tignon of Colonial Louisiana." Media Nola. Accessed November 2, 2014. http://medianola.org/

McMullen, R., and J. Jachowicz. "Thermal Degradation of Hair. I. Effect of Curling Irons." *Journal of the Society of Cosmetic Chemistry* 49 (1998): 223-44.

Merriam-Webster. "Natural." Accessed November 2, 2014. http://www.merriam-webster.com/dictionary/natural

Milczarek, P., M. Zielinski, and M. L. Garcia. "The Mechanism and Stability of Thermal Transitions in Hair Keratin." *Colloid and Polymer Sciences* 270 (1992): 1106-1115.

Mirmirani, P. and Nonhlanhla P. Khumalo. "Traction Alopecia: How to translate study data from Education—Closing the KAP Gap?" Dermatology Clinics 32 (2014) 153–161.

Quadflieg, Jutta Maria. "Fundamental Properties of Afro-American Hair as Related to Their Straightening/Relaxing Behaviour." PhD diss., RWTH Aachen University, 2003.

Robbins, C. R., and C. Kelly. "Amino Acid Analysis of Cosmetically Altered Hair." *Journal of the Society of Cosmetic Chemistry* 20 (1969): 555-64.

Robbins, C. R., and C. Kelly. "Amino Acid Composition of Human Hair." *Textile Research Journal* 40 (1970): 891-95.

Swift, J. A. "The Histology of Keratin Fibres." In *Chemistry of Natural Protein Fibres*, edited by R. S. Asquith, 81-146. New York: Plenum Press, 1977.

Syed, A. N., and A. R. Naqvi. "Comparing the Irritation Potential of Lye and No-Lye Relaxers." *Allured's Cosmetic Toiletries Magazine* 2 (2000): 115.

Vocabulary.com. "Transition." Accessed November 2, 2014. https://www.vocabulary.com/dictionary/transition

Wise, Lauren A., et al. "Hair Relaxer use and Risk of Uterine Leiomyomata in African-American Women."American Journa of Epidemiology 175 (5) (2012): 432-40. First published online January 10, 2012. doi:10.1093/aje/kwr351

Wong, Michael, Gabriela Wissurel, and Joseph Epps. "Mechanism of Hair Straightening." *Journal of the Society of Cosmetic Chemistry* 45 (1994): 347-52.

Product Ingredients Glossary

If you have ever scanned the back of your favorite shampoo or conditioner bottle, you know that trying to make sense of the ingredients in hair-care products can be next to impossible. Very few products today contain easily recognizable ingredients. This ingredients glossary will help you navigate the complex, tongue-twisting chemical compounds and shed some light on some of the more common chemical product ingredients you may encounter in the quest for a healthier head of hair. To simplify the look-up process, ingredients have been grouped by function. Additionally, since the list of ingredients is ever changing, this glossary lists key words rather than lengthy chemical names.

Cleansing Ingredients

Used to lift and remove product build up from the hair

Look for these key words:
Ingredients ending in *-sulfate, -sulfonate, -isethionate, -xylenesulfonate, -sulfosuccinate, -sarcosinate, -sulfoacetate.*

Look for these common ingredients:
Ammonium lauryl (or laureth) sulfate
Cocamidopropyl betaine
Cocoamphoacetate
Cocoamphodipropionate
Decyl glucoside
Sodium lauryl (or laureth) sulfate
Sodium tricedeth (or myreth) sulfate
TEA-Dodecylbenzenesulfonate

Moisturizers & Humectants

Used to increase the moisture content of hair

Look for these common ingredients:
Acetamide MEA
Alanine
Aloe vera
Carbamide/urea (also an antistatic)
Cocotrimonium chloride
Glycerin/glycerol
Honey
Inositol
Panthenol
Propylene glycol
Potassium PCA
Sodium PCA
Sorbitol

Proteins

Used to temporarily strengthen and rebuild the hair fiber

Look for these key words:
Ingredients ending in *amino acid* and ingredients starting with *hydrolyzed.*

Look for these common ingredients:
Amino acids
Collagen
Keratin
Silk protein
Soy protein
Vegetable protein
Wheat protein

Thickeners/Emulsifiers/Stabilizers

Used to thicken, stabilize, and provide some conditioning benefits

Look for these key words:
Ingredients ending with *-chloride, -stearate, -ceteareth.*

Look for these common ingredients:
Beeswax
Caprylic succinate
Carbomer

Castor oil
Cellulose
Cetyl alcohol
Cetrimonium chloride
Decyl glucoside
Dicetyldimonium chloride
Dicocodimonium chloride (also an antistatic)
Glycol distearate
Hydroxyethylcellulose
Lecithin (also antistatic)
Polysorbate

Lipids/Oils/Emollients

Used to improve hair manageability and ease comb through

Look for these key words:
Ingredients ending in *-cone, -conol, -col,* or *-xane* or the words *butter, oil.*

Look for these common ingredients:
Amodimethicone
Aluminum stearate
Behenic acid
Behentrimonium chloride
Cetyl alcohol
Cyclopentasiloxane (cyclomethicone)
Glyceryl monostearate
Glycol distearate
Lanolin
Polyquaternium
Tocopherol

pH Balancers

Used to adjust the acid balance of hair products

Look for these ingredients:
Ascorbic acid
Citric acid (also a chelating agent)
Lactic acid
Sodium hydroxide
Triethanolamine

Preservatives

Used to extend the shelf life of hair products

Look for this key word:
Ingredients ending in *-paraben.*

Look for these common ingredients:
Benzalkonium chloride
Benzoic acid
Carbamide/urea (also an antistatic)
Cocotrimonium chloride
Hydantoin
Paraben
Methylchloroisothiazolinone
Methylisothiazolinone
Sodium benzoate
Stearalkonium chloride (also an antistatic)

Index & Glossary of Selected Terms

B

Banding a heat-free method of lengthening and stretching out natural hair to combat shrinkage. Covered elastics or bands are placed at 1/2 to 1 inch intervals along a section of hair to stretch the hair. (p. 128)

Bantu Knots a protective hairstyle that is created by twisting small sections of hair into "mini-buns" or knots. The knots are secured with a bobby pin.

Big Chop (BC) the act of cutting off all relaxed hair to reveal newly grown-in natural hair. Also known as the "Big Cut."

Breakage the premature loss of a hair strand due to physical stressors.

Buildup the accumulation of hair product, oils or debris on the hair shaft.

Butter a solidified oil or wax-like substance.

C

Chelator (*pronounced key-lator*) a product (usually a shampoo) that is chemically formulated to remove mineral buildup from the hair. (p. 50)

Clarifying Shampoo similar to a chelating shampoo. A shampoo that cleanses and removes oil and hair styling products from the hair, but cannot remove mineral deposits. Diluted baking soda is a natural clarifier. (pp. 54-55)

Coconut Oil a natural, penetrating oil that binds to our hair's proteins and offers a light seal for moisture. Solid at room temperature.

Conditioner a water-based product that is applied to the hair after shampooing to improve its look and condition. Conditioners temporarily bond split ends, fill in missing material along the cuticle and add a layer of protection against further assault.

Conditioner Washing (Co-washing) a method of using conditioner in place of a shampoo to cleanse the hair and impart moisture. (pp. 78, 82, 133)

Cortex the innermost layer of the hair strand.

Mostly found in conditioners, they provide slip and softness to the hair. Some silicones can build up over time. (p.54-55, 60, 127, 157)

Stretching deferring or spacing out the time between relaxer services to improve the quality of the hair.
  definition 42-43
  shedding, and 70

Styling
  bantu knots 141, 148-149
  braided headband 140
  coils 139
  frohawk 148
  pineapple 149
  puff 142-144
  side pinup 140, 142
  top knot 145
  trimming 44, 65, 71, 78, 97, 118-119, 135, 154-155
  twists 143-147
  twistout 75, 146
  Twa 138

Sulfates harsh detergents found in many shampoos. (p. 54, 127, 168-171)

T

Transitional Hair a combination of wiry, dry and semi-straight natural hair that does not have a defined curl or coil pattern. This transitional hair is usually isolated to the first few inches of new growth that emerge after chemical relaxing has been stopped. (p. 8-9, 122)

Transitioning growing in your natural hair while your relaxed hair remains, and then cutting off your relaxed ends slowly over time.
  definition xv, 24-27,
  mental 36-37, 100-112
  physical 36-37, 41-98
  stages 7-27

TWA teeny, weeny Afro (p. 125-126, 133-134, 138)

Lightning Source UK Ltd.
Milton Keynes UK
UKOW07f0828080715

254799UK00005B/8/P

9 781938 266072